Developing and Sustaining Play Therapy Clinics

Erin M. Dugan
LSU Health New Orleans, USA

Krystal Vaughn
LSU Health New Orleans, USA

Kellie Camelford
LSU Health New Orleans, USA

A volume in the Advances in Psychology, Mental Health, and Behavioral Studies (APMHBS) Book Series

IGI Global
DISSEMINATOR OF KNOWLEDGE

Published in the United States of America by
IGI Global
Medical Information Science Reference (an imprint of IGI Global)
701 E. Chocolate Avenue
Hershey PA, USA 17033
Tel: 717-533-8845
Fax: 717-533-8661
E-mail: cust@igi-global.com
Web site: http://www.igi-global.com

Library of Congress Cataloging-in-Publication Data

Names: Dugan, Erin M., 1978, editor. | Vaughn, Krystal, 1977, editor. | Camelford, Kellie, 1984, editor.
Title: Developing and sustaining play therapy clinics / Erin M. Dugan, Krystal Vaughn, and Kellie Camelford, editors.
Description: Hershey, PA : Medical Information Science Reference, [2019] | Includes bibliographical references.
Identifiers: LCCN 2018052236| ISBN 9781522582267 (hardcover) | ISBN 9781522582274 (ebook)
Subjects: | MESH: Play Therapy--organization & administration | Health Facility Administration
Classification: LCC RC489.P7 | NLM WX 150.1 | DDC 616.89/1653--dc23 LC record available at https://lccn.loc.gov/2018052236

This book is published in the IGI Global book series Advances in Psychology, Mental Health, and Behavioral Studies (APMHBS) (ISSN: 2475-6660; eISSN: 2475-6679)

British Cataloguing in Publication Data
A Cataloguing in Publication record for this book is available from the British Library.

Advances in Psychology, Mental Health, and Behavioral Studies (APMHBS) Book Series

ISSN:2475-6660
EISSN:2475-6679

Editor-in-Chief: Bryan Christiansen, Global Research Society, LLC, USA & Harish C. Chandan, Argosy University, USA

MISSION

The complexity of the human mind has puzzled researchers and physicians for centuries. While widely studied, the brain still remains largely misunderstood.

The **Advances in Psychology, Mental Health, and Behavioral Studies (APMHBS)** book series presents comprehensive research publications focusing on topics relating to the human psyche, cognition, psychiatric care, mental and developmental disorders, as well as human behavior and interaction. Featuring diverse and innovative research, publications within APMHBS are ideally designed for use by mental health professionals, academicians, researchers, and upper-level students.

COVERAGE

- Mental Health & Disorders
- Counseling & Therapy
- Cognition
- Addiction
- Psychiatry
- Treatment & Care
- Socialization
- Human Interaction
- Developmental Disorders
- Eating Disorders

The Advances in Psychology, Mental Health, and Behavioral Studies (APMHBS) Book Series (ISSN 2475-6660) is published by IGI Global, 701 E. Chocolate Avenue, Hershey, PA 17033-1240, USA, www.igi-global.com. This series is composed of titles available for purchase individually; each title is edited to be contextually exclusive from any other title within the series. For pricing and ordering information please visit http://www.igi-global.com/book-series/advances-psychology-mental-health-behavioral/110200. Postmaster: Send all address changes to above address.

Titles in this Series

For a list of additional titles in this series, please visit:
https://www.igi-global.com/book-series/advances-psychology-mental-health-behavioral/110200

Ethical Problem-Solving and Decision-Making for Positive and Conclusive Outcomes
Penelope D. Keough (National University, USA)
Information Science Reference • ©2019 • 326pp • H/C (ISBN: 9781522575825) • US $195.00

Chronic Stress and Its Effect on Brain Structure and Connectivity
Ana Starcevic (University of Belgrade, Serbia)
Medical Information Science Reference • ©2019 • 318pp • H/C (ISBN: 9781522575139) • US $225.00

Analyzing the Role of Cognitive Biases in the Decision-Making Process
Verónica Juárez Ramos (International University of Rioja, Spain)
Information Science Reference • ©2019 • 262pp • H/C (ISBN: 9781522529781) • US $190.00

The Mental Health Effects of Informal Caregiving Emerging Research and Opportunities
Debra Gavin Ware (Argosy University, USA) and Tarnue Johnson (Argosy University, USA & Kirkwood Community College, USA)
Medical Information Science Reference • ©2019 • 131pp • H/C (ISBN: 9781522574521) • US $195.00

Virtual and Augmented Reality in Mental Health Treatment
Giuliana Guazzaroni (Università Politecnica delle Marche, Italy)
Medical Information Science Reference • ©2019 • 329pp • H/C (ISBN: 9781522571681) • US $265.00

Multicultural Counseling Applications for Improved Mental Healthcare Services
Anasuya Jegathevi Jegathesan (HELP University, Malaysia) and Siti Salina Abdullah (University Malaysia Terengganu, Malaysia)
Medical Information Science Reference • ©2019 • 302pp • H/C (ISBN: 9781522560739) • US $265.00

For an entire list of titles in this series, please visit:
https://www.igi-global.com/book-series/advances-psychology-mental-health-behavioral/110200

IGI Global
DISSEMINATOR OF KNOWLEDGE

701 East Chocolate Avenue, Hershey, PA 17033, USA
Tel: 717-533-8845 x100 • Fax: 717-533-8661
E-Mail: cust@igi-global.com • www.igi-global.com

Editorial Advisory Board

Table of Contents

Detailed Table of Contents

the importance of establishing play therapy laboratories in the classroom setting when providing graduate play therapy instruction. Additional recommendations will be made for the 2019 Play Therapy Best Practices published by the Association for Play Therapy.

Developing, growing, and maintaining a sustainable play therapy training clinic involves creating meaningful contact within the clinic's targeted community. How the play therapist developing the training clinic goes about creating contact within a community reflects that clinic's overall identity or brand. Counselors are often not trained regarding business practices, brand development, or marketing in their graduate programs. This chapter focuses on providing play therapists with information regarding branding a business and tools for promoting that brand in a manner that aids in the development, growth, and maintenance of a play therapy training clinic. Ethical considerations, as well as thought-provoking questions specific for the development and promotion of a play therapy training clinic are included.

Section 2
Advancing the University's Mission

Play therapy clinics are typically established to support the university mission of teaching, service, and research. As faculty members, we may choose to focus on any one of those areas. As teachers, we train undergraduates (child development), graduates (mental health professionals), and advanced therapists who seek certification (registered play therapists). This education may include observation, general office work, formal courses, and continuing education units. Service in the university may include service to the university, profession, and community. The university gains when faculty members are active in their chosen fields of study and students benefit from faculty who remain abreast of the current happenings in the field. Professionally, play therapy clinics allow for the continued advancement of one's career while educating the next generation of professionals on the benefits of play therapy. Clinics also are an arena for researchers to gather data and continue to advance the research in the field of play therapy. Additionally, registered play therapy supervisors remain up-to-date of the latest research and best practices in the field. Thereby offering quality supervision for the incoming play therapists. The community often benefits from play therapy clinics as they service the public in ways that other clinics may not be able to. For example, due to university funding, grant funding, or private funding, a university play therapy clinic may be able to offer services to those who are under-insured and would otherwise be unable to receive play therapy services. The following chapters provide rich detail into ways that faculty members may focus their activities in a university play therapy clinic.

More beginning graduate students and new mental health professionals are seeing children and families in their therapeutic work, creating a growing need for play therapy-specific training and supervision. Training students and professionals in the art of play therapy is critical to the wellbeing of children, families, and the future profession. A university-based approved center of play therapy education aims to fulfill this growing need while undertaking a momentous amount of responsibility. Training skilled play therapists is a complex endeavor requiring a combination of foundational knowledge, advanced clinical and conceptual skills, and supervision that surpasses classroom coursework requirements. The authors describe the evolution of Georgia State University's Center of Play Therapy Education and Play Therapy Training Institute to provide readers with a comprehensive model for play therapy training and supervision.

Play therapy training clinics are vital to the success of the field of play therapy, as they serve as the foundation for play therapists' education and clinical training. Furthermore, play therapy training differs depending on the developmental level of the play therapist. In this chapter, the authors present a clinical educational program for graduate level students designed to prepare play therapists through practicum experiences based in a play therapy training clinic. The authors address the structure of beginning and advanced play therapy trainings as well as practicum and internship courses, and provide detailed information regarding supervisors, potential course assignments, scheduling, play therapy skills, play therapy rooms, and supervision.

that promote awareness and empathy. Play therapy services offered in university clinics also offer opportunities for interns to increase understanding of social justice advocacy through client interactions and clinical supervision. Clinic directors promote social justice advocacy through managing just organization procedures and coordinating advocacy and outreach initiatives.

Experiential and contextualized learning experiences are essential for facilitating play therapy supervisees' skills development, understanding of play therapy, and self-insight necessary for growth. University-based training clinics have the capacities to provide such experiential learning opportunities; this setting, which often serves diverse community client populations, offers live supervision opportunities. To date, there is limited information available describing the process and procedure for providing live supervision in university-based play therapy training clinics. Therefore, the authors will discuss the functions of live supervision, the process and formats of live supervision, developmental stages of play therapy supervisees in live supervision, theoretical orientation and its impact on the play therapy live supervision process, additional considerations, and advantages and disadvantages of providing live supervision in this chapter all within the context of university-based training programs.

Section 3
Contemporary Applications

This section offers contemporary applications to setting up supervision as well as a specified focus populations in setting up play therapy clinics in the university setting as well as outside the university. Considerations, set up, and facilitation methods are reviewed and offer the reader essential aspects when developing a play therapy clinic.

In this chapter, the author introduces live play therapy supervision as a complementary method to the traditional ways in which play therapy supervision is done, particularly in the context of play therapy training clinics. As conceived here, live play therapy supervision represents a valuable addition to the clinical supervision practices

Foreword

As someone who has spent nearly 30 years in careers centered on helping others (30 years in healthcare settings such as pharmacies, clinics, and hospitals and nearly 17 years in mental health settings such as a university counseling center, a nonprofit play therapy center, and a private practice), *I can say that establishing and maintaining a clinic is not simple*. Wanting to establish a clinic is one thing; having the knowledge and ability is another. The processes involved in establish a clinic remind me of Prochaska and DiClemente's Transtheoretical Model of Change (TTM; 1982). The stages of this model resemble the process one goes through when establishing, running, and maintaining a clinic. In the case of establishing a clinic, instead of change, one is trying to make things happen and keep them happening.

As such, TTM is a multidimensional model developed from therapy and self-change research. The model has five distinct stages that occur in a cyclical pattern rather than the linear fashion described by older theories of change. If you were to take Prochaska and DiClemente's (1982) original model and substitute *make things happen* for *change,* the five stages might look like:

1. **Precontemplation:** Can be described as the stage when there is no observable desire to make things happen as well as an unawareness of any need for anything to happen.
2. **Contemplation:** Can be described as the stage of awareness and desire, yet no commitment to make things happen.
3. **Preparation:** Can be described as the stage of present intent, yet no attempts have been made to make things happen.
4. **Action:** Can be described as the stage when an individual is actively engaged in making things happen.
5. **Maintenance:** Can be described as the stage when an individual gathers strength from actions and make efforts to keep things happening.

The model is cyclical in that an individual's involvement and dedication to the process will determine whether there is progression or regression. In four dimensions, TTM also represents an effort to conceptualize and provide further detail of the process of change. The dimensions include:

1. **Stage of Change:** This dimension includes the five stages of change and is at the core of the other dimensions (Prochaska, DiClemente, Norcross, 1992).
2. **Process of Change:** This dimension is more abstract and consists of tasks individuals utilize in establishing the clinic (Prochaska & DiClemente, 1983).
3. **Decisional Balance:** This dimension involves the cognitive process of weighing the pros and cons of initiating a task to make the clinic a reality (Prochaska et al., 1994).
4. **Self-Efficacy:** This dimension is an underlying confidence that increases as the clinic begins to take shape (DiClemente, Prochaska, & Gilbertini, 1985).

To further describe the processes of change, Prochaska and DiClemente (1982) delineated 10 possible processes each of which is associated with a stage of change. If applied to establishing a clinic, the process(es) might look like:

1. **Precontemplation:** (a) Consciousness raising, gather information about the needed clinic (b) Dramatic relief, expressing and experiencing affect around the needed clinic, and (c) Environmental reevaluation, noting how the lack of a clinic affects the environment in which it would exist.
2. **Contemplation:** Self-reevaluation, considering how one sees him or herself involved in establishing a clinic.
3. **Preparation:** Self-liberation, a choice commitment to the ability to establish a clinic.
4. **Action:** (a) Reinforcement management, internal or external rewards for making the clinic a reality, (b) Helping relationships, openness and trust to share the establishment process with others, (c) Counter conditioning, replacing obstacles, (d) Stimulus control, resisting events that initiate the obstacles.
5. **Maintenance:** Social Liberation, increasing possible support from those available in society.

In order to visualize this model, consider that the stages of change are occurring in a cyclical, spiraling pattern with the decisional balance inspiring the processes of making the clinic possible (e.g., initiated tasks) as self-efficacy acts as an underlying confidence for the process. Considering this and what has been stated, *I can say that establishing and maintaining a clinic is not simple.*

As mental health practitioners, in a research and/or assessment course, we likely covered topics like *needs assessments*, *program development*, and *program evaluation*. We also likely learned about the necessary environment for counseling and play therapy to take place. We learned about the core components needed to establish a therapeutic relationship. However, it is highly unlikely that topics like *How to Establish a Clinic*, much less, *How to Establish A Play Therapy Clinic in a University Setting*, ever made it into any of our textbooks or lectures. With all of this said, what we did learn gave us the foundational understanding of what might be involved in establishing a clinic; yet, many of us have never put this knowledge to work.

Developing and Sustaining Play Therapy Clinics adds to our foundation and provides us with robust examples of nearly everything one might encounter when trying to establish a play therapy clinic in a university setting. This text brings the expertise of a team of editors in chief, section and chapter editors, and authors together to provide comprehensive coverage of topics related to establishing a play therapy clinic. *Developing and Sustaining Play Therapy Clinics* is appropriately divided into three sections: Developing Play Therapy Clinics, Fulfilling University Missions, and Applications. The objective of the text accurately lists the areas necessary for consideration as: education/instruction requirements, degree(s)/certificate(s), student accessibility, scholarship, policy and procedures, supervision, roles and responsibilities, and other criteria such as resource centers, play therapy playrooms, and professional development and continuing education training opportunities.

As a play therapist, educator, and university administrator, I challenge readers to find a text similar to *Developing and Sustaining Play Therapy Clinics* that is as comprehensive, practical, and beneficial. There can never be a *how to manual* for establishing a play therapy clinic, because each situation and location brings about its own unique challenges. However, with this text, the development and maintenance process will be much easier. I encourage readers to take advantage of what *Developing and Sustaining Play Therapy Clinics* offers.

Edward (Franc) Hudspeth
Southern New Hampshire University, USA

REFERENCES

DiClemente, C. C., Prochaska, J. O., & Gilbertini, M. (1985). Self-efficacy and the stages of self-change of smoking. *Cognitive Therapy and Research*, *9*(2), 181–200. doi:10.1007/BF01204849

Prochaska, J. O., & DiClemente, C. C. (1982). Transtheoretical therapy: Toward a more integrative model of change. *Psychotherapy (Chicago, Ill.)*, *19*(3), 276–288. doi:10.1037/h0088437

Prochaska, J. O., & DiClemente, C. C. (1983). Stages and process of self-change of smoking: Toward and integrative model for change. *Journal of Consulting and Clinical Psychology*, *51*(3), 390–395. doi:10.1037/0022-006X.51.3.390 PMID:6863699

Prochaska, J. O., & DiClemente, C. C. (1992). Stages of change in the modification of problem behaviors. *Progress in Behavior Modification*, *28*, 184–218. PMID:1620663

Prochaska, J. O., Velicer, W. F., Rossi, J. S., Goldstein, M. G., Marcus, B. H., Rakowski, W., ... Rossi, S. R. (1994). Stages of change and decisional balance for 12 problem behaviors. *Health Psychology*, *13*(1), 39–46. doi:10.1037/0278-6133.13.1.39 PMID:8168470

Preface

A university based play therapy training center or play therapy training clinic should be housed in an academic institution or university setting that offers not only direct play therapy services to children and families, but also provides quality education, training, research, and supervision. The Association for Play Therapy (APT), houses detailed information on becoming an Approved Play Therapy Center. This text will offer guidelines to professionals and institutions wishing to develop a setting which houses such an entity.

Play therapy trainings clinics are an important aspect of the clinical mental health field. While each setting may have a set of contractual standards for teaching, training, conducting research and providing supervision, few offer advice for setting up such university based play therapy training clinics. Areas for consideration in training clinics may include: education/instruction requirements, degree(s)/certificate(s), student accessibility, scholarship, policy and procedures, supervision, roles and responsibilities, resource centers, play therapy playrooms, professional development, and continuing education training opportunities.

Policy and procedures in a university based play therapy clinical setting may guide practitioners and trainees in multiple areas, including emergency and crisis situations, meeting required play therapy certification hours, paperwork requirements not limited to registration guidelines or clinic forms, and mandated reporting requirements set forth by the clinic. While these topics may be administrative in nature and may be addressed in policy and procedure manuals, they may also require attention in the clinical supervision realm.

Clinical supervision is required by many university training programs, state licensure boards, and accrediting bodies. Clinical supervision may be grounded in a multitude of theories, but also may include areas required by training programs. For example, training programs may require mid-term and final evaluations that may not be supported by some supervision theoretical orientations. These types of requirements may require a discussion between supervisor and supervisee of roles and responsibilities in the supervisory relationship during graduate level training as this relationship may evolve into supervision for licensure or certification.

Roles and responsibilities in training programs may seem endless; and may include roles such as administrative supervisor, clinical supervisor, clinic director, clinicians, interns, clinic managers, and staff. Each of these roles may have individual responsibilities or requirements within specific clinics. At times these roles may overlap and require one individual to hold more than one role at differing times in the training program. These multifaceted relationships may require open discussions, consultations, supervision, and clear boundaries.

This book offers an overview of establishing, developing, and sustaining a university based play therapy training clinic. Topics included in the book include the establishing a play therapy clinic, advancing the university's mission, and contemporary applications.

Acknowledgment

The editors would like to acknowledge the help of all the people involved in this project, and, more specifically, acknowledge the authors who contributed chapters and to the editorial review board that took part in the review process. Without their support, this book would not have become a reality.

Our sincere gratitude goes to the chapter authors who contributed their time and expertise to this book. It is our hope that *Developing and Sustaining Play Therapy Clinics* will provide our fellow and future colleagues educational and training opportunities.

Section 1
Establishing a Play Therapy Clinic

The notion of creating a play therapy clinic can be an overwhelming undertaking for a mental health professional. The following chapters provide considerations for play therapists in the planning and beginning stages of developing a play therapy clinic to help guide mental health professionals from playroom space design to marketing and branding their clinic to the community.

Chapter 1
Considerations for Setting Up Play Therapy Training Clinics:
Recommended Play Therapy Toys, Materials, and Other Professional Considerations

Nicola Shea Hughes-Brand
University of Central Florida, USA

Julie A. Clifton
University of Central Florida, USA

Columbus Edward Brand
University of Central Florida, USA

ABSTRACT

When setting up a play therapy training clinic, there are many considerations to explore regarding designing a therapeutic space, selecting toys and other materials, exploring the rationale for the toy selection and examining the cultural considerations in play therapy settings. This chapter will review the different types of play therapy clinics and the specific toys recommended based on the fourteen primary play therapy theoretical orientations. General considerations will be reviewed when utilizing art media and other materials, books and bibliotherapy, puppets and puppet theaters, sandtrays and miniatures, and psychotherapeutic games. Recommendations will be made for establishing community and university-based play therapy training sites offering clinical and mock play therapy services. Suggestions will be made regarding the importance of establishing play therapy laboratories in the classroom setting when providing graduate play therapy instruction. Additional recommendations will be made for the 2019 Play Therapy Best Practices published by the Association for Play Therapy.

DOI: 10.4018/978-1-5225-8226-7.ch001

INTRODUCTION

Considerations for Setting Up Play Therapy Training Clinics: Recommended Play Therapy Toys, Materials, and Other Professional Considerations

There are many unchartered, yet important, considerations for setting up a play therapy training clinic given the limited available literature. In the process of researching factors to consider when setting up a university-based or a community-based play therapy training clinic for this chapter, the authors reviewed the play therapy literature; reflected upon over their 25 years each of clinical practice in multiple settings including university-based, community out-patient, school-based, in-home counseling, hospital, residential, and inpatient /psychiatric care; and considered their teaching experiences at multiple universities, both at Approved Centers of Play Therapy Education, as defined by the Association for Play Therapy (APT), and universities lacking the approval status.

This chapter will highlight considerations for setting up university-based and community-based play therapy training clinics due to the limited available research on this important topic. Much thought and research are required in order to create an appropriate therapeutic space for providing play therapy services. Play therapy clinics need to create spaces that accommodate various cultural considerations, clinician's theoretical orientations, and even technological considerations. Clinicians must carefully select, acquire, and organize toys and materials in the play therapy room based on evidence-based practices, including the use of art media and other materials, books and bibliotherapy, puppets and puppet theaters, sandtrays and miniatures, and psychotherapeutic games. Specifically, this chapter is divided into five sections: 1) the different types of play therapy clinics, 2) the cultural considerations regarding the play therapy setting and toys, 3) the method for selecting toys and materials; 4) the limitations of this research review; and 5) the recommendations for setting up a community-based and a university-based play therapy training site providing clinical services and services for mock clients.

The APT is the national professional organization that standardizes the field of play therapy and offers national credentialing in play therapy. The organization developed *The Play Therapy Best Practices* as an on-line publication with the goal of establishing clinical, professional, and ethical guidelines for the field (APT, 2016). When researching considerations for setting up a play therapy clinic, the authors reviewed the APT best practices publication as a starting point; however, recommendations for structuring a play therapy room were not addressed in this document. This online publication further did not address the recommended play therapy room size, diverse settings in which play therapy occurs, playroom characteristics, cultural considerations when selecting toys and providing clinical services, the rationale for selecting play therapy toys and materials, and the playroom set-up including the toy organization and display (APT, 2016). The authors then researched available play therapy literature to find appropriate best practices for the field to create recommendations for setting up appropriate play therapy clinics.

TYPES OF PLAY THERAPY CLINICS

Whether one is establishing a university-based play therapy training clinic, a community-based play therapy clinic, or a university-based training site serving mock clients, there are many factors to consider. Before setting up a play therapy clinic or training site, one must consider the location of the clinic (university-based or community-based) and the purpose of the playroom. Some playrooms will be used solely to provide clinical services to community members, some may act as a training room for mock play therapy sessions, or some may serve clients and trainees. General recommendations will be reviewed for all play therapy sites, including specific recommendations for university-based, community-based, non-traditional training sites offering clinical services to the community, and university-based play therapy training sites offering mock play therapy services.

General Recommendations for All Play Therapy Clinics

General recommendations for all play therapy rooms, sites, or clinics will be discussed with a focus on the ages of the populations being serviced, the type of services being offered, and the specifications of the play therapy space. Additional considerations will include the recording or observation options, the accessibility of the play therapy clinic or room, and the ability level of all individuals being served.

First, when setting up a play therapy clinic or room, it is important to consider the age(s) of the client(s) being served and the type of services being offered. If clients will be seen in the playroom, it is important to determine the ages of the clients who may receive services (children ages two to 12, adolescent ages 13 and up, and/or adults and other family members seeking family therapy) so that the appropriate toys and materials are present for all populations being served (Landreth, 2012). One should also consider the type of services being provided such as individual, family, or group therapy.

Play therapists will benefit from not only working directly with youth when providing play therapy services, but also from gaining the experience of working with clients' parents, grandparents, and other caregivers to better understand the client and offer assistance to the clients' support systems. According to Gil (2015), the benefits of having the family members join the play therapy session are to offer insight to the play therapist on the family's dynamics, as well as to the family members. The therapist can observe the family's communication styles, levels of cooperation and organizational skills, levels of affective and physical contact, levels of enjoyment while interacting with one another, levels of spontaneous insight, the hierarchies and boundaries, and possible coalitions that may be present.

In order to provide appropriate play therapy services or instruction, there are multiple factors to consider when designing a therapeutic space. Landreth (2012), Kottman (2011), and Carmichael (2006) offered many recommendations for the play therapy space. The room size of the play therapy room should be approximately 12 feet by 15 feet with an area of between 150 and 200 square feet so that the child is never too far away. The room should be large enough to allow the child space to explore the room and toys, and to allow space for multiple children to play, but not too large that the trainee or therapist is unable to observe or track the child because the child is too far away from the trainee or play therapist. When providing group play therapy services, Landreth (2012) recommended a playroom approximately 300 square feet and O'Connor (2000) recommended a play therapy room to be approximately 15 feet by 25 feet.

Further considerations for the room itself include ensuring confidentiality and privacy during the session. The playroom needs to have a door that closes to ensure confidentiality. The room needs to be absent of any windows or inside walls to decrease any possible distractions or interruptions that may occur (Landreth, 2012; Carmichael, 2006). If windows are present in the play therapy room, the windows should be covered with curtains or blinds (Landreth, 2012; Kottman, 2011). The playroom needs to be located away from the main flow of traffic in the building so that caregivers in the lobby cannot hear the child in the session and other clients in the office will not be disturbed (Carmichael, 2006). All sessions, supervision meetings, and consultations should remain private. Sound proof walls may assist in preventing others in the hallway or lobby from overhearing conversations, as well as having a white-noise making device that may prevent conversations from being heard outside the play therapy room (Landreth, 2012). If possible, acoustical tiles should be fitted on the ceiling to reduce noise (Kottman, 2011). Further, no client's artwork should be displayed in the play therapy room, hallways of the office, or any other counseling or staff office (Landreth, 2012). All clients' artwork should be viewed as part of their medical record; therefore, displaying any artwork is seen as a violation of the clients' confidentiality and privacy. Also, all artwork from the prior client should be removed from the play therapy room and all toys should be returned to their original location before the next client enters the play therapy room.

Regarding the play therapy room flooring, the initial costs, replacement cost, durability, and ease of cleaning should be considered. Landreth (2012), Kottman

(2011), and Carmichael (2006) recommended that the playroom floors be durable and easy to clean, such as vinyl tile squares instead of carpet or solid sheet vinyl. Carmichael (2006) also recommended newer waterproof floors that have a wood appearance but warns against having carpet. Carpet may help keep the noise down in the room, but may be difficult to clean and may restrict painting and sand activities.

Like the floors, the walls of the playroom should be designed with ease-to-clean in mind and have washable enamel (Landreth 2012; Kottman, 2011; Carmichael, 2006) and be stain resistant (Carmichael, 2006). An off-white color (Landreth, 2012), neutral color (Kottman, 2011), or shades of white to cream (Carmichael, 2006) for the walls is recommended so that it provides a cheerful atmosphere, whereas vibrant, dark, or somber colors should be avoided (Landreth, 2012). The play therapy room is supposed to have a neutral and gender-neutral presence so that the room itself does not influence the child's feelings, behaviors, or cognitions. Carmichael (2006) recommended refraining from wall murals or non-neutral colors because this may change the child's mood for behaviors. Also, if artwork or other decorations are displayed in the room, it is recommended that the items need to be displayed at the child's eye level (Landreth, 2003).

Further physical space considerations include ensuring that the room has adequate air conditioning and heating. The lighting in the room needs to be adequate with preferred recessed lighting with protective guards. Recessed lighting, flush mount lights, or fluorescent ceiling lights may be safer if a child were to throw an object toward the ceiling, the light bulbs, or the light fixtures (Carmichael, 2006).

One should also consider the accessibility of the play therapy clinic or room and the ability level of all individuals being served. It is essential that the front door to the clinic, the clinic lobby, the hallway, the door to the play therapy room, and the room layout itself meet the Department of Justice (2010) Americans with Disabilities Act of 1990 requirements. If the site is an older building, renovations should be made to accommodate all clients in the building and the playroom. The toy set-up and the toys themselves should also accommodate the clients in terms of the weight, overall size, and height of the toys and furniture so that the needs of all clients can be met.

Safety considerations in the play therapy room include ensuring the room is both an emotional and physically safe place (Barnes, 1996; Carmichael 2006). Play therapists need to ensure all electrical outlets have outlet plug covers, and all bookshelves are attached to the wall and secured so that if a child tries to climb any large piece of furniture in the room, it will not fall over (Landreth, 2012; Kottman, 2011, Carmichael 2006). The room needs to be checked for sharp corners, objects, protruding nails, or another other possible hazardous material that may harm a child. If windows or window fans are present in the play therapy room, they need to have screens or locks in place to ensure the child cannot hurt him or herself. Space heaters should not be present in the play therapy room due to possible electrical fires or child burn hazards. Play therapists are recommended to contact their local fire marshal if they have any concerns about the room itself or the contents in the room (Carmichael, 2006). The chapter authors further recommend that all cleaning and flammable materials are not accessible to the clients, and all food and beverages are not allowed into the play therapy room in case another child may have food allergies.

An optional recommendation is to have water or bathroom access in or connected to the playroom. A sink in the play therapy room, at the child's height, with cold running water may be used for painting, cleanup, and play in the sandbox or sandtray. Hot water is not needed due to potentially burning the child's hands. If a sink cannot be present, the therapist may place a pitcher of water in the playroom for painting and sand play. It is further helpful to have a small bathroom in the play therapy room with a door that closes or a bathroom within close proximity of the play therapy room (Landreth, 2012; Kottman, 2011; Carmichael, 2006).

Another optional consideration is whether or not the play therapy clinic needs recording equipment or observational tools. Landreth (2012), Kottman (2011), and Carmichael (2006) recommended having a one-way mirror so that trainees or therapists can be observed while providing play therapy services. A one-way mirror also allows videotaping of the session, peer reviews, and the possible observation of the parents or caregivers during the play therapy session. It is also suggested to have recording equipment available so that the play therapy sessions can be recorded. Play therapists or trainees can go back and watch the recorded sessions to identify their strengths and areas to work on. Landreth (2012) recommended to not have a video recorder in the play therapy room due to the child possibly altering his/her behavior, becoming more animated, or being distracted by the equipment.

Ray (2011) further discussed the importance of having video-recording equipment in the play therapy space at university-based play therapy training clinics. Ray noted that self-report by play therapy trainees are notoriously inaccurate and audio recordings limit the play therapy instructor or supervisor's ability to observe the child's and the trainee's nonverbal communication. By video recording the play therapy session, the therapist or trainee can also re-experience the session in the presence of the supervisor or instructor, as well as re-connect with the trainee/therapist's and the child's or client's feelings. Enhanced emotional connections may assist the trainee or therapist in increasing his/he level of empathy and understanding of the child or client, as well as improve the trainee/therapist's level of self-reflection and awareness. Further, the chapter authors noted that any other occurrences that may have knowingly or unknowingly influenced the play therapy session, such as environmental factors, either inside the play therapy room or outside the room or hallway can be identified and addressed.

Researchers further provided items and pieces of furniture that may be beneficial in the play therapy room. A chalkboard mounted approximately 21 inches from the floor with a tray across the bottom with colored chalks or a dry erase board with non-toxic erasable markers with different colors is recommended (Landreth, 2012; Kottman, 2011; Carmichael, 2006). A polished metal mirror mounted to the wall may be helpful (Landreth, 2012). Sturdy wooden book shelves at the child's height (the top shelf should be no higher than 38 inches) with a long-lasting finish should be mounted to the wall to allow the display of toys, as well as ensure the child is safe if the child tries to climb in the shelves or on top of the shelves. A sturdy, wood, or hard-surfaced child-sized table and chairs need to be present in the playroom with an adult-sized chair for the therapist (Landreth, 2012; Kottman, 2011; Carmichael, 2006). Fabric chairs for the child or therapist are not recommended due to possible health concerns and the possible difficulty keeping them clean (Carmichael, 2006). A storage container may be present to store additional art supplies or could be used as a small sandbox or sandtray (Landreth, 2012; Carmichael, 2006). Landreth (2012) and Kottman (2011) also suggested having a storage cabinet to store art materials with a countertop to paint and display artwork. Kottman (2011) further recommended having a small desk if a table and chairs were not available, a pillow for the therapist if a chair could not be present, and additional furniture to accommodate parents or caregivers if they were to attend the session.

NON-TRADITIONAL PLAY THERAPY SPACES

Many universities and play therapy training programs offer practicum and internship experiences in non-academic settings. These diverse community-based and non-traditional counseling sites may include hospitals, community agencies, schools, churches, and in-home settings. In order to provide appropriate play therapy services, there are many factors to consider when designing a therapeutic play therapy space in non-traditional settings.

In medical settings, toys used in play therapy practice present a challenging cross-contamination issue when used in toy rooms or in portable medical play practices due to the pathogenicity. According to the Occupational Safety and Health Administration (OSHA, 2019), universal precautions are defined as "an approach to infection control to treat all human blood and certain human body fluids as if they were known to be infectious for HIV, HBV and other bloodborne pathogens" (p.1). Universal precautions are always recommended according to the World Health Organization (2007) and the United States Department of Labor (2019) standard precautions in health care. By finding ways to sterilize the toys and materials and by having child-specific toys per session, this can avoid cross contamination. Carmichael

(2006) recommended only selecting toys that can be washed in disinfectant. She further recommended not having puppets or stuffed animals in the playroom unless they can be washed or dry-cleaned often.

When providing play therapy services in a community, school, or non-traditional counseling settings, it is important that the agency, school, or hospital supervisor have basic knowledge of play therapy services, the recommended play therapy space, and the play therapy toys required to offer play therapy in a therapeutically conducive environment. Many non-traditional counseling settings may have toys at the site, but they are disorganized or broken. The toys made available may also be considered non-therapeutic based on the rational for selecting play therapy toys. The play therapy space may not be a safe and secure environment. Further, play therapy services may be offered at sporadic locations, for example in schools, playgrounds, empty offices, storage rooms, hallways, and media centers. In these cases it is difficult to ensure confidentiality when meeting in open spaces, and meeting in different places at different times with different toys does not ensure continuity or consistency in the clinical services provided.

In order to offer support to non-traditional counseling settings, the authors recommend that university-based play therapy supervisors offer play therapy workshops and trainings to the community supervisors and staff so that everyone at school-based and community-based agencies will better understand the necessity and requirements of a proper play therapy space. Play therapy supervisors could also offer agency consultations so that when students are placed in these non-traditional settings, if the agency is amenable to setting up a play therapy room, the therapeutic space could be established before the play therapy trainee begins his or her practicum or internship experience.

When play therapy services are offered in non-traditional sites, but the site does not have a play therapy room or the required toys, Landreth (2002, 2012) and Landreth and Bratton (2006) recommended the play therapist bring a play therapy toy tote bag with three primary categories of toys: 1) real-life toys, 2) acting-out aggressive toys, and 3) creative and emotional expression toys. *Real-life toys* include: a small baby doll, a nursing bottle, a doctor kit (with stethoscope), toy phones (at least two), a small dollhouse, a bendable doll family that is ethnically representative of the client's family, play money, a couple of domestic and wild animals, a car and truck, and kitchen dishes. Optional toys include: puppets (one aggressive and one gentle), doll furniture (for a bedroom, bathroom, and kitchen), and dress up items. *Acting-out aggressive toys* include: dart guns with a couple of darts and a target, a rubber knife, a rope, aggressive animals such as a snake, shark, lion or dinosaurs, small toys soldiers with two different colors (around 12-15), inflatable bop bag, a mask, and an optional set of toy handcuffs with a key. *Toys for creative/emotional expression* include: Play-Doh, crayons, plain paper, scissors, transparent tape, egg carton and Styrofoam cup or bowl, ring toss game, deck of playing cards, soft foam ball, two balloons per play session, an optional selection of arts and craft materials in a Ziplock bag, Tinker Toys or building blocks, binoculars, and a tambourine, drum or other small musical instruments, and a magical wand (Landreth, 2002, 2012; Landreth & Bratton, 2006).

University-Based Training Site Serving Mock Clients

The purpose of a play therapy training site serving mock clients is to allow play therapy trainees the opportunity to interact with the recommended toys, practice play therapy skills, receive immediate feedback and supervision from both the student counseling cohort and the supervisor, and process the session afterwards. If the playroom or clinic will not be utilized to provide services to real clients, it is important to explore what will be the purpose of establishing a play therapy playroom. Will the room be used for graduate students or play therapy trainees to practice their play therapy skills with each other during role plays? Will the students practice their play therapy skills with a non-clinical population such as friends or family members who may give consent to work with their children or adolescents? Will the instructor role play with students or vice versa to demonstrate the play therapy skills? What type of supervision will be provided if any to monitor the student's progress? Will supervision include live supervision in the playroom, supervision using a one-way mirror, or will an electronic recording device be present to record all sessions and role-plays so that the students will be able to go back and review their sessions at a later date?

It is recommended to have laboratory experiences (i.e. practicum or internships) including: observing play therapy sessions of other trainees; observing the instructor provide play therapy services live or reviewing a recording of a play therapy session; conducting a recorded role play session both with the instructor and fellow trainees; and conducting play therapy sessions with non-clinical populations such as children enrolled in daycares or nursery schools (Landreth, 2012).

For training sites, it is suggested to install electronic equipment to video record the sessions for later playback and viewing. If this is not possible, it is recommended to install a one-way mirror in the playroom (Landreth, 2012). Typically, graduate students enrolled in graduate counseling programs are required to record counseling sessions, review the sessions with their instructor and fellow classmates, and provide a formal case staffing or case conceptualization of their clients. Many university digital recording systems may only retain the counseling session for two to four weeks depending on the system. It is necessary to ensure the recorded sessions are kept for a minimum of four to eight weeks to allow the students the ability to discover themes and patterns of play after reviewing and reflecting upon their play therapy sessions.

It is further recommended by the authors to employ two full-time state licensed Registered Play Therapist Supervisors (RPT-S) to provide all supervision of the play therapy trainees at the university and community-based training sites and to provide graduate play therapy instruction. This number may vary based on the size of the student population and/or university; however, when applying for play therapy certification, all graduate play therapy coursework has to be taught by two different play therapy instructors (APT, 2019). Having only licensed RPT-S clinicians provide the play therapy supervision and teach the play therapy graduate courses, ensures a qualified professional has met the requirements for APT and can provide appropriate supervision and oversight for all play therapy instruction being provided. Further, it is important that the play therapy room be set up according to the theoretical-based clinical recommendations. If the play therapy room is not set up correctly, it will be difficult to provide play therapy supervision, address mistakes made, or discuss possible areas of improvement during the play therapy session that may occur when inappropriate toys are present in the room or the toys are displayed chaotically.

CULTURAL CONSIDERATIONS REGARDING THE PLAY THERAPY SETTING

Professional organizations such as the National Association of Social Workers (NASW) *Code of Ethics* (2017) and the American Association for Marriage and Family Therapy (AAMFT) *2015 Code of Ethics* deem multicultural competency and diversity as an ethical responsibility for the practitioner, as does the American Counseling Association *2014 ACA Code of Ethics,* the National Board for Counselors (NBCC) *Code of Ethics* (2016), and the American Psychological Association (APA, 2017) *Ethical Principles of Psychologists and Code of Conduct.* Cultural awareness and service interventions in play therapy education and in supervision of trainees will be described in the section.

Findings from three studies noted play therapy practitioners are predominantly Caucasian females from middle to upper class strata in the United States (Parikh, Ceballos, & Post, 2013; Gil, 2005; Baggerly, 2006; Phillips & Landreth, 1995). It has been theorized that most play interventions and playrooms were geared to Western European approaches representative of the play therapy education and supervision the registered play therapist received (Gil, 2005; Kranz, Ramirez, Flores-Torres, Steele, & Lund, 2005). O'Conner (2005) suggested that discord exists between basic play therapy theory and practice. Further, O'Conner (2005) recommended three ways play therapists may use to learn culturally appropriate skills: by pursuing information about the specific multicultural norms, the play materials used by that culture, and play interventions deemed most appropriate for that multicultural group.

Multiculturalism is a dynamic and real aspect of play therapy today. In the ever-increasing globalization of modern society, more children and families enter play therapy practices from wide arrays of primary cultures or blends of cultural heritages. These clients come with constellations of beliefs derived from their family systems, self-identities, and ways of communicating related to their upbringing by members of their own multicultural group (Post & Tillman, 2015). This shift in caseload composition is evolving. The shift from a predominantly Western Europe extracted demographic is reflected in many play therapy caseloads. By 2050, our multicultural population is likely to increase to 62% of the total US population (U. S. Census Bureau, 2010). Accompanying this shift in population and caseloads, clients and families are expected to come with a wide range of cultural issues including a likely lower socioeconomic status (Abramsky, 2012), cultural differences related to trust, religion and spirituality, language, self-identity, customs (Sue & Sue, 2003), within-group differences (Haidt, Koller, & Dias, 1993), immigration status, (Carmichael, 2006), and multicultural norms. Play therapists have a responsibility to provide informed evidence-based play interventions sensitive to the client's culture (Hinman, 2017; "National Association for," 2017; "Association for Play," 2018) and level of acculturation to their host country (Sue & Sue, 2003).

To provide services for this anticipated changing demographic in play therapy caseloads, graduate programs need to provide multicultural and additional social justice concepts in a variety of courses prior to graduation (Brubaker, Puig, Reese, & Young, 2010; Burnes & Singh, 2010; Dixon, Tucker, & Clark, 2010). Play therapists first learn about multicultural competency and diversity in their undergraduate and graduate programs, as well as during their clinical experiences in supervised play therapy. Traditionally, graduate school programs incorporate the Council for Accreditation of Counseling and Related Programs (CACREP) and the Council on Social Work Education (CSWE) standards. As a specialty, play therapy education, according to APT, requires specific education and supervised practice in addition to the professional practice license from the applicant's state (APT, 2019). Coverage of multicultural issues in play therapy primarily depends upon the trainee's education and supervision.

Additionally, play therapy training clinics need to consider incorporating multicultural concepts and discussions including social justice advocacy (Baggerly, 2006) in play therapy courses taught at the university level, practicum in multicultural settings, and culturally-informed supervision of trainees by sensitive trained play therapy supervisors (Burnes & Singh, 2010). Such informed discussion during practicum is thought to increase trainee self-assessment of one's own biases, cultural identification, and areas of prejudice (Baggerly, 2006; O'Connor, 2005).

Also, professional organizations such as APT should provide continuing education in multiculturally sensitive areas at national and state association conferences (Ceballos, Parikh, & Post, 2012) to best serve play therapy practitioners who work with children and families to keep ahead of the trends.

Play Therapy Settings: A Multicultural Context

In considering respectful services in a multicultural context, the space where play therapy is offered is often ignored or overlooked (Hinman, 2003). The office and playroom set up; however, provide a welcoming experience if selections of culturally specific decorations depict the demographic population served in a respectful manner. Multicultural equipment includes toys, books, games, and furniture.

Play therapists have long understood that play is a developmentally apt way for children to express themselves (Axline, 1969) where it is core to children on a daily basis (VanFleet, Sywulak, & Sywulak, 2010). Various cultures have specific and discreet qualities that play therapists are best served to become familiar with as caseloads reflect multicultural societal evolution.

As a way to familiarize themselves with clients from multicultural backgrounds, play therapists are encouraged to attend community events outside of the therapeutic relationship such as going to religious services, attending synagogues and churches, theater events, community group offerings, and eating in ethnic restaurants (Coleman, Parmer, & Barker, 1993). As well, therapists are encouraged to discover the community supports such as religious groups, social services, and other agencies available to the children and families in their community (O'Connor, 2005).

To provide culturally-appropriate and ethnically-informed play interventions, therapists have embraced approaches to ally or join with families from the early stages of rapport building and assessments (Hinman, 2003; VanFleet et al.,2010). With joining, noticing specific cultural distinctions may be taught both in graduate play therapy programs and in supervised play practicum. In order to effectively practice in a multicultural context, therapists are tasked to understand each child's cultural manifestations such as eye contact, respect for authority, and verbal and nonverbal communication and within-group differences (Killian, Cardona, & Hudspeth, 2017). Specific considerations related to working with African American, Arab American, Asian American, Mexican American, Muslim, and Refugee populations in play therapy are specifically highlighted below for considerations.

African American Populations

African American children and families generally do not voluntarily disclose information in the course of treatment, according to O'Connor, which is consistent with their multicultural group values (2005). This makes spontaneous discussion with the play therapist challenging but consistent with cultural norms (O'Connor, 2005). African-American children experience levels of poverty (Patterson, Stutey, & Dorsey, 2018). Odom, Pungello, and Gardner (2012) reported that African American infants and toddler levels of poverty measured by the national poverty levels was 42% where White infants and toddler poverty rates were 15%. Some African American children, according to O'Connor, experience violence and hatred at school and cautioned play therapists against assuming all black children have similar experiences that require interventions in play therapy (2005). He also recommended that clinicians attend to subgroup differences for children from rural and urban areas, for example.

Arab American Populations

Arab American families view therapeutic services as a treatment for a mental disorder (Sayed, 2003). According to the author, families view submission to Allah's will is linked to stable mental health, making mental illness a lack of moral consistency. This culture is more likely to pursue pharmacological therapy rather than talk therapy.

Asian American Populations

When working with Asian-American children and families, use of their name is tantamount to how the family member is tied to their family. For example, the common practice of using a first name in the therapeutic process is acceptable only for the child, but not for the parents. Using their title and last name is preferred (Vargas & Koss-Chioino, 1992). Not all Asian cultures view seeking therapeutic help in the same way. For example, families of Cambodian or Vietnamese descent feel seeking professional help incur a debt. They view their debt owed to the therapist as a great cost. So, these families may wish to know the cost and benefit of services sought and suggested by the therapist. In this culture, therapists have to present a clear treatment approach and expectations as the parents weigh their financial and emotional costs to family (Huang, 1998). When designing and setting up a playroom for Japanese and Japanese-American children, one should consider their cultural identity when selecting items to provide a strong bond between children and their parents. When designing the environment, the therapist is mindful of the client's acculturation process due to within-group differences (Hanson, 2004).

Japanese children and families often enter play therapy services with feelings of shame, as the family's inability to solve their own problems is representative of a parenting failure. In this culture, joining with the client and family is prioritizing confidentiality within the therapeutic relationships. According to Hinman (2003), learning about the family structure and later returning to their feelings of shame aid in conveying how the therapeutic process works. During the process, as trust is being developed, the therapist aids parents by providing therapeutic techniques they may perform at home to facilitate hope and diminish loss of control and feelings of failure by seeking therapeutic help.

Mexican-American Populations

Kranz, Ramirez, Flores-Torres, Steele, and Lund (2005) provided culture specific setting recommendations for play therapy with Mexican-American children such as painting waiting rooms in bright welcoming colors and using 12 inches by 12 inches red floor tiles. The indoor playroom dimensions were suggested to be approximately 150 to 200 square feet for individual play therapy sessions and approximately 300 to 400 square feet for group play therapy sessions. Kranz et al. (2005) also recommended having culturally appropriately sized small, sturdy furniture, colorful baskets, castanets, and colorful wall coverings. As Mexican-Americans play outdoor games, Moncada (1962) suggested offering an outdoor play yard including a play house structure, tree house with ladder, dirt, a tunnel, fence, table with benches, and basketball with hoop.

Muslim Populations

Muslim families tend to solve their own problems and eschew working with non-Muslim professionals (Baggerly & Abugideiri, 2010). For these children, many of whom have faced oppression, discrimination, and trauma, a move to a new country is fraught with many changes in their family systems and having to adjust to new school and home environment. For non-Muslim professional, Baggerly and Abugideiri (2010) suggested consulting Islamic leaders in the child and family's community to learn about Islam's role in family life. Baggerly and Abugideiri (2010) also suggested including both culturally-sensitive play materials and toys such as dolls with hijabs to create a culturally-appropriate play space for the child and the family.

Refugee Populations

Stauffer (2008) claimed cultural understanding was the key to providing appropriate play therapy interventions for refugee children. Further, to practice responsibly, the therapist must have knowledge of those multicultural considerations specific to the client (Killian, Cardona, & Hudspeth, 2017). For example, the act of seeking therapeutic services is not common with Somali refugees (Killian, Cardona, & Hudspeth, 2017). Refugees who have lived through oppression and prejudice have a bigger need for familiar toys that resemble those of their own culture (O'Connor, 2005). Additionally, when language may be a barrier, the use of Child Centered Play Therapy techniques and interventions have been suggested as therapists put into words what the child is expressing in their use of toys and materials in the playroom (Kottman, 2011). The authors acknowledge the nature of international immigration of refugees and their movement across borders. The United Nations Refugee Agency (UNHCR, 2018) estimated that 68.5 million people have been displaced. Of that number, 25.4 million were refugees with half estimated to be children under age 18 ("Figures at a Glance," 2018). The authors were unable to locate any current measure of refugee children seeking play therapy services at the time of this publication.

SELECTING TOYS AND MATERIALS

When practicing as a play therapist, it is important to explore the rationale for selecting toys and materials; deciding if one is going to provide mostly directive or non-directive play therapy services; deciding on one's theoretical orientation and selecting the corresponding toys recommended based on the theoretical orientation; and examining general considerations when using art media and other materials; puppets and puppet theaters; sandtray and miniatures; and psychotherapeutic games.

According to Landreth's *Play Therapy: The Art of the Relationship* (2012) and the University of North Texas Play Therapy Institute training video, *Toys and Materials* (Landreth, 2002), there are 14 considerations when determining the rationale for selecting toys and materials, including: 1. Toys and materials should be selected, not collected.; 2. Do the toys and materials facilitate and create a wide range of creative expression?; 3. Do the toys and materials facilitate and create a wide range of emotional expression?; 4. Do the toys and materials facilitate and allow for expressive and exploratory play?; 5. Do the toys and materials allow for exploration and expression without verbalization?; 6. Do the items allow success without prescribed structure?; 7. Toys should facilitate contact with an adult.; 8. Toys should permit reality testing.; 9. Toys should allow children to express their needs symbolically.; 10. Toys should provide for emotional release.; 11. Toys should allow for insight.; 12. Toys should engage the children's interests.; 13. Toys should allow for noncommittal play.; and 14. Toys should have study construction for active use.

If a play therapy room is present and play therapy services can be offered to individuals in the community or school settings, one must first decide if he/she may predominantly provide directive or non-directive play therapy. The length of treatment provided, and the setting or location of the play therapy services being offered, may determine this. Nondirective play therapy implies that the child is in the lead.

According to the *Glossary of Play Therapy Terms* published in the *Play Therapy Magazine* by APT, Schaefer and Peabody (2016) defined nondirective play therapy as being "based on the belief that children have an innate drive towards health and healing, this approach leaves the responsibility and direction of the play sessions to the child." In directive play therapy, the therapist is in the lead. Directive play therapy is defined as "an intervention wherein the therapist assumes responsibility for initiating and structuring the client's play activities in order to promote healing" (Schaefer & Peabody, 2016, p. 23).

Highlighting Toys by Theoretical Orientation

After deciding if one is going to practice predominantly as a directive or non-directive play therapist, one must further decide on his or her primary theoretical orientation when working with children ages two to 12 and adolescents ages 13 and up. According to Carmichael (2006), the purpose of a theory is to provide an underpinning for the interventions a counselor might use with the client. The theoretical orientations may serve as a coat rack that supports the philosophical coats of personality development, major assumptions of the client and his or her support system, the role of the therapist and client, model of pathology, and treatment goals and interventions. The theoretical orientation will determine what categories of toys are required, how many toys are present during the session, how the toys will be displayed, and how will the play therapy room be set-up (Carmichael, 2006; O'Connor & Braverman, 2009).

The primary fourteen play therapy theoretical orientations include: Psychoanalytic Play Therapy, Adlerian Play Therapy, Jungian Analytical Play Therapy, Child-Centered Play Therapy, Gestalt Play Therapy, Relationship Play Therapy, Cognitive-Behavioral Play Therapy, Child Developmental Play Therapy, Ecosystems Play Therapy, Child Parent Relationship Training, Filial Play Therapy, Family Play Therapy, Theraplay, and Prescriptive Play Therapy (Carmichael, 2006; O'Connor & Braverman, 2009). Based on all of the diverse play therapy theoretical orientations, there are similar categories found among the fourteen primary theoretical orientations or approaches with also very distinct differences. To ensure a play therapy training clinic center is prepared to adequately teach and demonstrate specific play therapy interventions from different theoretical models, specific toys and materials must be present in the graduate classroom or the play laboratory. The clinical setting also needs to be equipped with the appropriate toys to provide play therapy instruction and to provide clinical play therapy services to children, adolescents, and families.

The recommended toys and set-up for each theoretical orientation will be discussed, as well as general considerations for utilizing art media and other materials; books and bibliotherapy; puppet and puppet theaters; sandtrays and miniatures; and psychotherapeutic games. This will not be an exhaustive discussion of all of the recommended toys and materials. The authors will provide a general recommendation when setting up a play therapy training clinic, preparing a play therapy graduate classroom environment or play therapy laboratory, and offering graduate play therapy instruction on the different theoretical approaches.

Psychoanalytic Play Therapy Toys

Psychoanalytic play therapists select different toys specifically for the child he or she is working with. For each child, the toys are brought to each play therapy session in a private box by the therapist so that the toys are not shared by all of the children. The toys are kept safe from other children and the play is considered private. The box becomes a symbolic container for the child's feelings and expressions and is only shared between the therapist and the child. Children are able to symbolically represent their thoughts, feelings and wishes lending to their interpretative work in play therapy (Klein, 1955; Carmichael, 2006; Lee, 2009).

The materials utilized by a psychoanalytic play therapist include dolls, doll clothing, blankets, dollhouses, and family dolls representing mothers, fathers, and other children. Additional toys include transportation vehicles, domestic and wild animals, animal and people puppets, soldiers, guns, action figure, games, blocks, soft balls for basketball and baseball, a small house, and fences. Art materials may include paper, clay string, Play-Doh, pencils, markers, paints, finger paints, crayons, and construction materials to build things. A sandbox may also be present for younger children. Different toys are selected so that the items can be used in different ways to represent realistic everyday interactions and fantasy play (Klein, 1955; Carmichael, 2006; Lee, 2009). According to Lee (2009), depending on the tolerance level of therapist, the office furniture such as the couch, chair, desk, or bookshelves may also be used as part of the child's fantasy play.

Adlerian Play Therapy Toys

When providing Adlerian Play Therapy (AdPT), Kottman (2011) recommended five basic groups of toys including family/nurturing toys, scary toys, aggressive toys, expressive toys, and pretend-fantasy toys. Family/nurturing toys include a dollhouse, several different ethnically diverse families of dolls (with removable clothing and bendable bodies if possible), baby dolls, a cradle, a soft blanket, baby clothes, and baby bottles. Additional family/nurturing toys include pots, pans, dishes, silverware, empty food containers, and play kitchen appliances such as a sink and a stove. Animal families, stuffed toys, ethnically diverse people puppets, and sand in a sandbox are also included.

The scary toy category includes: snakes, rats, insects, sharks, alligators, dinosaurs, dragons, plastic monsters, and fierce animal puppets such as a wolf, bear, or an alligator. For children who have experienced a vehicle trauma, cars, trucks or ambulances may be considered a scary toy. Aggressive toys include a bop bag, weapons such as a play gun, swords, knives, a foam bat, plastic shields, handcuffs, toy soldiers, military vehicles, and small pillows for pillow fights. Expressive toys and materials include an easel and paints, watercolors, finger paints, crayons, markers, newsprint, glue, scissors, tape, egg cartons, feathers, Play-Doh or clay, materials for making masks, and pipe cleaners for crafts (Kottman, 2011).

The pretend/fantasy toy category includes masks, costumes, magic wands, hats, jewelry, purses, a doctor kit, telephones, blocks, and other building materials. Other toys items include people figures, zoo and farm animals, puppets and a puppet theater, a sandbox, trucks, construction equipment, kitchen appliances, pots, pans dishes, silverware, and empty food containers. Kottman (2011) further included a wide range of miniatures to be used in a sand tray as recommended by Homeyer and Sweeney (2017). These toy miniature recommendations will be reviewed in the general sandtray and miniature collection section.

Jungian Analytical Play Therapy Toys

When providing Jungian Analytical Play Therapy, the traditional play therapy room includes a dollhouse, doll family, art center with supplies, wet and dry sand, a collection of miniatures, a water source, nursing bottle, telephones, puppets, small bed, construction toys, and areas designated for construction activities and for board games (Allen & Levin, 1993). Allen (1994) utilized many art and drama activities while providing counseling services. Examples of the interventions include: spontaneous and directed drawings; serial drawings and serial story writing; creative drama involving activity group therapy and developmental drama; and sandplay therapy using eight categories of miniatures. The recommended miniatures include: 1. *People* (domestic, military, fantasy, and mythological); 2. *Buildings* (houses, schools, churches, and castles; 3. *Animals* (tame, wild, zoo, prehistoric, and marine; 4. *Vehicles* (land, air, water, space, and war machines); 5. *Vegetation* (trees, shrubs, plants, and vegetables); 6. *Structures* (bridges, fences, gates, doorways, and corrals); 7. *Natural objects* (shells, driftwood, stones, bones, and eggs); and 8. *Symbolic objects* (wishing wells, treasure chests, and jewelry).

Child-Centered Play Therapy Toys

Landreth (2002, 2012) and Landreth and Bratton (2006) recommended three broad categories of toys including real-life toys, acting-out aggressive-release toys, and toys for creative expression and emotional release when providing Child-Centered Play Therapy. *Real-life toys* include: dolls, a nursing bottle, a bendable doll family that is ethnically representative of the client's family, a dollhouse, doll furniture (for a bedroom, bathroom, and kitchen), diverse puppets with at least one aggressive and one gentle puppet, a couple of domestic and wild animals, a doctor kit (with stethoscope), toy phones (at least two), and a nondescript figure such as Gumby who could represent any person or family member in the child's life. Other real-life toys include a car, truck, boat, cash register, chalkboard, kitchen dishes, groceries, play money, dress up items, and a broom and a dust pan.

The *acting-out aggressive-release toys* include: small toy soldiers with two different colors (around 12-15), alligator puppet, guns (space or dart gun with a couple of darts and a target), a rope, rubber knives, set of toy handcuffs with a key, pounding bench, a bobo or bop bag, a mask, and wild and aggressive animals such as a snake, shark, lion or dinosaurs. Creative and aggressive toys can include Play-Doh that may be used for pounding, smashing, pinching or rolling. Aggressive-release toys may also include items that can be destroyed, torn or broken in the play therapy room such as egg cartons, paper and popsicle sticks (Landreth, 2002, 2012; Landreth & Bratton (2006).

Toys utilized for *creative expression and emotional release* include: sand, water, Play-Doh, crayons, easel paints, plain and newsprint paper, blunt scissors, transparent tape, egg carton and Styrofoam cup or bowl, ring toss game, deck of playing cards, soft foam ball, two balloons per play session, an optional selection of arts and craft materials in a Ziplock bag, Tinker Toys or building blocks, a magical wand, and binoculars, a tambourine, drum or other small musical instruments. Landreth recommended to not include in the play therapy room any mechanical toys that may limit the child's creativity (Landreth, 2002, 2012; Landreth & Bratton, 2006).

Gestalt Play Therapy Toys

The founder of Gestalt Play Therapy is Violent Oaklander. Oaklander first published her book, *Windows to Our Children: A Gestalt Therapy Approach to Children and Adolescents*, in 1988. In this book, Oaklander described the process of integrating Gestalt Therapy with play therapy and reviews the necessary toys and activities recommended. Oaklander (1988) selected toys and other materials based on the five senses to appeal to the child's sense of hearing, taste, touch, seeing, and smelling when practicing Gestalt Play Therapy. Oaklander (1988) also recommended music instruments, storytelling, poetry, and puppets to assist the child in creative and fantasy exploration.

Suggested art materials may include paper of all sizes, colored pencils, crayons, pastels, felt-tip pens, finger-paints, a pair of scissors, glue, paste, stapler, paper fasteners, scotch tape, masking tape, hole puncher, and diverse collage materials. Collage materials may include tissue paper, construction paper, gift wrapping paper, old greeting cards, newspaper, paper sacks, corrugated paper, poster board, butcher paper, cardboard cartoons, doilies, wallpaper, magazine pictures from old and new magazines, calendars, date books with images, coloring books, children's activity books, and old story books. It is also useful to have pre-cut images and words from magazines and newspapers (Oaklander, 1988).

It is further recommended to have both soft and rough or hard items, as well as items with various textures. Various textures of cloth are recommended such as cotton, wool, burlap, flannel, silk, and lace. Soft items include feathers, cotton, and furry pieces of material. Rough or hard items include pieces of steel, glass, wood, wool, sandpaper, sponges, and pieces of plastic. Other craft items that may lend to creative building and expression are yarn, string, buttons, ribbons, and mosquito netting. Examples of household, kitchen, bathroom, or outdoor items are aluminum foil, cellophane, orange sacks, egg cartons, noodles and macaroni, plastics, bottle caps, chicken wire, tongue depressors, and cotton swabs. Naturally found and food items include leaves, shells, driftwood, cork, pebbles, and seeds of all kinds. Any other additional items that are lightweight and can be attached, pasted, or fastened to a flat surface in any manner are also considered to be a good collage material (Oaklander, 1988).

Relationship Play Therapy Toys

According to Moustakas (1959, 1997), when practicing Relationship Play Therapy, the number of toys in the play therapy room is not important. The attitude of the therapist and the relationship with the child are considered to be the most important factors of therapy. It is also important that the child be able to play with any toy in the manner he or she chooses without the child feeling pressured to play with a specific toy in a specific way. The toys are purposely not displayed in a specific manner to identify their use or context.

Moustakas (1959, 1997) described the toys present in the play therapy room as structured or unstructured items. Unstructured items such as sand, water, paints, crayons, finger paint, paper, scissors, steel vises, tools, and clay allow the child to express pent-up feelings and tension. Structured items such as guns, knives, swords, darts, and a punching toy or bobo allow the child to express hostility. Other recommended toys to express emotions include family dolls and a large dollhouse, dollhouse furniture, puppets, stuffed animals, and other items representing human figures. Cars, trucks, tractors, boats, airplanes, checkers, paper, and pencils allow noncommittal play activities. Additional recommended toys include bowls, spoons, nursing bottles, plastic aprons, telephones, soldiers, shovels, jump rope, masks, blocks, balloons, and a bop toy (Moustakas, 1959, 1997).

Cognitive-Behavioral Play Therapy Toys

When proving Cognitive-Behavioral Play Therapy (CBPT), Knell (1995, 1998, 2009) recommended similar toys to be utilized when providing Child-Centered and Adlerian Play Therapy. Additional items recommended are books to be used in bibliotherapy, child prepared stories and books, stories both made up by the therapist and published, structured workbooks, recordings of stories, music that depicts various moods, board and card games, pictures of faces depicting various feelings, charts, art materials, sculpting materials, dolls, puppets, stuffed animals, and action figures. Additional information regarding the use of puppets and bibliotherapy can be found under the specific play therapy toy selection discussion.

Developmental Play Therapy Toys

Brody (1997) did not have toys available in the play therapy room when providing Developmental Play Therapy. The core therapeutic component of Developmental Play Therapy is a dialogue between the therapist and the child using touch. Toys are considered a distraction to the relationships with the therapist. Brody recommended having a large rug big enough for an adult and a child to sit on comfortably, a rocking chair, a table and chair, a bottle of lotion, and paper with basic art materials such as crayons and pencils (Brody, 1992; 1997; Carmichael, 2006).

Ecosystemic Play Therapy Toys

In Ecosystemic Play Therapy, O'Connor (1994, 2009) described the therapist as the primary material or therapeutic agent of change with limited play therapy toys present. When providing Ecosystems Play Therapy, it is recommended to have three to five toys present at a time during the play therapy session. O'Connor (2009) recommended that three toys are selected based on the child's developmental functioning. One toy is selected based on the child's current developmental functioning. One toy is selected that is below the child's developmental level and one toy is selected that is above the child's developmental level requiring a higher level of functioning. An additional two toys may be selected based on the toys' possible symbolic value to the child based on the child's presenting problems, current situation, or the child's treatment goals (O'Connor, 1994, 2009).

CPRT, Filial Therapy, and Family Play Therapy Toys

When providing Child Parent Relationship (C-P-R) Training, the same suggested toys utilized in Child-Centered Play Therapy are recommended in the *Child-Parent Relationship Therapy (CPRT) Treatment Manual: A 10-Session Filial Therapy Model for Training Parent* (Landreth & Bratton, 2006; Bratton, Landreth, Kellam, & Blackard, 2006). Landreth and Bratton (2006) cautioned against the use of mechanical toys that may inhibit the children's creativity. When preparing for the filial play therapy in-home session, parents were instructed to arrange the toys on an old blanket or quilt that serves as the boundary for the play area. This blanket would also protect the carpet if spills occurred. Further, a cookie sheet or a similar flat and easy-to-clean surface could be used for drawing on and for play with Play-Doh. After the play sessions were completed, Landreth and Bratton (2006) recommended the parents have a special playtime box to store the toys in.

When providing Family Play Therapy, Gil (2014) recommended using therapeutic games and diverse art supplies to provide family art therapy. These art supplies and craft materials included: pencils, pens, markers, chalk pastels, drawing and construction paper, large poster board, easels and easel paper, scissors, glitter glues, beads, feathers, pompoms, buttons, small tiles, sand, plastic eyes and mouth, and additional craft materials. She further recommended having sandtrays (one wet and one dry) with many diverse miniatures. She also suggested that clinicians should have approximately 30 diverse and similar puppets to conduct family puppet interviews.

In Filial Therapy, similar to Child-Centered Play Therapy, the toy selection is comparable (VanFleet, 2014). Playrooms contain toys that facilitate expressions of feelings including aggressive toys, such as dart guns that do not look similar to real guns, a bop bag, flexible rubber knives, and ropes. In playrooms, a full array of nurturing toys including dollhouses, nuclear family figures, infant dolls, puppets, food-making and food-eating toys, water, and bowls are found. Games and toys used to build and construct allowing competition, cooperation, and mastery are also seen in filial therapy playrooms along with blocks, play money, and toss games. Expressive art materials such as sand, crayons, paint materials, and markers as well as dress-up clothing, toy medical kits with masks, round out many filial playrooms.

VanFleet (2014) encouraged filial therapists consider three aspects when deciding to include certain toys in their playroom: a) is the item safe, b) does it's use facilitate children's feelings, and c) does it provide the child with avenues for imagination or projection? Further, VanFleet (2014) encouraged the use of less elaborate and costly playroom materials, suggesting instead use of moderate-cost useful toys that parents may find in their own homes. As older children frequent filial playrooms,

VanFleet (2014) recommended expanding this toy list to include more toy options. She recommends board games for child-family play outside of the filial playroom. In filial therapy, home toy kits are recommended for parent and children. Additionally, VanFleet (2014) made "loaner toy kits" (p. 25) available for families who lack funds, including items from each toy area.

Theraplay Toys

Theraplay, founded by Dr. Ann Jernberg, focused on increasing attachment between Head Start mothers and their children. Theraplay is highly adaptable and does not use traditional play therapy toys. Activities are created to maximize the emotional and physical connection with caregivers, children, and the therapist. Materials such as cotton balls, nerf balls, ping pong balls, balloons, bean bags, beans, straws, bubbles, bubble wands, water pistols, plastic garbage bags, band-aids, small books for balancing, small pillows, large floor pillows, beanbag chairs, scarves, chairs or hoops, small hand towels, and a blanket are used in the activities. Art and craft materials provided are Play-Doh, felt pens, finger paints, white drawing paper, newspaper, construction paper, crepe paper strips, and paper towels. Snacks are also provided such as apples, seedless grapes, or other piece of fruit, raisins, slices of watermelon without seeds or with seeds for spitting out, potato chips, pretzels, M&M and other small candies, doughnuts, popsicles, Jell-O, popcorn, lollipops, licorice, bubble gum, soda, and a baby bottle or juice cartoon filled with juice or milk. Hygiene, hair and make-up products are also provided including lotion, shaving cream, liquid soap, baby powder, hair brushes and combs, hair ribbons, ties, headbands, clasps, and barrettes. Dress up items may include necklaces, bracelets, sunglasses, hats, neckties, and make-up for older children (Munns, 2000; Carmichael, 2006).

Prescriptive Play Therapy Toys

When providing Prescriptive Play Therapy, toys and play therapy activities were selected and provided based on the individual child's presenting problem or symptom, diagnosis, and/or goal for treatment to create a comprehensive, tailor-made treatment program. Play therapy toys and materials may include paper, drawing materials, books, videos, dollhouses (multiple houses if working with children whose parents are separated or divorced), and miniatures representing the child's family members (Schaefer 2001; Gil & Shaw 2009).

Highlighting Specific Play Therapy Toys and Materials

Art Media and Materials

Many play therapists may use art or employ art-based activities during their play therapy session; however, they may not consider the possible health hazards that may occur by the actual art media itself and the unsafe storage practices of media and other art supplies. Further, play therapists may use inappropriate art materials based on the client's age, medical background, or ability. They may overlook the therapeutic qualities of the art media and may not consider the importance of selecting a least to most controlled media referred to as the Media Dimension Variables (Graves-Alcorn & Green, 2014).

MDV). When processing the art activity, play therapists may also not consider the kinesthetic, sensory, perceptual, affective, cognitive, symbolic, and creative level of the media referred to as the Expressive Therapies Continuum (Landgarten, 1987; Kagan & Lusebrink, 1978; Lusebrink, 1990; Lusebrink, 1992; Graves-Alcorn & Green, 2014).

Safety Considerations of Art Media and Other Materials

When reviewing the recommended toys and materials for the primary play therapy theoretical orientations, thirteen theoretical orientations recommended art materials. These play therapy approaches included: Psychoanalytic (Klein, 1955; Carmichael, 2006; Lee, 2009), Adlerian (Kottman, 2011), Jungian Analytical (Allen & Levin, 1993; Allen, 1994), Child-Centered (Landreth, 2012), Gestalt (Oaklander, 1988), Relationship (Moustakas, 1959, 1997), Cognitive-Behavioral (Knell (1995, 1998, 2009), Child Developmental (Brody, 1992; Brody, 1997; Carmichael, 2006), Child Parent Relationship Training (Landreth & Bratton, 2006; Bratton, Landreth, Kellam, & Blackard, 2006, Filial (VanFleet, 2014), Family (Gil, 2014), Theraplay (Munns, 2000; Carmichael, 2006), and Prescriptive Play Therapy (Schaefer 2001; Gil & Shaw 2009). The categorizations or qualities of the art materials were not discussed possibly due to the scarcity of evidence-based literature in the field of play therapy. By play therapists becoming more aware of the safety considerations of art media and materials and the media dimension variables, play therapists can better prepare for their sessions and provide directive or non-directive art activities to better meet the needs of their clients.

When providing art materials to clients, it is important to be aware of the properties of the materials, abilities of the clients, as well as possible safety precautions when using certain materials. The chapter authors have noted possible safety considerations based on their personal and professional practice. Safety considerations of art materials include being mindful of the expiration date of paints, aerosols, and glue. Some art materials may also be flammable and cannot be stored in direct sunlight or rooms with elevated temperatures. Some materials must be stored in open, ventilated rooms due to possible toxic fumes. When using markers, it is also preferred to use washable and non-toxic markers and dry erase markers (Carmichael, 2006).

When working with art media and sand, the play therapist must always consider possible medical problems the client may have such as asthma, allergies, diabetes, or other chronic illnesses. Clients who are sensitive to dust or may have any respiratory problems may not be able to use chalk (CDC, 2019; Carmichael, 2006) or play with sand. Non-dust play sand is always recommended. Also, many materials may carry a Proposition 65 Warning that indicates any exposure to chemicals that may cause cancer, birth defects, or other reproductive harm. Materials such as silica and some paints have cancer-causing agents that result in a Proposition 65 Warning (Office of Environmental Health Hazard Assessment, 2019).

Many clients with severe asthma or allergies cannot tolerate smells found with certain paints, aerosols, markers, dry erase markers, Play-Doh, plasticine, clay or other materials that may have a strong odor (CDC, 2019). Further, many odors of art materials may linger in the room for an hour or hours; therefore, the play therapist should not only consider the needs of the current client they are working with but also future clients. Clients with major chronic illnesses may be very hypersensitive to certain smells, both art materials and food. If clients ingest any hazardous materials, the therapist needs to have a safety protocol in place with access to a fresh water source (CDC, 2019).

When working with children or clients who present with self-harming thoughts or behaviors or have a history of substance abuse, blunt scissors should be available, however all sharp objects (Rubin, 1999) or other hazardous materials, such as toxic markers, aerosols, X-ACTO knives or detailed knives, box cutters, or a cut-off wire or wire, should be removed. When working in an individual and group setting, the play therapist should ensure the return of all art materials and supplies by having an updated inventory list available and count all items before and after distributing the supplies to the clients.

Selection of Art Media

According to Landreth, toys should be carefully selected and not collected (2012). When using art media and other materials, media should also be purposefully selected. According to Wadeson (1980), art media should be purposefully selected based on the needs of the client and the goals of the session. When determining what art media to use in session, the therapist should consider the amount of space needed to complete the activity, how much preparation is required to set up the art media in the play therapy room, and how much time it will take to clean up after the session. If the client presents with difficulties either holding or controlling the media or has problems with gross and/or fine motor control such as young children or senior adults, it is recommended to use media that can be easily manipulated lending to more control. A sufficient variety of media and colors are needed, as well as an adequate size and amount of paper, canvasses, and other media such as clay or plasticine. Too much media can be overwhelming to clients; however, too little media can be restrictive and frustrating to clients. Wadeson (1980) suggested that when therapists are choosing art media, they should be aware of the possible feelings and reactions the media may elicit, as well as the properties of the media.

Media Dimension Variables (MDV)

According to the Media Dimension Variables, this concept was developed based on four factors including: "a) the reinforcement value of making art is inherently a therapeutic process; b) all individuals can be creative to some degree; c) dimensions of art media are discernable and can be classified; and d) media dimensions can be therapeutically applied." The continuum of least controlled media to most controlled media is referred to as the Media Dimension Variables (MDV). Beyond classifying materials as least to most controlled media, other aspects of the physical properties of the media were examined such as the media's fluidity, malleability, indestructibility, expansiveness, unpredictability, and adaptability. Three variables were delineated to include: a) structure, b) task complexity, and c) media properties. Unstructured activities or goals were left up to the client and the instructions were simple such as "Paint anything you wish." Structured activities provided little choice by the client with specific directions provided by the art therapist. Easy to complete tasks were classified as having a low-complexity versus complicated level. More difficult to complete tasks were classified as having a high-complexity level (Graves-Alcorn & Green, 2014, p. 4-5).

Art materials and media were either categorized as less restrictive and fluid in nature or more restrictive and complex in nature. Least controlled materials or media are soft, aqueous, malleable, and easy to manipulate. Examples of fluid media include finger paints, watercolors, soft or wet clay, soft plasticine, polymer acrylics, oil pastels, and thick felt markers. More controlled and restrictive materials are hard, brittle, slightly pliable to nonmalleable, and difficult to manipulate. Examples of more restive media include hard or highly gorged clay, hard plasticine, metal, wood, poster boards, heavier papers, collage materials, lead pencils, colored pencils, and felt markers. The medium based on more controlled or least controlled properties can heighten or lower the client's affective state, influence the freedom of expression, and can circumvent defenses (Graves-Alcorn & Green, 2014, Landgarten, 1987)

Expressive Therapies Continuum (ETC)

The Expressive Therapies Continuum (ETC) describes a systems-oriented approach to the expressive therapies. The ETC consists of three hierarchical levels, including the kinesthetic/sensory (K/S), the perceptual/affect (P/A), and the cognitive/symbolic level (C/S). These levels are based on "the sequence of increased complexity in cognitive and emotional development." The fourth level is that of creativity which can cross all of the levels. A reflective distance that "denotes the time span between the impulse or stimulus and the reaction to it" characterizes each level of the ETC. The reflective distance increases with the consecutively higher levels of the ETC from the first level of the kinesthetic/sensory to the cognitive/symbolic level (Landgarten, 1987, p.395; Kagan & Lusebrink, 1978; Lusebrink, 1990; Lusebrink, 1992; Graves-Alcorn & Green, 2014).

The *kinesthetic* component focuses on releasing energy and expressing it through bodily action such as pounding clay or scribbling on paper. The *sensory* component focuses on inner sensations and tactile experiences, including interacting with different media such as exploring finger-paints. The *perceptual* component focuses on the formation of schematic forms and representational images. Examples might include focusing on the formal elements of a form, color, or pattern. Experimenting with different media, such as highly structured media (pencils and markers) versus fluid media (watercolors and paints), allows the person to perceive the media differently and to enhance the *affective* component by applying intense color or using fluid media, thereby enhancing the expression of one's affect. The *cognitive* component emphasizes the analytical and logical thought required for information processing. The *symbolic* component emphasizes the metaphorical and intuitive nature of the art process whereby one can view problems differently and enhance problem solving and decision-making skills. The *creative expression* can be experienced on all three levels and can enhance all three components, thus encouraging new experiences though perceptual openness and enhanced receptiveness to inner and outer stimuli (Landgarten, 1987; Kagan & Lusebrink, 1978; Lusebrink, 1990; Lusebrink, 1992; Graves-Alcorn & Green, 2014).

Books and Bibliotherapy

Many play therapists use modern and older fictional and non-fictional books in play therapy. Bibliotherapy, as defined by Carmichael (2006), is the use of books, structured workbooks, stories, and recordings that address a specific topic. According to Knell (1995, 1998), bibliotherapy has been used as an adjunct to Cognitive-Behavioral Play Therapy. Children's literature offers messages and morals, but also serves as a storytelling approach. Many children's books may address specific clinical issues such as divorce, relocation, dying, or other traumas. By reading a story in which the character is experiencing the same problem as the child, the child may experience the sense that he or she is not alone and that other children may have experienced the same problem as the child. Secondly, bibliotherapy allows children to see that they are not alone in their feelings and if the character has learned to cope with whatever the presenting problem may have been, so can the child learn to cope with the problem or event. Finally, stories describing characters dealing with possible problems or traumas also provide a means of desensitizing the child to the presenting problem.

In many stories used in bibliotherapy, a message is conveyed more indirectly with the hopes that the child will learn something through the book characters through an indirect form of psychoeducation. The characters in the story will model for the child healthy ways of coping with life events. Many play therapists may also write a children's story particularly for a child dealing with a stressful event. The story may be read to the child several times over multiple sessions and sent home with the child so that the caregivers could continue to the read the story. The child may then be able to personalize the story and utilize the same healthy coping skills described in the story by the main character (Knell, 1995).

Selection of Books

Oaklander (1988) specifically recommended the use of fairy tales and folk tales to help children tap into the basic universal emotions of love, hate, fear, rage, loneliness, isolation, worthlessness, and deprivation. Children are able to gain meaning from the stories based on the individual person, as well as at various moments in the person's life. Regarding suggesting a list of recommended books to use in bibliotherapy, there are many different types of books and resources that may be helpful. Suggested topics by Pardeck and Pardeck (1994) included: changing role models, blended families, separation and divorce, child abuse, foster care, adoption, and childhood fears. Doll and Doll (1997) provided a list of recommended novels, picture books, poetry, and audiovisual materials to address building friendships for fourth-graders. Stanley (1999) further offered a recommendation of fiction, nonfiction, self-help books, and poetry with sample reading plans to address 36 diverse topics.

In Davis' (1996) *Once Upon a Time: Therapeutic Stories that Teach and Heal*, 108 therapeutic stories with a variety of themes were provided in twelve categories. These categories included: 1) stories that empower and treat symptoms of trauma and Post-Traumatic Stress Disorder; 2) stories that empower and treat symptoms of child abuse; 3) stories that develop healthy emotional reactions, thinking, perceptions, beliefs, self-image, and social skills; 4) stories to aid in the disclosure of traumatic experiences and/or abuse; 5) stories for children who must testify in court proceedings; 6) stories to reduce and eliminate nightmares; 7) stories for children who have not followed a normal developmental path; 8) stories to help with death, loss and illness; 9) stories to help with problems related to parents, siblings, adoption, foster care, and divorce; 10) stories for adolescents and adults; 11) stories for school-related problems; and 12) modern day fairy tales.

Kottman and Meany-Walen (2018) provided a list of recommended books to address 14 diverse topics in the publication, *Doing Play Therapy: From Building the Relationship to Facilitating Change*. These topics included: 1) maladaptively perfectionistic children; 2) children whose parents are divorcing; 3) anxious children and children with specific fears; 4) children who struggle with problem solving; 5) children with low self-esteem/self-confidence or need help with self-doubts/believing in themselves; 6) children who have experienced trauma; 7) foster and adopted children; 8) children being raised by grandparents; 9) children who steal and/or lie; 10) children with ADHD/impulsive behavior; 11) children who are uncomfortable about being different/struggle with belonging; 12) children with social skills and friendship issues; 13) children who need help with recognizing and expressing feelings; 14) angry and aggressive children; and 15) children with behavior problems.

Additionally, books about counseling and specifically play therapy may be helpful for clients to understand the process of counseling. The authors recommend Nemiroff and Annunziata's picture book published in 1990 entitled *A Child's First Book About Play Therapy,* Rashkin's (2005) book entitled *Feeling Better: A Kid's Book About Therapy,* and Zilberstein and Abel's (2014) book entitled *Calming Stormy Feelings: A Child's Introduction to Psychotherapy.*

Puppets and Puppet Theaters

Puppets are recommended in almost every play therapy theoretical orientation and are a staple in the field of play therapy. According to Landreth (2012), puppets can promote a wide range of feelings for children so that the child and the puppet may express a negative or positive feeling. Puppets provide a safe way for children to express their innermost emotions and thoughts without feeling threatened or judged. Children may also need a safe place to hide or escape from the therapist. The puppet theater allows the child the space to hide from the therapist and gain emotional distance and separation if needed.

Use of Puppets

Puppets can be used in both directive and non-directive therapy. They can be used in the assessment process as part of a structured or semi-structured interview (Knell, 1995) or as a clinical intervention with either only the child playing with puppets or the child and the therapist playing with the puppets simultaneously (Gil, 1994).

According to Oaklander (1988), it is easier for the child to talk through the puppet than it is for the child to say something directly to the therapist or caregiver.

The therapist can also utilize puppets for modeling purposes in CBPT. The therapist, through the voice of the puppet, can model adaptive coping skills for the child. As therapy progresses, the child may then incorporate these skills into the child's stories and puppet play. Eventually, the child may integrate the coping skills discussed and learned into his or her daily routines at home or school (Knell, 1998).

Selection of Puppets

Carter and Mason (1998) found the following guidelines useful when selecting puppets: 1) Choose puppets which are easy to manipulate for both children and adults; 2) Choose puppet figures that do not carry universal symbolism; 3) Choose puppets that will fit in both children's and adult's hands; 4) Choose puppets that are soft and cuddly as opposed to firm and rigid; 5) Choose puppets that are washable or can be dry cleaned; and 6) Choose puppets with personality that engage the child's and the therapist's imagination and can express a diverse range of feelings and behaviors. Bromfield (1995) also recommended choosing puppets with mouths to enhance verbal expression to allow additional behaviors such as eating, licking, sucking, and biting to occur. The chapter authors recommend choosing puppets with mouths and tongues to make it is easier to manipulate the puppets to kiss, sing, yell, whisper, cough, and yawn. If the child may be experiencing inappropriate touch, a medical illness, or needs to express a secret or intense feelings, having well-defined mouth movements will allow the child to express more verbal and nonverbal information through the use of puppetry.

Based on the work of Irwin (1993), Carter and Mason (1998), and Sweeney, Baggerly, and Ray (2014), it is recommended to have a wide range of puppets with at least 15 to 25 puppets. Gil (1994) recommended having at least 30 puppets present to include duplicates of selected puppets. When providing group therapy to more than five children, it is suggested to have more than a five to one ratio of puppets to children.

The puppets need to represent a wide range of affects including neutral, friendly, and aggressive puppets. The selection needs to include real and fantasy puppets, realistic and ethnically diverse family puppets, and royal family puppets including a puppet to represent mothers, fathers, children, a queen and king puppet, and a princess and prince puppet. Occupational puppets are recommended to include doctors, nurses, policemen, and teachers. Symbolic puppets are recommended to include a ghost, witch, devil, skeleton, and pirate. Animal puppets are recommended to include both wild or predatory or domestic or tame animals (Irwin 1993; Carter & Mason, 1998).

Gil (1994) recommended having duplicates of selected puppets to symbolically represent blurred boundaries, sibling rivalry, or a lack of differentiation among family members. When working with children with abuse or neglect issues, children may need to retreat symbolically when sharing their thoughts or feelings. Additional recommended animal puppets may include a turtle puppet with a shell so that the turtle can retreat and hide. Other recommended hand or finger puppets utilized by the authors include an armadillo, clam, or snail with a shell for hiding or other animal or people puppets that are housed or can hide in a tree, house, shelter, box, or can. Gil (1994) further recommended possible aggressive or neutral puppets such as a tarantula, other spiders, or sharks that may have the ability to intimidate others and can make a quick entrance and exit. Other aggressive puppets used by the chapter authors include puppets with large teeth such as a monster, dinosaur, alligator, crocodile, tiger, lion, wolf, bear, Tasmanian devil, piranha, or barracuda puppet.

Gil (1994) proposed having a caterpillar puppet that can turn into a butterfly to represent a state of metamorphosis, a fairy godmother who can grant wishes, a judge who can make decisions, police puppets who can maintain the law, and reversible puppets who can be turned over to uncover another character. Additional cultural considerations for a puppet selection may include having an indigenous healer, priests, or mariachi puppets. The chapter authors recommend having puppets available to represent family pets such as a cat, dog, bird, fish, rabbit, guinea pig, gerbil, hamster, ferret, hedgehog, small turtle, lizard, and a snake. Additional family puppets to be considered may include having a grandmother, grandfather, or a senior or aged puppet to represent an older family or community member. Many children often come into therapy to deal with grief or loss issues. They may need specific people or animal puppets to represent the family member or pet they have lost. They may further need religious or spiritual puppets such as a priest, minster, or angel to help them deal with their loss.

The authors further suggest having people puppets that represent the children and families we serve with puppet clothing and other items to represent the child's family heritage. It is also recommended by the authors to have animal puppets from the child's geographical background such as a Tasmanian devil or a camel puppet so that the child may experience a closer connection to his or her home environment. The authors also suggest having selected puppets from popular fairytales and storybooks including an elf, gnome, unicorn, genie, troll, jester, magician, dragon, monster, alien, and prehistoric animals such as a sabretooth tiger, mastodon, or wooly mammoth for the purpose of fairytale and folktale enactments. Please see *Appendix A* for a list of puppet artists and retailers listed alphabetically.

Basic Skills of Puppet Use

Carter and Mason (1998) acknowledged that many play therapists may be apprehensive to use puppets due to possibly appearing foolish in front of their clients. Hand puppets are noted to be the most popular type of puppet due to their ease of use and weight. When therapists are using puppets in counseling, there are some points to remember when using hand puppets. A puppet should hold the interest of the audience and should look directly at the audience. Many puppeteers or therapists make the mistake of having the puppet either look up towards the ceiling or down towards the floor. When using puppets, it is recommended to keep the puppet moving; do not keep the puppet still and staring into space. It is also important that the movements of the puppets should mimic human-like movements such as talking and walking. When talking using the puppet, one should manipulate only the lower jaw, not the upper jaw or both. The therapist should keep the upper jaw fixed since all humans and most animals only move the lower jaw. To wrinkle the face of the hand puppet, the therapist can move the thumb to emphasize different emotions. When practicing with puppets, the therapist can practice in the front of a mirror tailing, walking, or singing. The child will be more likely to respond to the puppet if the puppet acts more lifelike and engaging with the child.

Further, if the play therapist can take a puppetry course or workshop and learn more about the manipulation of hand and rod puppets, the therapist will have an additional avenue to emotionally and physically connect with the caregivers and children served. By using rod puppets, the puppets are not only able to establish an emotional connection with the child, therapist, and/or caregivers, but also a physical connection with other people or puppets through the use of hand or foot rods. For families that may have difficulty expressing physical intimacy or appropriate physical boundaries, connection, or contact among the family members, the caregivers and children may be able to initiate and receive physical contact in a safe and appropriate manner.

Sandtrays and Miniatures

Sand and some variation of a use of sandtray in therapy is another common approach utilized among various play therapists of diverse theoretical orientations. Sandtray as defined by Homeyer and Sweeney (2017), is "an expressive and projective mode of psychotherapy involving the unfolding and processing of intra and inter-personal issues through the use of specific sandtray materials as a nonverbal medium of communication, led by the client or therapist and facilitated by a trained therapist" (p. 5).

Based on the clinician's theoretical orientation, one may practice from a variety of recommendations including, but not limited to, The World Technique (Lowenfeld, 1939,1950), The World Test (Buhler, 1951); The Picture World Test (Buhler & Manson, 1956); Sandplay Therapy (Bradway, 1979; Kalf 2004), Sandrama (Toscani, 1998); Sandplay-Worldplay (De Demenico, 2000), or Sandtray Therapy (Homeyer & Sweeney, 2017). Sandtray containers may vary by number, size, color, shape, and type of sand based on diverse theoretical orientations. The above play therapists and researchers are merely a partial list of contributors associated with the use of sand and sandtray as an assessment tool or as the primary clinical intervention; however, having an extensive sandtray miniature collection is required to assist the client in exploring one's thoughts, feelings, behaviors, and wishes.

Selection of Sandtray Miniatures

Different types of sandtrays may be used, along with various types of miniatures lending to diverse theoretical interpretations, and distinctive forms of processing the activity (Lowenfeld, 1950; Buhler, 1951; Buhler & Manson, 1956; Bradway, 1979; Allan, 1994; Toscani, 1998; De Demenico, 2000; Kalf, 2004; Sweeney, Baggerly, & Ray, 2014; Homeyer & Sweeney, 2017). According to Lowenfeld (1950), miniatures are viewed as the words, symbols, and metaphors for the client's nonverbal communication. The figures can be used to express thoughts, beliefs, feelings, and desires that may be too overwhelming or challenging for the clients to express in words. It is recommended that therapists have a great number and a wide variety of miniatures with multiples of many objects. The size of the miniatures should vary with some miniatures being smaller than others so that not all of the miniatures are in scale with one another. The composition of miniatures should also vary. The miniatures may be made of wood, plastic, and metal with different shapes, colors, weights, and textures. There should include a wide array of category of miniatures including people, animals, buildings, vegetation, boundary structures, natural items, fantasy, spiritual/mystical, landscaping, household items, vehicles, and additional miscellaneous items.

Lowenfeld (1939; 1950), a British pediatrician who was first documented using sandplay as a counseling technique, recommended clinicians possess people miniatures including: 1) Ordinary: farmers, workers, policeman, country/city (sitting and standing); 2) Military: soldiers, guns, tanks, some from county not known to children (some lying down); and 3) Special: circus, witches, gnomes, and other cultures. The miniature collection should also include *houses* (both large and small, shops, stations, churches, schools). Tree sizes should vary with large and small variations, as well as bushes, hedges, and jungle trees. A large quantity of fences should be included in the miniature selection with gates and different types of bridges. The *animal selection* should include wild animals (both timid and fierce animals with wild birds), and tame animals such as farm animals and birds, horses, and other domestic animals. The age (both young and old) and the sex of the animals should differ.

Transport miniatures may include: 1) Road (most usual on child's country's roads), 2) Rail (open and closed rail cars and coal cars), and 3) River and Sea (ordinary and military). Street signs should include gas pumps and telephone boxes. Lastly, a *miscellaneous category* should include garden equipment, flowers, domestic equipment such as vacuums, school desks, lavatories (interior thought), planks, blocks, broken parts of objects and people, sticks, and stones (Lowenfeld, 1950).

Homeyer and Sweeney (2017) offered suggestions for intentionally selecting sandtray miniatures and not just collecting miniatures. Many sandtray miniatures are made from plastic; they are both durable and inexpensive. Plastic miniatures are easier to select; however, the miniatures should be diverse in size, type and composition. Sandtray miniatures should be small so that they can fit in the sandtray; however, the miniatures do not have to be to scale as found in railroad miniatures. It is also important to have some miniatures such as predatory animals or creatures (e.g. rats, spiders, snakes) to represent a power differential between the client and a possible perpetrator. The miniature people figures should be representative of the client's world with varying ethnicities and occupations. The vegetation should vary with different trees, bushes, and grass. Diverse living accommodations such as single-family housing, multi-family housing, and apartment buildings should be included. The buildings and structures should reflect regional and geographical differences. The miniatures should also vary based on a variety of materials such as natural materials (e.g. wood, minerals, rock, sea shells) either shaped or in the original or carved form. It is also important to have heavy and light items that may be textured.

Homeyer and Sweeney (2017) published a suggested list of 300 required miniature toys in 11 categories. These categories are listed below: 1. *People* (diverse families, babies with different poses if possible); bride and groom; occupational figures (police, firemen, construction workers, etc.); 16 or more army solders; and astronauts or knights; 2. *Animals* (four different dinosaurs, and zoo animals (lions, giraffes, zebra, and elephants), domestic animals such as cows, horses, sheep, insects, spiders, snakes, and sea animals; 3. *Vegetation* (trees, plants, and flowers); 4. *Buildings* (houses, school, lighthouse, castle fort, teepee, or jail); 5. *Vehicles* (cars, trucks, airplane, boat, helicopter, police car, ambulance, and other rescue vehicles; 6. *Fences and Signs* (fences, traffic signs, and barricades); 7. *Natural Items* (sea shells, vegetation, twigs, rocks that are plain and polished, Fools gold, and crystal; 8. *Fantasy* (wizard, fairy godmother, dragons, monsters, cartoon figures, and space aliens); 9. *Spiritual Mystical* (angels, cross Buddha, Madonna, Star of David, and menorah) and small mirrors; 10. *Landscaping and Other Accessories (*wishing well, bridges, treasure chest, treasure, gold coins, cannon, and various flags); and 11. *Household Items* (furniture, tools, garbage can, mailbox; windmill, and food).

Psychotherapeutic Games

There are many therapeutic games that may be useful in therapy, both currently and no longer manufactured or published. Dr. Richard Gardner's first developed therapeutic game, *The Talking, Feeling, and Doing Game* (Creative Therapeutics, Cresskill, NJ) was first developed in 1968 and later published and made available to mental health professionals in 1973. Since then, there have been approximately 100 additional therapeutic games published. Shapiro (1993) published *The Book of Psychotherapeutic Games: A Review of the Most Popular Games Used in Psychotherapy* to describe 70 psychotherapeutic games. He describes each game according to five primary categories with additional subcategories. The categories are as follows: 1) age considerations of the players; 2) numbers of recommended players; 3) types of games; 4) who the game is designed for such as mental health professionals, mental health professionals with at least a master's degree, parents, teachers, or a general audience; and 5) the major theme of the game or the recommended theoretical orientation. For the major themes or theories, classifications were determined by the editors and not by the original authors.

Each game may address a specific skill such as communication, cooperative, diagnostic/therapeutic, skill-oriented, theory-oriented, and theme oriented. Communication games are designed primarily to teach and/or stimulate communication skills. Cooperative games demonstrate the benefits of cooperation among the players with no winners or losers. Everyone wins the game together. Diagnostic/ therapeutic games a have a broader purpose of diagnosing and treating the problem. Skill-oriented games teach specific psychological and/or social skills. Theory-oriented games indicate a specific theory of psychology or counseling. Theme oriented games are designed to address a specific psychoeducational problems or concerns (Shapiro, 1993).

LIMITATIONS

When conducting the literature review for this chapter, the chapter authors either found limited information on certain topics or a vast amount of information on other topics that were well researched and published. Therefore, the authors chose to provide limited, more general, or detailed information based on the available research gathered. The authors also reflected upon over 25 years each of clinical practice in multiple settings and over 15 years each of teaching experiences at multiple universities and other professional settings teaching diverse art and play therapy, community mental health and substance abuse counseling, marriage and family therapy, and human services and social work coursework. Many recommendations were based on professional practice, teaching, and supervisory experiences. The authors attempted to review multiple considerations to explore when setting up university-based and community-based play therapy clinics offering clinical services to the community, as well as many considerations when establishing a university-based play therapy training site providing mock play services to play therapy trainees. Acknowledging the current fluid nature of global immigration, the authors were unable to locate recent professional peer-reviewed data reflecting children and adolescent refugees seeking play therapy services.

Recommendations

Due to the limitations of this chapter, the chapter authors have made several recommendations related to considerations when designing a play therapy space or clinic. There is still more room for further research on the multicultural refugee needs and settings. In the community-based agencies, the authors recommend play therapists to consider the multicultural groups they serve by providing a milieu consistent with their demographic groups' cultural norms and values when setting up their play therapy clinics.

It is further recommended that university and community-based settings provide opportunities for direct clinical experiences to work with children, adolescents, and families under the direct supervision of a licensed professional who is a qualified Registered Play Therapist-Supervisor (RPT-S). If an RPT-S is not available at community-based sites, it is recommended to have an RPT-S from the university-based training site provide on-site supervision and trainings for the agencies or sites.

Mock play therapy experiences are helpful at university-based sites; however, play therapy trainees need as many opportunities as possible to work with diverse clinical populations. Further, it is necessary to create play laboratories in the classroom setting when providing graduate play therapy instruction for play therapy trainees, as well as ensure the university-based play therapy training sites are well equipped with play therapy toys and materials to correspond to the primary fourteen play therapy theoretical orientations or approaches discussed in the chapter. It is also recommended that all play therapy clinics have the basic play therapy toys and supplies to include: art media and other materials; books for use in bibliotherapy; puppets and puppet theaters; sandtrays and miniatures; and psychotherapeutic games.

It is also suggested that when APT updates the Association for Play Therapy publication, *The Play Therapy Best Practices*, in 2019, these areas reviewed in this chapter are included: a) recommendations for toys and materials based on diverse theoretical orientations, cultural sensitivity, and specific considerations for popular materials; b) play therapy space and technology; c) considerations for specific settings and multicultural practice, d) the need for consistent play therapy supervision by a RPT-S for all students completing a practicum or internship placement either at a university setting or off-site community-based setting; and e) the need and possible benefits for a consistent playroom laboratory in all graduate classroom settings. By developing and sustaining quality play therapy clinics and training sites, as well as conducting research in our field to guide our clinical practice, this will promote the field of play therapy and ensure we are providing the most efficacious treatments according to *The Play Therapy Best Practices.* In light of the ever-evolving nature of global immigration, studies are needed to reflect emerging needs, interventions, and trends of children and teens who are refugees seeking play therapy services.

CONCLUSION

This chapter presented the required toys based on one's theoretical orientation, and the therapeutic space necessary to provide quality play therapy services based on the available research and the authors' professional experiences within the field of play therapy. A detailed discussion about toy selection specific to the wide-variety of theoretical orientations provided information necessary for both trainees and supervisors designing and practicing in university and community-based play therapy clinics. The authors presented considerations for most-represented multicultural groups including play space, toys, and values to be acknowledged when working with children, adolescents and their families. Trainees and play therapy supervisors face a myriad of issues in today's play practices. Having current information is more than helpful. It is critical to providing best practice to our children, adolescents, families and groups.

Presently, there is limited research and/or practical application literature available regarding prudent and effective preparation and set-up of a play therapy training clinic. Many perspectives and considerations went into the development of this chapter, as well as review of the existing research and literature. In addition, using a filter of having over 25 years of teaching and therapeutic application in a variety of settings, the authors reflected upon their personal experiences and offered a pragmatic direction that may be followed by those who wish to establish their own play therapy training clinic using this as a guide.

The chapter offers guidance to creating an appropriate therapeutic space for providing play therapy services. Emphasis is placed on the importance of cultural sensitivity and accommodating for the various client cultural therapeutic needs, setting up for clinical theoretical orientations that are appropriate and match the specific client populations, being mindful of safety concerns, and discussing technological and/or mechanical enhancements that better serve the clients' needs. Given this, clinicians are guided to be mindful and intentional when they select, acquire, and organize toys and materials in the play therapy room based on evidence-based practices, including the use of art media and other materials, books and bibliotherapy, puppets and puppet theaters, sandtrays and miniatures, and psychotherapeutic games.

A discussion was provided on the required toys based on theoretical orientation, the therapeutic space necessary to provide quality play therapy services from the available research, and the authors' professional experiences within the field of play therapy. A detailed discussion about toy selection specific to the wide-variety of theoretical orientations provided information necessary for both trainees and supervisors designing and practicing in university and community-based play therapy clinics. The authors presented considerations for most-represented multicultural groups including play space, toys, and values to be acknowledged when working with children, adolescents and their families.

Trainees and play therapy supervisors face a myriad of issues in today's play practices. Having current information is more than helpful and critical to providing best practice to our children, adolescents, families and groups. The authors make suggestions and recommendations that illuminate and pave the way for needed research in the future and open discourse between clinicians and researchers that may positively heighten the play therapy experience and provide more efficacious treatment outcomes.

REFERENCES

Abramsky, S. (2012). The other America 2012. *Nation, 294*(20), 11-18. Retrieved from https://login.ezproxy.net.ucf.edu/login?auth=shibb&url=https://search-ebscohost-com.ezproxy.net.ucf.edu/login.aspx?direct=true&AuthType=ip,cookie,shib,sso,uid&db=ulh&AN=74602403&site=eds-live&scope=site

Allan, J. (1994). *Inscapes of the child's world: Jungian counseling in schools and clinics*. Dallas, TX: Spring Publications, Inc.

Allen, J., & Levin, S. (1993). Born on my bum: Jungian play therapy. In T. Kottman & C. Schaefer (Eds.), *Play therapy: A casebook for practitioners* (pp. 209–243). Northvale, NJ: Aronson.

American Association for Marriage and Family Therapy. (2015). Retrieved August 5, 2018 from https://www.aamft.org/Legal_Ethics/Code_of_Ethics.aspx

American Counseling Association. (2014). *2014 ACA Code of Ethics - As approved by the ACA Governing Council.* Retrieved August 5, 2018 from ttps://www.counseling.org/resources/ aca-code-of-ethics.pdf

American Psychological Association. (2017). *Ethical Principles of Psychologists and Code of Conduct.* Retried on August 5, 2018 from http://www.apa.org/ethics/code/ethics-code-2017.pdf

Association for Play Therapy. (2016). *Play Therapy Best Practices: Clinical, Professional, and Ethical Issues.* Retrieved August 2, 2018 from https://cdn.ymaws.com/www.a4pt.org/ resource/resmgr/publications/Best_Practices__-_Sept_2016.pdf

Association for Play Therapy. (2019). Retrieved from https://www.a4pt.org/ page/ Credentials Homepage

Association of Play Therapy. (2019). *Approved provider guide.* Retrieved from https://cdn.ymaws.com/www.a4pt.org/resource/resmgr/education_&_training/approved_ provider_guide_-_au.pdf

Axline, V. M. (1969). *Play therapy.* New York, NY: Ballantine Books.

Baggerly, J. (2006). Service learning with children affected by pervert: Facilitating multicultural competence in counseling education students. *Journal of Multicultural Counseling and Development, 34*(4), 244-255. Retrieved from https://login.ezproxy.net.ucf.edu/login?auth=shibb&url=https://search-ebscohost-com.ezproxy.net.ucf.edu/login.aspx?direct=true&AuthType=ip,cookie,shib,sso,uid&db=tfh&AN=23054881&site=eds-live&scope=site

Baggerly, J., & Abugideiri, S. E. (2010). Grief counseling for Muslim preschool and elementary school children. *Journal of Multicultural Counseling and Development, 38*(2), 112–124. Retrieved from https://login.ezproxy.net.ucf.edu/login?auth=shibb&url=https://search- ebscohost-com.ezproxy.net.ucf.edu/login.aspx?direct= true&AuthType= ip, cookie,shib,sso,uid&db=eric&AN=EJ881625&site=eds-live&scope=site

Barnes, M. A. (1996). *The healing path with children: An exploration for parents and professionals.* Kingston, Ontario, Canada: Viktoria, Fermoyle, & Berrigan.

Bradway, K. (1979). Sandplay in psychotherapy. *Art Psychotherapy, 6*(2), 85–93. doi:10.1016/0090-9092(79)90003-6

Bratton, S. C., Landreth, G. L., Kellam, T., & Blackard, S. R. (2006). *Child parent relationship therapy (CPRT) treatment manual: A 10-session filial therapy model for training parents*. New York, NY: Routledge Taylor and Francis Group. doi:10.4324/9780203956793

Brody, V. (1992). The dialogue of touch: Developmental play therapy. *International Journal of Play Therapy, 1*(1), 21–30. doi:10.1037/h0090232

Brody, V. (1997). *The dialogue of touch: Developmental play therapy*. Northvale, NJ: J. Aronson.

Bromfield, R. (1995). The use of puppets in play therapy. *Child & Adolescent Social Work Journal, 12*(6), 435–444. doi:10.1007/BF01875812

Brubaker, M. D., Puig, A., Reese, R. F., & Young, J. (2010). Integrating social justice into counseling theories pedagogy: A case example. *Counselor Education and Supervision, 50*(2), 88–102. Retrieved from https://login.ezproxy.net.ucf.edu/login?auth=shibb&url= https://search-ebscohost-com.ezproxy.net.ucf.edu/login.aspx?direct= true&AuthType=ip,cookie, shib,sso,uid&db=eric&AN=EJ911809&site=eds- live&scope=site

Buhler, C. (1951). The world test, a projective technique. *Journal of Child Psychiatry, 2*, 4–23.

Buhler, C., & Manson, M. (1956). The picture world test: A new projective technique. *The Journal of Psychology, 42*(2), 303–316. doi:10.1080/00223980.1956.9713043

Burnes, T. R., & Singh, A. A. (2010). Integrating social justice training into the practicum experience for psychology trainees: Starting earlier. *Training and Education in Professional Psychology, 4*(3), 153–162. doi:10.1037/a0019385

Carmichael, K. (2006). *Play therapy: An introduction*. Upper Saddle River, NJ: Pearson Education, Inc.

Carter, R., & Mason, P. (1998). The selection and use of puppets in counseling. *Professional School Counseling, 1*(5), 50–53.

Cattanach, A. (2003). *Introduction to play therapy*. Hove, NY: Brunner-Routledge.

Ceballos, P. L., Parikh, S., & Post, P. B. (2012). Examining social justice attitudes among play therapists: Implications for multicultural supervision and training. *International Journal of Play Therapy, 21*(4), 232–243. doi:10.1037/a0028540

Centers for Disease Control and Prevention. (2019). *Workplace Safety and Health Topics*. Retrieved from https://www.cdc.gov/niosh/index.htm

Centers for Disease Control and Prevention. (2019). *Asthma: Management and treatment*. Retrieved from https://www.cdc.gov/niosh/index.htm

Chang, C., Ritter, K., & Hays, D. (2005). Multicultural trends and toys in play therapy. *International Journal of Play Therapy*, *14*(2), 69–85. doi:10.1037/h0088903

Coleman, V., Parmer, T., & Barker, S. (1993). Play therapy for multicultural populations: Guidelines for mental health professionals. *International Journal of Play Therapy*, *2*(1), 63–74. doi:10.1037/h0089381

Davis, N. (1996). *Once upon a time: Therapeutic stories that teach and heal*. Royal Oak, MI: Self-Esteem Shop.

De Domenico, G. (2000). *Sandtray-Worldplay: A comprehensive guide to the use of sandtray in psychotherapy and transformational settings*. Oakland, CA: Vision Quest Images.

De Domenico, G. (2000). *An experiential Sandtray-Worldplay home study course for individuals and groups (Module 1)*. Oakland, CA: Vision Quest Images.

Department of Justice. (2010). *2010 ADA standards for accessible design*. Retrieved from https://www.ada.gov/regs2010/2010ADAStandards/2010ADAStandards.pdf

Dixon, A. L., Tucker, C., & Clark, M. A. (2010). Integrating Social Justice Advocacy with National Standards of Practice: Implications for School Counselor Education. *Counselor Education and Supervision, 50*(2), 103–115. Retrieved from https://login.ezproxy.net.ucf.edu/login?auth=shibb&url=https://search-ebscohost- com.ezproxy.net.ucf.edu/login.aspx?direct=true&AuthType=ip,cookie,shib,sso,uid&db=e ric&AN=EJ911810&site=eds-live&scope=site

Doll, B., & Doll, C. (1997). *Bibliotherapy with young people: Librarians and mental heath Professionals working together*. Englewood, CA: Libraries Unlimited, Inc.

Figures at a Glance. (2018, June 19). Retrieved from http: //www.unhcr.org/figures-at-a glance.htm

Fontes, C., Coral, T., & Toso, L. (2015). The therapeutic toy in a pediatric critical care environment: Integrative Review. *Journal of Nursing*, *9*(8), 8899–8907.

Gardner, R. (1973). *The Talking, Feeling, and Doing Game*. Cresskill, NJ: Creative Therapeutics.

Gardner, R. A. (2001). The talking, feeling, and doing game. In C. E. Schaefer & S. E. Reid (Eds.), *Gameplay: Therapeutic use of childhood games* (2nd ed.; pp. 78–105). New York: Wiley.

Gil, E. (2005). From sensitivity to competence in working across cultures. In E. Gil & A. A. Drewes (Eds.), *Cultural issues in play therapy* (pp. 3–25). New York, NY: Guilford Press.

Gil, E. (2006). *Helping abused and traumatized children*. New York: Guilford Press.

Gil, E. (2015). *Play in family therapy* (2nd ed.). New York: The Guilford Press.

Gil, E., & Shaw, J. A. (2009). Prescriptive Play Therapy. In K. O'Conner & L. Braverman (Eds.), *Play therapy theory and practice: comparing theories and techniques* (2nd ed.; pp. 451–487). Hoboken, NJ: John Wiley & Sons, Incorporated.

Graves-Alcorn, S. L., & Green, E. J. (2014). The Expressive Arts Therapy Continuum: History and Theory. In E. J. Green & A. A. Drewes (Eds.), *Integrating expressive arts and play therapy with children and adolescents* (pp. 1–16). Hoboken, NJ: John Wiley & Sons, Incorporated.

Haidt, J., Koller, S. H., & Dias, M. G. (1993). Affect, culture, and morality, or is it wrong to eat your dog? *Journal of Personality and Social Psychology*, *65*(4), 613–628. doi:10.1037/0022-3514.65.4.613 PMID:8229648

Hanson, M. J. (2004). Ethnic, cultural, and language diversity in service settings. In E. E. Lynch & M. J. Hanson (Eds.), *Developing cross-cultural competence: A guide for working with with children and their families*. Baltimore, MD: Brookes Publishing Company.

Hinman, C. (2003). Multicultural considerations in the delivery of play therapy services. International Journal of Play Therapy, 12, 107-122. doi:10.1037/h0088881

Homeyer, L., & Sweeney, D. (2017). *Sandtray: A practical manual* (3rd ed.). New York, NY: Routledge.

Huang, Ln. N. (1998). Southeast Asian refugee children and adolescents. In J. T. Gibbs & L. N. Huang (Eds.), Children of color: Psychological interventions with culturally diverse youth (pp. 264-304). San Francisco, CA: Josey-Bass Publishers.

Hudak, D. (2000). The therapeutic use of ball play in psychotherapy with children. *International Journal of Play Therapy*, *9*(1), 1–10. doi:10.1037/h0089437

Irvin, E. C. (1993). Using puppets in assessment. In C. E. Schaefer & D. M. Cangelosi (Eds.), *Play therapy techniques* (pp. 69–81). Northvale, NJ: Jason Aaronson.

Kagan, S., & Lusebrink, V. (1978). The expressive therapies continuum. *Art Psychotherapy*, *5*(4), 171–180. doi:10.1016/0090-9092(78)90031-5

Kalff, D. M. (2004). *Sandplay: A psychotherapeutic approach to the psyche.* Cloverdale, CA: Temenos Press.

Killian, T., Cardona, B., & Hudspeth, E. F. (2017). Culturally responsive play therapy with Somali refugees. *International Journal of Play Therapy, 26*(1) 23-32. https://doi-org.ezproxy.net.ucf.edu/10.1037/pla0000040

Klein, M. (1955). The psychoanalytic play technique. *The American Journal of Orthopsychiatry, 25*(2), 223–237. doi:10.1111/j.1939-0025.1955.tb00131.x PMID:14376493

Knell, S. (1998). Cognitive-behavioral play therapy. *Journal of Clinical Child Psychology, 27*(1), 28–33. doi:10.120715374424jccp2701_3 PMID:9561934

Knell, S. M. (1995). *Cognitive-behavioral play therapy.* Northvale, NJ: Jason Aronson Inc.

Knell, S. M. (2009). Cognitive-Behavioral Play Therapy. In K. O'Conner & L. Braverman (Eds.), *Play therapy theory and practice: comparing theories and techniques* (2nd ed.; pp. 203–236). Hoboken, NJ: John Wiley & Sons, Incorporated.

Kottman, T. (2011). *Play Therapy: Basics and beyond* (2nd ed.). Alexandria, VA: American Counseling Association.

Kottman, T., & Meany-Walen, K. K. (2018). *Doing play therapy: From building the relationship to facilitating change.* New York: The Guilford Press.

Kranz, P. L., Ramirez, S. Z., Flores-Torres, L., Steele, R., & Lund, N. L. (2005). Physical settings, materials, and related Spanish terminology recommended for play therapy with first-generation Mexican-American children. *Education, 126*(1), 93-99. Retrieved from https://login.ezproxy.net.ucf.edu/login?auth=shibb&url=https://search-ebscohost- com.ezproxy.net.ucf.edu/login.aspx?direct=true&AuthType=ip,cookie,shib,sso,uid&db=e ric&AN=EJ725160&site=eds-live&scope=site

Landgarten, H. (1987). *Family art psychotherapy: A clinical guide and casebook.* New York, NY: Brunner/ Mazel Publishers.

Landreth, G. (2003). *Toys & materials for play therapy.* Denton, TX: Play Therapy Institute.

Landreth, G. (2012). *Play therapy: The art of the relationship* (3rd ed.). New York, NY: Routledge Taylor and Francis Group. doi:10.4324/9780203835159

Landreth, G., & Bratton, S. (2006). *Child parent relationship therapy (CPRT): A 10-session filial therapy model.* New York, NY: Routledge Taylor and Francis Group.

Lee, A. C. (2009). Psychoanalytic Play Therapy. In K. O'Conner & L. Braverman (Eds.), *Play therapy theory and practice: comparing theories and techniques* (2nd ed.; pp. 25–81). Hoboken, NJ: John Wiley & Sons, Incorporated.

Lowenfeld, M. (1939). The world pictures of children: A method of recording and studying them. *The British Journal of Medical Psychology*, *18*(1), 65–101. doi:10.1111/j.2044-8341.1939.tb00710.x

Lowenfeld, M. (1950). The nature and use of the Lowenfeld World Technique in work with children and adults. *The Journal of Psychology*, *30*(2), 325–331. doi:10.1080/00223980.1950.9916070

Lusebrink, V. (1992). A systems-oriented approach to the expressive therapies: The expressive therapies continuum. *The Arts in Psychotherapy*, *18*(5), 395–404. doi:10.1016/0197-4556(91)90051-B

Lusebrink, V. B. (1990). *Imagery and visual expression in therapy*. New York, NY: Plenum Press.B. doi:10.1007/978-1-4757-0444-0

Moncada, F. (1962). *Asi juegan los ninos: Recopilacion de juegos infantiles*. Mexicao, D. F., Mexico: Editorial Avante.

Moustakas, C. E. (1959). *Psychotherapy with children*. Harper and Row.

Moustakas, C. E. (1997). *Relationship play therapy*. Northvale, NJ: Jason Aronson Incorporated.

Munns, E. (2000). *Theraplay: Innovations in attachment-enhancing play therapy*. Northvale, NJ: Jason Aronson Incorporated.

National Association for Social Work. (2015). *Standards and indicators for cultural competence in social work practice*. NASW Press. Retrieved from https://www.socialworkers.org/ LinkClick.aspx?fileticket= 7dVckZAYUmk%3d&portalid=0

National Association of Social Workers. (2017). Retrieved August 3, 2018 from www.socialworks.org/About/ethics/Code-of-Ethics

National Board for Certified Counselors. (2016). Retrieved August 3, 2018 from http://www.nbcc.org/Assets/Ethics/NBCCCodeofEthics.pdf/

Nemiroff, M. A., & Annunziata, J. (1990). *A child's first book about play therapy*. Washington, DC: American Psychological Association.

O'Connor, K. (1994). Ecosystemic play therapy. In K. O'Connor & C. Schafer (Eds.), *Handbook of play therapy: Advances and innovations* (Vol. 2, pp. 61–84). New York: Wiley.

O'Connor, K. (2000). *The play therapy primer* (2nd ed.). New York, NY: Wiley.

O'Connor, K. (2005). Addressing diversity issues in play therapy. *Professional Psychology: Research and Practice, 36*(5), 566-573. https://doi-rg.ezproxy.net.ucf.edu/10.1037/0735-7028.36.5.566

O'Connor, K., & Braverman, L. (2009). *Play therapy theory and practice: Comparing theories and techniques* (2nd ed.). Hoboken, NJ: John Wiley and Sons, Incorporated.

O'Connor, K. J. (2009). Ecosystemic Play Therapy. In K. O'Conner & L. Braverman (Eds.), *Play therapy theory and practice: comparing theories and techniques* (2nd ed.; pp. 367–450). Hoboken, NJ: John Wiley & Sons, Incorporated.

Oaklander, V. (1988). *Windows to our children: A Gestalt approach to working with children and adolescents*. Gouldsboro, ME: The Gestalt Journal Press.

Odom, S. L., Pungello, E. P., & Gardner-Neblett, N. (Eds.). (2012). Translating contemporary developmental and health science: Designing an early childhood program for young children and their families living in poverty. In Infants, toddlers, and families living in poverty: Research implications for early child care (pp. 353–371). New York, NY: Guilford Press.

Office of Environmental Health Hazard Assessment (OEHHA). (2019). *Proposition 65 Warnings Website*. Retrieved from https://www.p65warnings.ca.gov/

Pardeck, J. T., & Pardeck, J. A. (1993). *Bibliotherapy: A clinical approach to helping children*. London: Gordon and Breach Science Publishers.

Parikh, S. B., Cebellow, P., & Post, P. (2013). Application: Theory to culturally competent practice: Factors related to play therapists' social justice advocacy attitudes. *Journal of Multicultural Counseling and Development, 41*(4), 240–252. doi:10.1002/j.2161-1912.2013.00039.x

Patterson, L., Stutey, D. M., & Dorsey, B. (2018). Play therapy with African American children exposed to adverse childhood experiences. *International Journal of Play Therapy, 27*(4), 215-226. https://doi-org.ezproxy.net.ucf.edu/10.1037/pla0000080

Post, P., & Tillman, L. S. (2015). Cultural issues in play therapy. In D. A. Crenshaw & A. L. Stewart (Eds.), *Play therapy: A comprehensive guide to theory and practice* (pp. 406–510). New York, NY: The Guilford Press.

Ramirez, O. (1998). Mexican American children and adolescents. In J. T. Gibbs & L. N. Huang (Eds.), *Children of color: Psychological interventions with culturally diverse youth* (pp. 215–239). San Francisco, CA: Josey-Bass Publishers.

Rashkin, R. (2005). *Feeling better: A kid's book about therapy*. Washington, DC: Imagination Press.

Ray, D. (2011). *Advanced play therapy: essential conditions, knowledge, and skills for child practice*. New York: Routledge Taylor and Francis Group. doi:10.4324/9780203837269

Ray, D., Lee, K., Meany-Walen, K., Carlson, S., Carnes-holt, K., & Ware, J. (2013). Use of toys in child-centered play therapy. *International Journal of Play Therapy, 22*(1), 43–57. doi:10.1037/a0031430

Rubin, J. (1999). *Art therapy: An introduction*. Philadelphia, PA: Brunner/Mazel.

Rubin, J. (2010). *Introduction to art therapy: Sources and resources*. New York: Routledge.

Sayed, M. A. (2003). Psychotherapy of Arab patients in the West: Uniqueness, empathy, and "otherness." *American Journal of Psychotherapy, 57*(4), 445–459. Retrieved from https://login.ezproxy.net.ucf.edu/login?auth=shibb&url=https://search-ebscohost-com.ezproxy.net.ucf.edu/login.aspx?direct=true&AuthType=ip,cookie,shib,sso,uid&db=l sdbip&AN=PREV200400136507&site=eds-live&scope=site

Schaefer, C. (2001). Prescriptive play therapy. *International Journal of Play Therapy, 10*(2), 57–73. doi:10.1037/h0089480

Schaefer, C. & Peabody, M. A. (2016, June). Glossary of play therapy terms. *Play Therapy*, 20-24.

Shapiro, L. (1993). *The book of psychotherapeutic games: A review of the most popular games use din psychotherapy.* The Center for Applied Psychology Incorporated.

Stanley, J. (1999). *Reading to heal: How to use bibliotherapy to improve your life*. Boston, MA: Element Books, Inc.

Stauffer, S. (2008). Trauma and disorganized attachment in refugee children: Integrating theories and exploring treatment options. *Refugee Survey Quarterly, 27,* 150-163. https://doi- org.ezproxy.net.ucf.edu/10.1093/rsq/hdn057

Sue, D., & Sue, D. (2003). *Counseling the culturally diverse: Theory and practice* (4th ed.). New York, NY: Wiley.

Sweeney, D., Baggerly, J., & Ray, D. (2014). Group play therapy: A dynamic approach. New York: Routledge: Taylor & Francis Group. doi:10.4324/9780203103944

Toscani, F. (1998). Sandrama: Psychodramatic sandtray with a trauma survivor. *The Arts in Psychotherapy, 25*(1), 21–29. doi:10.1016/S0197-4556(97)00058-0

Tsai, M.-H., & Ray, D. (2011). Play therapy outcome prediction: An exploratory study at a university-based clinic. *International Journal of Play Therapy*, *20*(2), 94–108. doi:10.1037/a0023441

United States Access Board. (1990). *Chapter 4: Entrances, Doors, and Gates.* Retrieved from https://www.access-board.gov/guidelines-and-standards/buildings-and-sites/about-the- ada-standards/guide-to-the-ada-standards/chapter-4-entrances,-doors,-and-gates

United States Census Bureau. (2010). *Poverty: 2008 and 2009-American survey briefs*. Retrieved from www.census.gov/prod/2010pubs/acsbr09-1.pdf

United States Department of Health and Human Services. (2019). *HIPAA for professionals*. Retrieved from https://www.hhs.gov/hipaa/for-professionals/index.html

United States Department of Labor. (2019). *Occupational Safety and Health Administration: Universal Precautions*. Retrieved from: https://www.osha.gov/SLTC/etools/ hospital/ hazards/univprec/univ.html

VanFleet, R. (2014). Selection of toys. In *Filial therapy: Strengthening parent-child relationships through play* (3rd ed.; pp. 23–25). Sarasota, FL: Professional Resource Press.

VanFleet, R., Sywulak, A. E., & Sniscak, C. C. (2010). *Child-centered play therapy*. New York, NY: Guilford Press.

Vargas, L. A., & Koss-Chioino, J. D. (1992). *Working with culture: Psychotherapeutic interventions with ethnic minority children and adolescents*. San Francisco, CA: Jossey- Bass, Inc.

Vernon, A. (2009). *Counseling children and adolescents* (4th ed.). Denver, CO: Love Publishing.

Wadeson, H. (1980). *Art psychotherapy*. New York: John Wiley and Sons.

World Healthcare Organization. (2007). *Standard precautions in health care*. Retrieved from http://www.who.int/csr/resources/publications/EPR_AM2_E7.pdf

Yuanhong, J., Ramirez, S., & Kranz, P. (•••). Physical settings and materials recommended for play therapy with Japanese children. *Journal of Instructional Psychology*, *34*(4), 53–61.

Zilberstein, K., & Abel, S. K. (2014). *Calming stormy feelings: A child's introduction to psychotherapy*. Bloomington, IN: AuthorHouse.

APPENDIX

Puppet Artists and Retailers (Hughes-Brand, Clifton, & Brand, 2019)

Puppet Artists and Retailers Listed Alphabetically

- **Alex Paper Bag Puppets:** https://www.alexbrands.com/product/arts-crafts/paper-bag-puppets/
- **All Hands Productions:** https://www.etsy.com/shop/AllHandsProductions?ref=search__shop_redirect_
- **Darice Foam and Sock:** https://www.joann.com/darice-foam-and-felt-kit-12pk-bug-finger-puppets/1619980.html#q=puppets&start=1
- **Folkmanis Puppets:** https://www.folkmanis.com/146/home.htm
- **Ikea:** https://www.ikea.com/us/en/search/?query=puppet
- **Kaplan Toys:** https://www.kaplantoys.com/shop/puppets
- **Lakeshore:** https://products.lakeshorelearning.com/search#w=puppet
- **Manhattan Toys:** https://www.manhattantoy.com/search?q=puppets
- **Melisa and Doug:** http://www.melissaanddoug.com/our-toys/puppets-and-puppet-theaters/puppets/
- **Oriental Trading Company:** http://www.orientaltrading.com/web/search/search Main?keyword=puppet
- **The Puppet Factory:** http://www.thepuppetfactory.com/puppets/pc/home.asp
- **Stage Struck Puppets:** https://www.facebook.com/StageStruckPuppets/
- **Sunny Toys:** https://www.sunnytoys.com/ecommerce/index.html

Chapter 2
Valuing Your Play Therapy Practice:
Using What You Know to Brand and Grow

Karen Taheri
Independent Researcher, USA

ABSTRACT

Developing, growing, and maintaining a sustainable play therapy training clinic involves creating meaningful contact within the clinic's targeted community. How the play therapist developing the training clinic goes about creating contact within a community reflects that clinic's overall identity or brand. Counselors are often not trained regarding business practices, brand development, or marketing in their graduate programs. This chapter focuses on providing play therapists with information regarding branding a business and tools for promoting that brand in a manner that aids in the development, growth, and maintenance of a play therapy training clinic. Ethical considerations, as well as thought-provoking questions specific for the development and promotion of a play therapy training clinic are included.

INTRODUCTION

Mental health professionals often graduate with little to no educational exposure to business knowledge and strategies. Entering into the business of setting up and growing a play therapy training clinic involves a steep learning curve for many. Play therapists establishing a training clinic must consider the laws regarding mental health practitioners and businesses within their state, all code(s) of ethics related to their primary licensing credentials, as well as the Association for Play Therapy's

DOI: 10.4018/978-1-5225-8226-7.ch002

Best Practices (APT, 2016). In addition to legal and financial basics for the training clinic, there are several aspects of business to consider: choosing a location for the clinic, hiring employees, providing human resources, structuring policies and procedures, offering continuing education, training, and maintaining a thriving practice, or continuing to grow, when initial goals have been met.

Once the legal, ethical and basic business foundations of the training clinic are set, then the acts of branding and marketing may be used to communicate with the public and grow the business. While there is an arguably wide gap between business education and mental health education, play therapists have many skills that can prove useful throughout the branding and marketing processes. Branding and marketing can be summarized as the core actions of establishing and maintaining authentic relationships with the people the professional seeks to provide services for. Play therapists are equipped with the attitudes and skills to build authentic relationships (Landreth, 2012; Ray, 2011). The objectives of this chapter are to introduce play therapists to information regarding brand development and promotion, to link branding and brand promotion to knowledge play therapists are familiar with, communicate ethical considerations regarding brand development and promotion, and to provide prompts for creating an action plan to begin brand development and marketing for a play therapy training clinic.

BACKGROUND

Perspectives vary as to whether or not the utilization of marketing and advertising for promotion of mental health services is beneficial. Though some professionals deem the use of advertising as going against the altruistic core of the counseling profession (Stadler, 1988), others perceive marketing processes as essential components for strengthening community outreach and thus the practitioner's business. Gilchrist and Stringer (1992) stated, "Counselors in all settings must understand marketing principles and be able to apply them ethically and effectively (p. 5)." Literature surrounding efficacy of incorporating branding and marketing methods into the development of a play therapy training clinic is deficient. Graham (2018) provided insight into developing a play therapy private practice, along with suggestions for identifying and using a mission statement to guide the growth of that clinic. The Association for Play Therapy provides marketing materials (free of charge) and clear definitions of play therapy terms via the association's website (APT, 2018). Play therapists who communicate with clear, accurate messages regarding services offered are informing the community of existing resources. It is useful for the community to understand what play therapy is, to be aware of the types of play therapy services available to them, as well as to understand the potential impact of such play therapy services. Accurately informed consumers can decipher whether or not those available play therapy services are a good fit for their needs.

The realms of advertising, marketing, and public relations often overlap. Distinguishing boundaries between these forms of business promotion can be complicated. For the purposes of this chapter, advertising is defined as "a paid, mass-mediated attempt to persuade" that "must be paid for", and "delivered to an audience via mass media (O'Guinn, Allen, Semenik, & Close Scheinbaum, 2015, p. 7)." While pursuing the traditional route of advertising (purchasing ads for distribution through television, radio, newspaper, or billboards) may prove effective for play therapists, it can also be costly and may not be as accessible or as effective as other methods of brand promotion. According to the American Marketing Association (AMA, 2013), marketing is defined as "the activity, set of institutions, and processes for creating, communicating, delivering, and exchanging offerings that have value for customers, clients, partners, and society at large." Public relations is similar to marketing in that it involves the sharing of information, yet differs because it "is a strategic communication process that builds mutually beneficial relationships between organizations and their publics" (Public Relations Society of America, n.d., p.1). Marketing and public relations may be combined under the umbrella of integrated brand promotion. Integrated brand promotion is defined as "the process of using a wide range of promotional tools that work together to create widespread brand exposure" (O'Guinn et al., 2015, p. 8). How widespread the goal for outreach is can vary greatly depending on the goals of the business. An example of a play therapist utilizing integrated brand promotion would be posting regularly on several different social media or web platforms, such as Instagram, video blogging via YouTube, and maintaining an active presence pinning on Pinterest. That same play therapist could additionally be strengthening outreach through face-to-face networking to build a referral system with pediatricians, psychiatrists, psychologists, school counselors, occupational therapists, and speech therapists practicing within the local community. The key is to figure out what works best for connecting with the target audience and then updating the promotional plan accordingly to maximize efforts. Basic marketing research can be used to accomplish evaluation of what is working most effectively. One simple way a play therapist can track how beneficial connections within the target community are being established is to include a question in the intake packet, such as: 'How did you first learn about our services?' This may be an open-ended, short answer type of question or a multiple choice question with specific answers based on the promotional tools the play therapist is evaluating.

The act of defining the brand of a play therapy clinic essentially occurs through distilling that clinic's identity down to its core mission and values, and honing what makes that company unique. Brand communication occurs anytime the essential identity, or brand, of the clinic is communicated to current or potential customers.

This chapter focuses on discovering the brand of a play therapy training clinic, how various forms of brand promotion can be used to create impactful community contact, ethical considerations for brand development and promotion, and prompts for creating an action plan to begin the brand development and promotion process for a play therapy training clinic.

BRANDING

The initial stage of the process for developing a marketing action plan is to discover the brand of the play therapy training clinic. A brand is defined as "a name, term, sign, symbol, or any other feature that identifies one seller's goods or services as distinct from those of other sellers" (O'Guinn et al., 2015, p. 383). A word used to describe this process is differentiation. One basic way to begin looking at play therapy and distilling the brand of a play therapy training clinic is to consider the who, what, where, when, and why of play therapy.

One essential question to answer is 'What is play therapy?' APT (n.d.a; n.d.b) defined play therapy as "the systematic use of a theoretical model to establish an interpersonal process wherein trained play therapists use the therapeutic powers of play to help clients prevent or resolve psychosocial difficulties and achieve optimal growth and development" (p.1). This definition is ripe with information useful to individuals that may not understand what play therapy is, who can provide play therapy, and what the purpose of play therapy is. Distinguishing characteristics that readily stand out are that play therapy is not simply offering the use of play materials in a talk therapy session. Play therapists are trained to establish and maintain therapeutic relationships with clients and caregivers throughout the course of play therapy services and to identify and utilize the therapeutic powers of play within and across play therapy sessions. Play therapists are uniquely trained professionals who provide specialized services, most often to children and their families (Bratton, Ray, Rhine, & Jones, 2005; Landreth, 2012; Ray, 2012). As such, a clinic providing play therapy services is already a distinguishable entity within the field of mental healthcare. Possessing the unique qualities, skills, and training for providing play therapy, along with the ability to offer specialized training for professionals seeking to become play therapists, will likely set the play therapy training clinic apart from other mental health clinics within the community. However, some communities may be more saturated with play therapists than others. Determining the identity, or brand, of a play therapy clinic involves discerning the defining features that set a particular play therapy training clinic apart. Discovering the unique aspects of a clinic can occur through reflection of the values and mission for the play therapy clinic, the needs of the clients served, needs of trainees, community goals, and the unique features of the play therapy clinic compared with surrounding play therapy training clinics.

The scope of promotional outreach in conjunction with the number of competing play therapy clinics can serve as a measuring stick for the depth of brand awareness necessary to discern what makes one play therapy training clinic stand out from another. For instance, in the event that the play therapy training clinic is seeking to create brand awareness and promotion on a national, or international level, the distinguishing characteristics of that brand may need to be more fully developed than those of a lone play therapy training clinic that is reaching out to compete with non-play therapy specific clinics within its surrounding city.

Individuals, or the 'who,' the play therapy clinic aims to connect with through brand promotion are that clinic's target audiences. Within the play therapy training clinic, play therapy training services are offered to individuals interested in enhancing their clinical acumen in relation to offering play therapy services (via education and supervision), and play therapy clinical services are provided to those experiencing some difficulty related to their mental health. Thus, the two basic audiences that a play therapy training clinic targets are clients and trainees. Considerations for each of these target audiences will be addressed (and overlap occurs), as development of a single action plan for branding and promotion is the intended outcome. In addition to contemplating target audiences, it is helpful to discern which aspects of the business being conducted are the desired primary sources for income. Reflecting on the target audiences, selecting focused sources of income, and deciphering the core values of the company can instigate the branding process.

Mission Statement

A clear mission statement aids in the identification of the base from which to build the brand of the play therapy training clinic (Graham, 2018). Sinke (2009) encouraged business owners to begin developing a deeper understanding of their drive to do what they do by considering why they are in their line of business. Sinke (2009) said,

When I say why, I don't mean to make money— that's a result. By why I mean what is your purpose, cause, or belief? Why does your company exist? Why do you get out of bed every morning? And why should anyone care? (p 39)

In short, what is the play therapist's passion for providing the services offered? What are the values that drive the business? How do these values shape the mission of the clinic and the services provided? What do clients stand to gain from the services they receive from the play therapists at the clinic? What do trainees stand to gain from the services they receive from the play therapists at the clinic?

Developing a Statement

Take a moment to consider each of the aforementioned questions and develop a list of values that come to mind. Try not to censor brainstorming efforts and instead include them all on one list. This can take as much or as little time as one is willing to allow. What themes are present amongst the values on the list? Choose two to three core values that resonate strongly with the objectives of the play therapy training clinic. Once the core values are identified, then try to clearly summarize those values in a concise mission statement (three sentences or less). This is an exercise that can be done individually or may be modified to create a team-based approach. If there are several individuals overseeing the clinic, a team-based approach is recommended to allow for increased consistency and a more thorough understanding of the values that drive and define the practice. Once this exercise is completed, write the mission statement down at the beginning of the integrated branding and promotion worksheet, see Figures 1, 2, and 3. An example mission statement is: The mission of this play therapy training clinic is to provide education and training to developing play therapists while discovering new and meaningful ways to utilize play throughout the supervisory and educational processes to facilitate trainee development.

While it is important for clients to buy into the process of play therapy and to at least begin to understand the purpose of play therapy, the play therapist must understand the 'why' behind their professional interest in providing play therapy services. Be prepared to share this with potential clients and trainees at a moment's notice. Communicating the mission of the training clinic effectively can aid in connecting with potential customers, as well as developing authentic relationships within the community.

Target Audiences: Clients and Trainees

The audiences that a play therapy training clinic will target, for the purpose of developing a branding and marketing action plan, are clients and trainees. Clients for play therapy services are those individuals who are seeking out play therapy services for their personal benefit, or for the benefit of their child or family. Clients may include caregivers, parents, legal guardians, and families. Trainees include graduate students, novice mental health professionals, and even seasoned mental health professionals seeking out fresh information, continuing education, or new perspectives within the field. The APT (n.d.d.) delineates specific types of approved education for individuals seeking out the Registered Play Therapist, School Based- Registered Play Therapist or Registered Play Therapist Supervisor credentials. "Individuals or organizations that have been approved to offer play therapy continuing education" may become "Approved Providers of Continuing Education" through the APT (APT,

Figure 1. Brand development and promotion worksheet, page 1

Branding and Marketing Action Plan

<u>Stage One, Branding</u>

Step 1: Develop A Mission Statement

List of Core Values:

Mission Statement (three sentences or less) using top two to three core values:

Step 2: Identified Target Populations

Describe your ideal client:

Describe your ideal trainee:

Step 3: Identifying a Niche

What makes this play therapy clinic special?

How does this clinic stand out from other clinics within the community?

List any desired niche(s):

Community Needs Addressed:

Qualifications of Clinicians:

Step 4: Primary Sources of Income:

Intangible services offered:

Tangible products offered, if any:

n.d.d., p.1). Similarly, play therapy training clinics "designated to generate more play therapy research, peer-reviewed publications, instruction, supervisor training, and supervised clinical experiences at universities" can become recognized by the APT as "Approved Centers of Play Therapy Education" (APT, n.d.d., p. 1). Most play therapy training clinics will probably offer education for topics related to services the clinic specializes in. However, this may not always be the case. A training clinic may include a separate educational department through which education concerning a variety of clinical topic areas is provided, even if clinical services to address such needs are not readily offered within the clinic. For instance, an Approved Provider of Play Therapy Continuing Education may offer a workshop wherein a guest lecturer who specializes in working with children who have been sexually abused educates attendees about providing play therapy services to this specific population, even if the training clinic hosting the workshop does not specialize in these services. Essentially, the business structure of the play therapy training clinic will drive the marketing plan. The idea is to cater the marketing efforts to the audiences who may satisfy their goals through the services the clinic provides.

Figure 2. Brand development and promotion worksheet, page 2

Stage Two, Promotional Strategies Internal Communication Plan:

Step 1: List the core values of the company and relate those values to each of the services provided to or by the following:

Play Therapy Supervisors- Educators-

Supervisees-

Trainees-

Consultees-

Clients-

Step 2: List the clinic's Policies and Procedures for communication and feedback:

Supervisor to Supervisee-

Supervisee to Supervisor-

Client to Supervisee-

Client to Supervisor-

Trainees to Educators-

Consultees to Play Therapist Consultant-

Clients

One purpose of marketing is to provide accurate information about the services offered so that individuals who may be interested in utilizing such services are aware of their existence. Understanding the needs of the people the play therapist hopes to serve will assist in developing appropriate information for marketing materials. The presenting issues the clinic will focus on addressing will shape the types of services the clinic provides. A professional niche may exist, in addition to play therapy, and that can also shape the types of services offered or potential client population(s) served.

Identifying Preferred Populations and Presenting Issues

Sanok (2018) encouraged practitioners to consider the clients they feel most excited about working with. Take a moment to do the same. What specific populations does the play therapist creating the training clinic enjoy working with the most?

Figure 3. Brand development and promotion worksheet, page 3

Stage 3. Promotional Strategies External Communication Plan:

Step 1: List the steps that you can take to make use of each of the following marketing tools for promotion of the play therapy training clinic. Skip those that do not seem relevant.

Logo:
Website:
Pamphlets/ Postcards/ Brochures:
Social Media Platforms:
Podcast:
Person-to-Person (including building a referral network):

Stage Four. Action Plan:

Create three action steps to accomplish within the next two weeks to begin branding and promoting the play therapy training clinic.

1.

2.

3.

Create three action steps to accomplish on a weekly, ongoing basis to consistently promote the play therapy training clinic.

1.

2.

3,

Create three action steps to complete within the next two months to further promote the outreach of the play therapy training clinic.

1.

2.

3.

For instance, perhaps they enjoy working with children experiencing anxiety and their families. Are there presenting issues that the play therapist, or their colleagues working within the clinic, are eager to gain as much information about as possible? Is there a theme throughout those preferences? If there is not, then are there strong preferences that might balance one another out? For instance, perhaps one play therapist enjoys counseling parents and one play therapist prefers providing individual play therapy services to children. Another example of complementary services is when one provider prefers to provide attachment-related services for adoptive families, whereas another provider in the same play therapy clinic chooses to work with families surviving divorce. Try and recognize all of the overlap in the interests and training as well as the differences. Document the areas of overlap and dissimilarities.

The goal is to discover the strengths of each clinicians' talents and to utilize those strengths to inform the overall identity and brand of the play therapy training clinic.

The play therapy training clinic may be a general clinic where the purpose is to target as many presenting issues and populations as possible. Perhaps each clinician has their own niche in a generalized practice setting. Or, the clinic may be a highly specialized clinic that is looking for very specific referrals, such as children coping with chronic medical conditions. Whether the services offered through the training clinic are specialized or general, the knowledge and understanding of the desired presenting issues and target populations allows for clarity in identifying the development of a niche.

Identifying a Niche

A niche may exist as a specific type of service offered or a collective of diverse services provided to treat a specialized area of concern. For the purposes of this chapter, a niche is relative to existing services within the community. If there is a dearth of services provided in the area, then a more targeted niche may not be as beneficial. Identifying a niche does not mean that clients with other presenting concerns are always referred out for services. The niche provides a means for identifying a specialty professional service to enhance pinpointing marketing strategies. The intent is to discover what sets the play therapy training clinic apart from other training clinics, or mental health agencies and practices, within the surrounding communities. Effectively, what does this training clinic offer that other mental health professionals in the area do not? What needs might this clinic be able to address that other clinics are not? How can this clinic reach those individuals who may not already resonate with the services being provided within their community?

Sanok (2018) encouraged practitioners to reflect on who their ideal client is. For instance, perhaps the play therapy training clinic's ideal client is a child who has recently received an Autism Spectrum Disorder diagnosis. One such client might be Peter, a five year old who has been diagnosed with Autism Spectrum Disorder. Using this imaginary ideal client as a guide, the clinician might decide to offer, in addition to individual play therapy services for Peter, parent training for Peter's caregivers and a possible support group for caregivers working to meet the needs of children with experiences similar to Peter. Referrals for supplemental services, such as occupational therapy and speech therapy, may also be likely. Perhaps there are certain pediatricians or psychologists in town that specialize in assessing and diagnosing individuals on the autism spectrum. Those might be wonderful places to send promotional materials for autism-related play therapy services.

Some considerations that may assist in discovering specific concerns the training clinic will treat, or who the ideal client is, are in Figure 4. Once the ideal client is established, creating marketing strategies can become more streamlined. Another outcome of considering the ideal client, is that a need for additional training and education may become apparent to enhance clinical acumen for working with certain populations or presenting concerns. In that case, steps may be taken to enhance counselor preparedness for providing effective services. An additional option may be to hire professionals who are already equipped to provide such services.

Trainees

A play therapy training clinic may provide any single service or combination from the following for trainees: education, clinical experience, and supervision. Depending on the type of training services offered and the location of the play therapy training clinic, the clinic may become an Approved Provider of Continuing Education or an Approved Center for Play Therapy Education through APT (n.d.d). Trainees seeking educational services from the clinic may include graduate students, pre-licensed professionals, and licensed clinicians from a variety of mental health backgrounds (social work, psychology, psychiatry, counseling, etc.). Assessing for the educational and developmental needs of the students and professionals in the community may assist in creating appropriate curriculum content for trainee development. For

Figure 4. Ideal client diagram

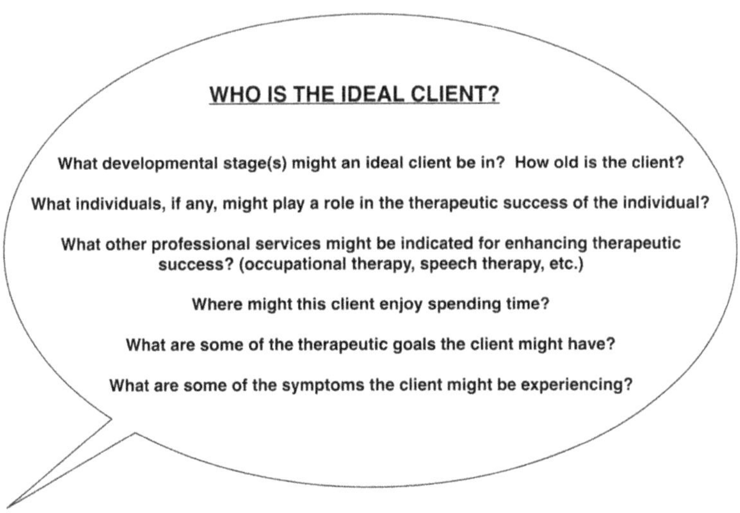

example, individuals working from a Child-Centered Play Therapy perspective seeking to enhance caregiver engagement throughout their play therapy services may benefit from training in Filial Therapy, Child-Parent Relationship Therapy, or Child-Teacher Relationship Therapy. Additional considerations to keep in mind are: whether or not trainees receiving education from the clinic are being prepared to provide play therapy clinical services to clients in the community as an intern or employee, and whether or not the primary supervisor of the trainees providing such clinical services is also an employee of the training clinic. For trainees providing clinical services within the training clinic, it makes sense that consistent educational messages (through education), as well as clinical accountability and modeling (through supervision), would be provided to trainees on-site. Consistency in information provided (or messages conveyed) would strengthen the overall communication of the brand and mission of the clinic internally (amongst employees and interns) and potentially externally (employees and interns to community members). However, there are additional ethical considerations, including multiple relationships that would be imperative to demystify in order to ensure each individual is entering such a professional relationship with awareness of potential boundary conflicts. Additional outside supervision, or consultation, could be suggested to new professionals in order to maintain a fresh flow of clinical information from outside professionals to create a healthy checks and balances system for enhanced clinical acumen and accountability at all levels.

Primary Sources of Income

A training clinic can earn income from a variety of sources: clinical services offered, professional education and workshops, supervision, and consulting. Clinical play therapy services may be offered to adults, but are most often provided to children and their families (Landreth, 2012). Play therapy services may include psycho-education, parent coaching for individuals or groups, assessments, caregiver consultations, and individual, group, and family therapy sessions. Further considerations may include whether or not the play therapy clinic will accept third party reimbursement, will target a self-pay population only, or will blend various payment methods. Training for play therapy professionals may occur in various forms: individual, triadic, or group play therapy supervision (including live supervision or video recordings of play therapy sessions), and professional consultation (including on an as-needed basis or as ongoing services) in face-to-face format or distance consultation (through use of HIPAA-compliant phone or videoconferencing technology). Ancillary forms of income may include resources created and provided to clients and trainees, such as: webinars, blogs, podcasts, speaking at engagements, and authoring or editing books.

Identifying primary avenues for income may prove helpful to discern the brand of the clinic and to develop a marketing plan. For instance, a training clinic that receives the majority of its revenue from educational workshops for professionals may seek to focus marketing efforts toward potential professional trainees. The mission statement for the play therapy training clinic should accurately reflect the goals of the clinic; in this case that may be to provide play therapy educational opportunities for professional trainees within the community. In terms of developing a marketing plan, it might prove helpful to consider the following questions: Is the education provided in person only, or is there also access to online educational formats? Is there a specific clinical niche, or population, that the education tends to be provided about? Or, is there a focus on providing a wide range of educational topics? Is there a certification program associated with the training services the clinic is offering? What types of supervision are provided?

Brand Clarity

Before moving on to the brand promotion section, take a moment to summarize the brand of the play therapy training clinic. At this point, there should be a clear, concise mission statement for the training clinic, a list of core values, easily identifiable target population(s), knowledge of how the play therapy training clinic differs from other mental health clinics in the community, and awareness of the primary sources of income. In order to accurately provide consistent marketing messages, a thorough understanding of the brand is essential. If there is uncertainty regarding the brand, then it is recommended to return to the aspect of the brand in question and further develop or discover that aspect of the brand before moving on.

BRAND PROMOTION

Brand promotion is any type of communication, whether internal or external, that is intended to relay information about the play therapy training clinic's brand. Sending consistent messages across promotional methods is key to engaging potential clients (O'Guinn et al., 2015).

Internal communication can occur between any individuals working within the training clinic. An example of internal communication is two interns discussing the mission of the training clinic and how the mission relates to the services they are providing within the clinic. External communication involves an individual working within the training clinic providing information to an individual within the community that does not work at the training clinic. An example of external communication is a trainee discussing the mission of the training clinic, or describing the clinical services offered, with a graduate school class member. Any messages provided to individuals outside of the training clinic, or external communication, is an opportunity for brand promotion. Attention in the following sections is focused on internal and external brand promotion through creation of the following promotional materials: a logo, having a web presence, policies and procedures, and use of person-to-person promotion.

Logo

If the creative ability or time to devote to creating a logo for the play therapy clinic is lacking, seek external help by hiring a designer to create the business logo. A quick online search for local logo designers should provide ample choices, and, if not, then there are online options for hiring designers. The use of a logo may not seem readily important, yet it can be a powerful marketing tool. The logo can serve as a distinct symbol that represents the brand of the play therapy training clinic. Brainstorm powerful images that coincide with the values list created in the branding section of the branding and promotion worksheet in Figures 1, 2, and 3. When working to create the logo, pay attention to colors and readability of fonts used within the logo. The purpose of the logo is to streamline communication. A well-communicated brand via a logo can easily indicate the play therapy clinic by image alone. Logos are often used on business cards, letterhead, and promotional materials (such as fliers, brochures, handouts, website, staff t-shirts, stress balls, etc.). A designer can also assist in the creation of banners with your logo for use on social media platforms or the clinic's website. An online presence with consistent imaging can reinforce the brand of the play therapy training clinic and can serve as a community-building tool.

Website and Internet Presence

The use of the Internet for marketing purposes is widespread. One only needs to check their e-mail, a social media site, or browse their favorite website to witness the inundation of marketing materials present online. Creating an impactful website or web presence involves empathizing with the consumer's experience. Content created and shared is often driven by the expressed needs of the target audiences. Relevant information draws consumers in and can instigate and assist in maintaining client to play therapist connection. One example of a play therapist effectively connecting with their target audience via their web presence is a play therapist creating a video blog post wherein that therapist acknowledges and normalizes caregivers' occasional feelings of frustration with their toddler's tantrums and provides helpful tips for emotional regulation that caregivers can use to self-regulate so they are able to effectively respond to their child's needs. Another example of a play therapist effectively reaching a target audience, this time trainees, through a web presence is a play therapist who is an approved provider of continuing education hosting a webinar discussing the history, purpose, rationale, and basic skills for providing Child-Centered Play Therapy (CCPT). It can prove useful to create a free resource for prospective trainees or clients that is offered through the training clinic's website. Providing a resource free of charge can serve as an opportunity to allow potential clients and trainees to experience a small sample of the information and services the play therapy training clinic offers. Blogging is another way to create a flexible space to provide information through sharing knowledge of various topics of choice that reflect the brand of the clinic. Blogging is a means that many Internet users are familiar with and can become an easy-to-connect-with platform due to consumers' comfortability with this method for receiving information.

In addition to contemplating applicability of content to facilitate connection with target audiences, consumer's ease of use is important to factor in when designing a web presence. Cole (2016) stated, "Research has shown that today's buyer values, beyond price and product functionality, are characterized by a universal interest in simplicity, emotional gratification and a frictionless experience" (p.1). The goal is to design a relatable, easy-to-connect-with presence online to attract clients and trainees interested in receiving play therapy clinical, educational, or training services. Take time to ponder the needs of the 'ideal client' or trainees the play therapist hopes to serve. Be as specific as possible. Become familiar with existing web platforms and imagine the type of content that would likely resonate with the 'ideal client.' Creation and use of a website for the play therapy training clinic provides a separate type of online presence for clients and trainees than that of a social media platform. Practice tools, such as intake materials, between appointment communications, and assessments can often be found on a training clinic's secured website. Additional in-depth information about specific play therapy services and trainings offered, as well as the qualifications of the play therapists and trainees providing services, allows for clients to receive important information regarding the services their child receives at the clinic. It is important to understand the culture of the target audiences (prospective clients and trainees) and to communicate and promote the brand across platforms that are relevant to the target audiences. Regular evaluation of which online platforms are most productive at creating connections to and maintaining contact with the target audiences can aid in shifting use of online promotional materials as needed to stay relevant.

Person-to-Person Promotion

There are methods of brand promotion that do not readily include the use of technology. Creating and disseminating brochures, fliers, face-to-face communication, word-of-mouth, and business cards are methods for brand promotion that do not require technology as the means for supplying information. Person-to-person promotion can occur through any individual who works in the clinic, or utilizes the services at the clinic. Satisfied employees, trainees, and even clients can become akin to serving as a brand ambassador for the training clinic. A brand ambassador is a person who spreads positive information regarding the play therapy clinic's brand to others and therefore promotes the business. The term brand ambassador is not an additional title necessary to provide to employees or volunteers. It is simply a natural occurrence due to the social nature of human beings and the desire for person-to-person communication. The hope is that a healthy, inspiring, enjoyable culture is created within the play therapy training clinic and that individuals experiencing clinical services, education, or training have such a positive experience that they begin to discuss their satisfaction with others. Offering clear, consistent messages regarding the mission, values, services, and overall brand of the training clinic to employees and volunteers who work at the clinic can help to ensure a thorough understanding of the clinic's brand. When those individuals decide they would like to share their positive thoughts and feelings about the training clinic they are prepared to use information that is succinct and streamlined and can easily become brand ambassadors for the clinic. Consider making free brochures, or informational pamphlets explaining play therapy and the services of the play therapy training clinic, available for trainees and supervisees to provide to individuals they would like to share their experiences with.

Community outreach, and strengthening connections with target audiences, can happen in many different forms of face-to-face interactions. One suggestion for creating contact with potential trainees is to speak as a guest lecturer for a child and adolescent counseling course, or a human development course, in a local graduate school program. Perhaps ongoing presentations can be provided at several local universities to educate graduate students in psychology, social work, and counseling programs (prospective trainees) about play therapy and the services offered at the play therapy training clinic. Additionally, play therapists can build strong referral networks with professionals within the community, such as psychiatrists, psychologists, school counselors, occupational therapists, and speech therapists. Hosting ongoing networking events at the play therapy clinic, and providing regular opportunities for community professionals to meet one another promotes a strengthening of the networking community and sets the play therapy clinic apart as the facilitator for building up those connections. Possibilities extend as far as one's access to creativity and resources. Take some time to get creative about methods that might work for creating memorable brand promotion for the play therapy training clinic.

ETHICS AND MARKETING

In a field that focuses on helping others, seeking to profit from providing that help can become a conflict of interest. The end goal of developing a marketing plan is not to manipulate clients into seeking out play therapy services; it is to provide accurate, transparent information about services offered and to connect individuals with play therapy services they may benefit from. The play therapy profession can also benefit from the dissemination of accurate information regarding the process of play therapy and the potential, realistic outcomes individuals seeking help can expect. Play therapy is not a panacea; however, research supports that there are many benefits individuals can experience from engaging in play therapy (Bratton, Ray, Rhine, & Jones, 2005; LeBlanc & Ritchie, 2001; Lin & Bratton, 2015; Ray, Armstrong, Balkin, & Jayne, 2015). Reporting research results in an easy-to-understand format can prove to be a useful marketing tool. Potential clients can gain information about play therapy from those reports and establish realistic personal goals. Play therapists can provide knowledge to the public regarding the wellness model and can aid in reducing the stigma surrounding mental health concerns and normalize individual experiences. Gilchrist and Stringer (1992) encouraged supervisors and educators to provide accurate information to counseling students and clinicians-in-training regarding ethical use of marketing, as well as the positive aspects of marketing to reduce negative stigma associated with seeking out help for mental health. Sanok (2018) said mental health professionals who struggle to sustain a healthy business may have to discontinue providing services, and a competent, non-practicing professional is a lost resource for the community. While it is unethical to manipulate, create false hope regarding treatment outcomes, or to take advantage of those in need, it is not unethical to create a business that is profitable and sustainable. A successful play therapy training clinic can provide valuable mental health training and services to many diverse individuals.

Gilchrist and Stringer (1992) stated that counselors who utilize marketing in an ethical way stand to benefit from the perks of marketing, such as increased brand awareness, while providing beneficial knowledge to the public. There are several ethical considerations to keep in mind while discovering a brand and carrying out a promotional marketing plan. This section of the chapter provides an overview of some key aspects of the Association for Play Therapy's *Best Practices* (APT, 2016) and the American Counseling Association's (ACA, 2014) *Code of Ethics* that readily pertain to the branding and marketing of a play therapy training clinic. For structural purposes, when overlapping guidelines occur, the ACA (2014) guideline is provided initially and the APT (2016) guideline is cited in the discussion portion below. The Registered Play Therapist credential is a secondary credential. As such, play therapists have a variety of training backgrounds and consideration of additional ethical codes may be necessary dependent upon the play therapist licensure or professional organization memberships.

All counselors are healthcare providers that enter into a helping relationship with clients. Within that relationship is an inherent power differential. Play therapists are aware of the power differential in their relationships with clients, clients' families, supervisees, and trainees and work to create safety within those relationships. The operations of a play therapy training clinic are functioning within the scope of the brand of the play therapy profession when the tone for relational dynamics throughout the clinic is positive, and communication is taking place in an effective, helpful manner. Feedback and receptivity to feedback are key in an effective play therapy supervisory relationship. Creating a safe space wherein the play therapist in training or supervisee can voice concerns, and those concerns are heard and responded to, promotes a therapeutic learning environment. Dismissing employees' or trainees' concerns and not allowing the voices of employees, trainees, supervisees, or clients a safe platform from which to be heard is not operating within the brand of the play therapy profession. Key ethical codes and questions for consideration are included throughout this section. The ethical considerations for developing, branding, and promoting a play therapy training clinic are grouped into the following categories: branding, marketing, and cultural considerations.

Branding

The idea of a company operating 'off-brand' is similar to that of a play therapist experiencing incongruence in professional and therapeutic relationships. A grocery store that specializes in offering natural foods, selling a highly processed, genetically modified, inorganic, high calorie food is akin to a play therapist supervisor becoming angry with a play therapist in training for making an inaccurate reflective response in session. This type of behavior is not congruent with the values of the play therapy profession. Play therapists strive to be mindful of their values and to intentionally and authentically contribute to relationships in a manner that facilitates actualization. From a training perspective, an effective supervisor is empathic, congruent, and authentic in relationship with trainees and clients. These relational dynamics can trickle down from supervisor to trainee, from trainee to clients. Similarly, the operations, policies, and procedures within the play therapy training clinic can affect the morale and experience of employees, trainees, and clients. A play therapy training clinic will be 'off-brand', or incongruent, and operating in an unethical fashion when not in accordance with the following guidelines addressing safety and quality of services.

Safety

At the most basic level, employees and trainees need to be safe physically and psychologically. In this section regarding branding and the workplace, attention is focused on creating positive, ethical conditions within the workplace environment. This includes freedom from punitive actions. Play therapist supervisors, play therapists, and play therapists in training work collaboratively to create an empathic and responsive environment. Openness to feedback regarding the clinic's policies and procedures can serve to enhance the workplace.

Negative Conditions

Counselors alert their employers of inappropriate policies and practices. They attempt to effect changes in such policies or procedures through constructive action within the organization. When such policies are potentially disruptive or damaging to clients or may limit the effectiveness of services provided and change cannot be affected, counselors take appropriate further action. Such action may include referral to appropriate certification, accreditation, or state licensure organizations, or voluntary termination of employment. (ACA, 2014, p. 10)

The policies and procedures of the training clinic serve to protect the play therapists, supervisors, trainees, and clients. Welcomed feedback through invited communication is essential to bringing awareness to any issues or concerns from clients, trainees, supervisees, play therapists, or supervisors. Some questions to consider are: How will the play therapy training clinic receive feedback from employees and trainees? How can the communication process for feedback be streamlined? What are some ways to facilitate an open-door structure for receipt of employee feedback on a regular, ongoing basis? Consider what types of procedures can be included in the structure of the play therapy clinic to encourage and facilitate regular check-ins with clients regarding their experiences of the services they are receiving. How can employees be assured that the play therapists overseeing the training clinic will be flexible if certain policies or procedures prove to be unhelpful (or even worse, harmful) to the clients, employees, or trainees? Modeling is a key component within effective supervision. The manner in which feedback and communication are shared and encouraged can serve as a beneficial opportunity for modeling. Policies and procedures surrounding communication and feedback are strengthened when clearly delineated and expectations are expressed early on. Employees and trainees need to feel safe to express their concerns to their supervisors and employers, and supervisors and employers need to provide constructive feedback and any necessary environmental changes for employees and trainees to thrive.

Protection From Punitive Action

Counselors do not harass a colleague or employee or dismiss an employee who has acted in a responsible and ethical manner to expose inappropriate employer policies or practices. (ACA, 2014, p.10)

A trainee that fears remediation, or termination, for expressing disagreement with a policy may choose not to speak up regarding inconsistencies within the training clinic. Trainees, as well as employees and play therapist supervisors each need to understand their rights to voice concerns as employees. While the responsibility to speak up regarding inconsistencies in the practices of the play therapy training clinic ultimately resides with the individual, the responsibility to create a safe space for employees and play therapists to share their voices resides with the director of the play therapy training clinic.

Play therapists work to create a safe environment to invite vulnerability, honesty, and transparency from employees and trainees. Some basic considerations for implementing safe communication and procedures surrounding protecting employees, trainees, and clients are: What measures can the clinic take to provide physical safety to clients, employees, and trainees? What measures can the clinic take to provide for psychological safety to employees, trainees and clients? If a complaint against an employee or trainee is brought up by a client, how will that complaint be addressed in a manner that allows for safety for both the client and the employee? What is the action plan to be followed to ensure the client continues to receive the upmost care if the complaint is about their own counselor? How will the employees be provided with feedback from clients regarding clients' experiences? What is the safest way to handle complaints to encourage continued, honest communication from staff, trainees, and clients? Transparency as early as possible is recommended to ensure employees, trainees, and supervisees understand and are in agreement with the policies of the play therapy training clinic.

Employer Policies

The acceptance of employment in an agency or institution implies that counselors are in agreement with its general policies and principles. Counselors strive to reach agreement with employers regarding acceptable standards of client care and professional conduct that allow for changes in institutional policy conducive to the growth and development of clients. (ACA, 2014, p. 10)

Play therapists strive to reach agreement with employers regarding these Play Therapy Best Practices that allow for changes in institutional policy conducive to the therapeutic relationship. (APT, 2016, p. 12)

Transparency is encouraged between the employer and employees regarding values that drive the business operations within the clinic, as well as the values and principles related to providing play therapy services to clients. Open conversations regarding values and principles are recommended during the hiring process, as well as throughout all stages of employment. Clearly defined policies in an easy-to-access format for potential hires, as well as current employees, are essential. Aspects of the identity of the organization are further delineated through policies for client care and communication. Policies and procedures for client engagement allow for clear communication of expectations and potential consequences for inappropriate client engagement or worse, harm. Clear communication and a healthy checks and balances system can allow for accountability at each level within the play therapy training clinic. When an inconsistency in the training clinic's policies and the needs of clients exists, then steps are taken to change internal policies to protect and enhance client development.

Quality of Services

Personnel Selection and Assignment

When counselors are in a position requiring personnel selection and/or assigning of responsibilities to others, they select competent staff and assign responsibilities compatible with their skills and experiences. (ACA, 2014, p. 10)

Ensuring that clients receive appropriate and competent care is essential. Play therapist supervisors and clinical directors are knowledgeable about the competencies of their supervisees and trainees, and are mindful of who they choose to work with. Play therapy supervisors are aware of their supervisees' development and strive to appropriately pair their supervisees with responsibilities commensurate to their abilities and strengths. Supervisee areas for growth are addressed within the supervisory relationship. Some considerations regarding personnel choice and supervise clinical assignments are: What measures will be in place to ensure play therapy trainees are competent to provide services upon their initial contact with clients? What considerations will occur when choosing employees to provide services within the organization? Once hired, how will employees' levels of competency be tracked? What are the play therapy training clinic's, or supervisors', required procedural steps to act upon when an inconsistency between self-perceived and actual competency levels exists? What considerations are necessary to discern whether or not a trainee's or employee's responsibilities are commensurate with their abilities and experience? How might plans to address inconsistencies in employee responsibilities change when considering a new hire versus a current trainee, or even a seasoned play therapist?

Marketing

Marketing professionals within the play therapy clinic appropriately involves accurately portraying the credentials of the trainees and professionals providing play therapy services, not engaging in exploitive relationships, considering all of the potential benefits and consequences for using testimonials, and veracity in communications.

Accurate Advertising

When advertising or otherwise representing their services to the public, counselors identify their credentials in an accurate manner that is not false, misleading, deceptive, or fraudulent. (ACA, 2014, p.9)

The APT (2016) upholds the importance of integrity in reporting a clinician's credentials. Falsely advertising the "Registered Play Therapist" credential is unethical and inconsistent with best practices. While it is possible for individuals to use the terms 'play therapy' or 'play therapist' without holding the credential of "Registered Play Therapist", this can be misleading. Incorporating toys or playful activities into therapy is not equivalent to providing play therapy services and is not automatically indicative that practitioner is a play therapist. Individuals who have not received appropriate education, training, and supervision should not be advertised as play therapists (APT, 2018). When play therapists become aware of individuals inaccurately utilizing the terms 'play therapy' or 'play therapist,' they are encouraged to provide the necessary information to help those professionals understand the appropriate use of such terms (APT, 2018). Supervisors are also responsible for maintaining awareness as to whether or not their supervisees are accurately communicating their credentials and capacity for independent practice.

Counselor Credentials

Counseling supervisors work to ensure that supervisees communicate their qualifications to render services to their clients. (ACA, 2014, pp. 12-13)

Counselors are required to be forthcoming about their credentials and capability for independent practice. Supervisors hold a responsibility to monitor individuals working under their supervision to ensure they are accurately portraying their qualifications and credentials to the public. It is recommended that all play therapy supervisees and trainees include their current credentials (and supervisor's credentials and contact information) in their disclosure statement to provide to clients with their intake paperwork. Face-to-face discussions during the initial stages of the intake process regarding the supervisee's status as a supervised clinician, is encouraged to ensure clients are accurately informed before beginning play therapy. Play therapists do not engage in counseling relationships that are not based on an informed consent process; clients without accurate information cannot make an informed consent regarding the play therapy process.

Exploitation of Others

Play therapists provide mental health services primarily to children, who are deemed a vulnerable population (Ray, 2011). Play therapists and play therapist supervisors are aware of the power differential within their professional relationships and are careful not to exploit their relationships with clients, clients' families, or trainees. While the ethical codes within this sub-section focus primarily on exploitation of professional relationships, play therapists are mindful not to be exploitive of clients.

Counselors do not exploit others in their professional relationships. (ACA, 2014, p.10)

Play therapists do not engage in exploitive relationships with supervisees, students, staff, or other subordinates. (APT, 2016, p. 11)

Play therapists understand the importance of the quality of dynamics within professional, and personal, relationships. Exploitation can leave relational trauma in its wake. As professionals who specialize in providing and encouraging physical and psychological safety in relationships, exploitation does not have a place within the play therapy profession. Prompts to consider for how exploitation might occur include: What does exploitation through marketing look like? What are some realistic changes or outcomes that individuals can expect from engaging in therapy? What sort of negative outcome is possible to come about through entering into play therapy services? One example of exploitation through marketing is using inaccurate, or embellished, information to persuade a client to engage in therapeutic services that may or may not prove beneficial in achieving the client's therapeutic goals. Play therapists strive to provide accurate information and expectations regarding the play therapy process.

Clients are not the only individuals who can be harmed through exploitive relationships; trainees and employees of the training clinic can also be harmed through an exploitive relationship. Supervisors and seasoned play therapists have a responsibility to model effective interpersonal skills and professional boundaries. A few considerations for play therapist supervisors and play therapy clinic directors are: Is hiring a post-master's level, unlicensed clinician without pay exploitive? If the master's level clinician is not receiving pay for the services they provide, particularly if the clinic is receiving income for those services delivered, what can that clinician expect to gain in exchange for their time and services provided? Transparency here is key in order to maintain clear boundaries and to avoid exploiting the clinician's time and efforts. There is also an ethical responsibility to ensure that any hired 'trainee' is receiving quality training.

Testimonials

Counselors who use testimonials do not solicit them from current clients, former clients, or any other persons who may be vulnerable to undue influence. Counselors discuss with clients the implications of and obtain permission for the use of any testimonial. (ACA, 2014, p. 9)

Some counselors use testimonials to advertise their work. Attention to who this benefits, and the potential for harm, is imperative in understanding the costs and benefits of using testimonials. How the testimonials are acquires is also of concern. The APT (2016) concurs that testimonials or reviews may not be solicited from current or former clients. There is an additional stipulation that "when such are freely offered by the client and/or legal guardian(s), the play therapist makes every effort to protect the client or guardian's identity" (APT, 2016, p. 10). The rationale for the use of testimonials from clients deserves in-depth exploration before its occurrence. Some prompts for exploration include: Who stands to gain from sharing this client's disclosure? Who was this information originally provided to and for what purpose was it shared? How does utilizing this shared information in a potentially new fashion shape the relational dynamics between the play therapist and the client, or former client that provided the testimonial? How can the play therapist best protect the client's, or former clients, identity? Does the potential benefit of using the testimonial outweigh the potential harm to the client or the therapeutic relationship? How would a play therapist supervisor advise a trainee to handle the use of testimonials?

Communicating with the public with veracity and accuracy is important. Play therapists represent their professional abilities and credentials to the public with trustworthiness. While play therapists do share in a common background of knowledge, skills, and training, all play therapists are not the same. Play therapists take precautions not to construe that they are speaking on behalf of the entire play therapy profession, or for all play therapists, when they provide presentations or address the public.

Media Presentations

When counselors provide advice or comment by means of public lectures, demonstrations, radio or television programs, recordings, technology-based applications, printed articles, mailed material, or other media, they take reasonable precautions to ensure that

1. *The statements are based on appropriate professional counseling literature and practice,*
2. *The statements are otherwise consistent with the ACA Code of Ethics, and*
3. *The recipients of the information are not encouraged to infer that a professional counseling relationship has been established. (ACA, 2014, pp. 9-10)*

The APT (2016) has a similar statement with the same three specifications included in its *Best Practices*. Play therapists are aware of the veracity of the information they provide to professionals, clients, and the public. Training materials disseminated are accurate and provide intentionally communicated information to enhance trainee knowledge of play therapy and play therapy services. Similarly, play therapist supervisors monitor the information trainees and supervisees provide to the public and model trustworthiness through their communications.

Consultant Competency

Counselors take reasonable steps to ensure that they have the appropriate resources and competencies when providing consultation services. Counselors provide appropriate referral resources when requested or needed. (ACA, 2014, p. 10)

It is likely that play therapy consultation services occur frequently within a play therapy training clinic. Employees and play therapy trainees may informally or formally consult with one another between sessions, during group consultation sessions, and throughout the play therapy supervision process. When issues arise that are beyond the competency levels of the play therapists within the organization, recommendations for outside consultation are provided. Appropriate informed consent measures are followed before engaging in formal consultation.

Informed Consent in Formal Consultation

When providing formal consultation services, counselors have an obligation to review, in writing and verbally, the rights and responsibilities of both counselors and consultees. Counselors use clear and understandable language to inform all parties involved about the purpose of the services to be provided, relevant costs, potential risks and benefits, and the limits of confidentiality. (ACA, 2014, p. 10)

Professional consultation services may be provided within the play therapy training clinic to employees, trainees, supervisees, and outside professionals. Formal consultation requires use of an informed consent process, often using a formalized document, wherein professional boundaries, confidentiality, and competencies are clearly delineated. Marketing professional play therapy consultation services through streamlined communication can enhance the portrayal of the brand of the play therapy clinic as being a leader within the field of child and adolescent mental health. Further considerations include: What specific measures can be taken to ensure consultation services are marketed in an ethical manner? What policies and procedures will be included within the play therapy training clinic for conducting professional consulting services in a transparent manner? It is recommended that a formal consultation contract, much like a play therapist supervisor would have for play therapy supervisees, is used to create consistency across all professional play therapists within the training clinic who offer professional play therapy consultation services. What are the established competencies within the training clinic for providing professional play therapy consulting services?

Trustworthiness and a desire to promote wellness through competent services are values consistent with the act of providing play therapy. Play therapists who offer competent services can enhance their client's capacity for actualization through providing a meaningful therapeutic relationship (Landreth, 2012). Facilitation of client movement toward wellness and growth is an essential component in play therapy. Competent play therapists are aware of their values, as well as their clients' values and cultural perspectives and collaborate throughout the play therapy process.

Cultural Considerations

Nondiscrimination

Counselors do not condone or engage in discrimination against prospective or current clients, students, employees, supervises, or research participants based on age, culture, disability, ethnicity, race, religion/spirituality, gender, gender identity, sexual orientation, marital/partnership status, language preference, socioeconomic status, immigration status, or any basis proscribed by law. (ACA, 2014, p. 9)

Play therapists are aware of the impact of cultural perspectives, experiences, and identities of the individuals they serve as clients, students and supervisees. Play therapists are also aware of their cultural identity, experiences and perspectives that have shaped the way they perceive others; they are mindful to take both their own cultural lens as well as the client's cultural lens into account throughout services. Engaging in play therapy with cultural sensitivity means gaining awareness of what is happening throughout society on personal, professional, and political levels. Play therapist supervisors and play therapists do not discriminate against potential employees, supervisees, or trainees. Prompts for consideration include: What are some ways discrimination might occur in branding and brand promotion? What steps may be taken to ensure marketing practices are not discriminatory? Consider who the potentially marginalized clients are within the target communities. What is the most effective way to connect with them?

Contributing to the Public Good (Pro Bono Publico)

Counselors make a reasonable effort to provide services to the public for which there is little or no financial return (e.g., speaking to groups, sharing professional information, offering reduced fees). (ACA, 2014, p. 10)

Play therapists are in a unique position to provide psychoeducation and relational skills building to caregivers during one of the most impactful times of growth and development. Play therapists understand that early relational dynamics become a core part of the way a child perceives self and self in relation to others and that those internalized beliefs can be carried forward throughout life (Solomon & George, 1999). This knowledge and the skills that play therapists are trained in can provide invaluable assistance to children and families. Play therapists also understand the impact of early childhood adverse experiences and how those negative or traumatic experiences can predispose a child to elevated risk for a variety of mental health concerns (Felitti et. al, 1998). Lower socioeconomic status is often correlated with increased stressors. Play therapists have an ethical obligation to provide their wealth of knowledge and skills to those individuals who can benefit from such services yet cannot afford them. Prompts for consideration include: How will the play therapy training clinic incorporate efforts to provide services to marginalized communities within your target audiences? How might marketing be tailored to incorporate the provision of such services? Some suggestions are to create workshops and informational sessions for the public that provide free, or at a greatly reduced cost, access to information regarding child development and the importance of early exposure to positive, healthy relational dynamics. Another option is to provide knowledge regarding access to services within the community for individuals who are unable to afford services at the play therapy training clinic. In the event the play therapy training clinic is unable to offer direct play therapy services or workshops without financial return, then perhaps a partnership with a non-profit organization to provide psycho-educational presentations or workshops for lower income individuals would be a possible avenue for sharing knowledge and expertise.

CONCLUSION

There are many aspects of providing play therapy clinical services and education to consider when developing the brand and planning promotional strategies for a play therapy training clinic. Focusing on the core values and mission, the target audiences and their needs, identifying a professional niche, and delineating the primary sources of income is essential to understanding the purpose of the training clinic. Reflective considerations of each of these aspects of the play therapy clinic are essential in distilling the overall brand of the play therapy training clinic. Once the brand is clear, then promotional strategies can be utilized to effectively reach target audiences. Methods for community engagement can include use of technology, person-to-person strategies, or a combination of both. Diversifying use of marketing strategies and conducting basic marketing research to determine the most effective use of efforts for client engagement is important for sustaining growth of the clinic's outreach. Data from simple measures regarding efficacy of marketing strategies can be used to update the marketing plan in terms of specific strategies to be used. Maintenance of community engagement is important once initial goals for outreach have been accomplished, particularly to sustain the desired level of business the play therapy training clinic conducts.

Branding and marketing can be simplified to understanding the identity of the training clinic (brand), and the needs of the training clinic's target audiences (clients and trainees), and working to provide knowledge that creates connections between the two (marketing) to promote a mutually beneficial engagement. Play therapists understand the importance and value of positive interpersonal dynamics and can utilize their skills and knowledge to foster productive professional relationships within the community. Ethical and cultural considerations play a key role in the development of a training clinic's brand as well as the promotional plan for the clinic. Research regarding the promotional practices, as well as efficacy of promotional strategies, of play therapists is scant. The creation of a database for play therapist use wherein effective strategies for use are shared can enhance the communication between play therapists and the public regarding services offered.

REFERENCES

American Counseling Association. (2014). *Code of ethics*. Alexandria, VA: Author.

American Marketing Association. (2013). *About marketing*. Retrieved from https://www.ama.org/AboutAMA/Pages/Definition-of-Marketing.aspx

Association for Play Therapy. (2016). *Play therapy best practices: Clinical, Professional and Ethical Issues*. Retrieved from https://cdn.ymaws.com/www.a4pt.org/resource/resmgr/ publications/Best_Practices__-_Sept_2016.pdf

Association for Play Therapy. (n.d.a). *About play therapy*. Retrieved from https://www.a4pt.org/ page/AboutAPT

Association for Play Therapy. (n.d.b). *Clarifying the use of play therapy*. Retrieved from https://www.a4pt.org/page/ClarifyingUseofPT

Association for Play Therapy. (n.d.c). *Find a play therapist*. Retrieved from https://www.a4pt.org/page/TherapistDirectory

Association for Play Therapy. (n.d.d.). *Education and training*. Retrieved from https:// www.a4pt.org/general/custom.asp?page=EducationTraining

Bratton, S., Ray, D., Rhine, T., & Jones, L. (2005). The efficacy of play therapy with children: A meta-analytic review of treatment outcomes. *Professional Psychology, Research and Practice*, *36*(4), 376–390. doi:10.1037/0735-7028.36.4.376

Cole. (2016). Can focusing on customer experience unify marketing and sales functions. *Marketing News*. Retrieved from https://www.ama.org/publications/MarketingNews/ Pages/experiential-view-unify-the-entire-prospect-to-customer-lifecycle.aspx

Felitti, V., Anda, R., Nordenberg, D., Williamson, D., Spitz, A., Edwards, V., & Marks, J. (1998). Relationship of childhood abuse and household dysfunction to many of the leading causes of death in adults: The adverse childhood experiences (ACE) study. *American Journal of Preventive Medicine*, *14*(4), 245–258. doi:10.1016/S0749-3797(98)00017-8 PMID:9635069

Gilchrist, L., & Stringer, M. (1992). Marketing counseling: Guidelines for training and practice. *Counselor Education and Supervision*, *31*, 154-162.

Graham, C. (2018). Developing the dream: Play in private practice. *Play Therapy*, *13*(3), 24–27.

LeBlanc, M., & Ritchie, M. (2001). A meta-analysis of play therapy outcomes. *Counselling Psychology Quarterly*, *14*(2), 149–163. doi:10.1080/09515070110059142

Lin, D., & Bratton, S. (2015). A meta-analytic review of child-centered play therapy approaches. *Journal of Counseling and Development*, *93*(1), 45–58. doi:10.1002/j.1556-6676.2015.00180.x

O'Guinn, Semenik, & Close Scheinbaum. (2015). Advertising and integrated brand promotion. Boston, MA: Cengage.

Public Relations Society of America. (n.d.). *About public relations*. Retrieved from https:// www.prsa.org/all-about-pr/

Ray, D. (2012). *Advanced play therapy: Essential conditions, knowledge, and skills for child practice*. New York, NY: Routledge.

Ray, D., Armstrong, S., Balkin, R., & Jayne, K. (2015). Child centered play therapy in the schools: Review and meta-analysis. *Psychology in the Schools*, *52*(2), 107–123. doi:10.1002/pits.21798

Sanok, J. (2018, January 17). *How to attract your ideal client* [Webinar]. Retrieved from: https:// 24b71c9a-dc9b-4e8e-b130-25cb723ebb1c.webinarninja.com/webinars/16578

Solomon, J., & George, C. (1999). *Attachment disorganization*. New York: Guilford.

Stadler, H. (1988). Marketing counseling: Caveat emptor. *Counselor Education and Supervision*, *27*(4), 320–322. doi:10.1002/j.1556-6978.1988.tb00774.x

KEY TERMS AND DEFINITIONS

Brand: The essential identity of an individual or company, particularly the aspects of the identity that individual or company desires to be associated with in others' minds.

Brand Promotion: The act of increasing awareness of a brand.

Branding: The act of discovering, or distilling, the essential elements of an individual or company into an easily discernible identity.

Integrated Brand Promotion: The act of utilizing various forms of brand promotion to increase brand awareness.

Mission Statement: The core values of the individual or company succinctly communicated, in three sentences or fewer.

Play Therapist: A mental health professional, or professional-in-training, who understands the developmental basis for play therapy, the utility of play therapy for addressing a variety of concerns, and accesses the therapeutic powers of play while working within their chosen theoretical framework for providing play therapy.

Play Therapy: A developmentally sensitive approach to mental health counseling wherein a trained mental health professional accesses the therapeutic powers of play, while remaining grounded within a chosen theoretical orientation, in order to facilitate client growth and development.

Section 2
Advancing the University's Mission

Play therapy clinics are typically established to support the university mission of teaching, service, and research. As faculty members, we may choose to focus on any one of those areas. As teachers, we train undergraduates (child development), graduates (mental health professionals), and advanced therapists who seek certification (registered play therapists). This education may include observation, general office work, formal courses, and continuing education units. Service in the university may include service to the university, profession, and community. The university gains when faculty members are active in their chosen fields of study and students benefit from faculty who remain abreast of the current happenings in the field. Professionally, play therapy clinics allow for the continued advancement of one's career while educating the next generation of professionals on the benefits of play therapy. Clinics also are an arena for researchers to gather data and continue to advance the research in the field of play therapy. Additionally, registered play therapy supervisors remain up-to-date of the latest research and best practices in the field. Thereby offering quality supervision for the incoming play therapists. The community often benefits from play therapy clinics as they service the public in ways that other clinics may not be able to. For example, due to university funding, grant funding, or private funding, a university play therapy clinic may be able to offer services to those who are under-insured and would otherwise be unable to receive play therapy services. The following chapters provide rich detail into ways that faculty members may focus their activities in a university play therapy clinic.

Chapter 3 The Evolution of a University-Based Center of Play Therapy Education

Tiffany McNary
Georgia State University, USA

Galina Kadosh Tobin
Georgia State University, USA

Sarah D. Stauffer
Association ESPAS, Switzerland

ABSTRACT

More beginning graduate students and new mental health professionals are seeing children and families in their therapeutic work, creating a growing need for play therapy-specific training and supervision. Training students and professionals in the art of play therapy is critical to the wellbeing of children, families, and the future profession. A university-based approved center of play therapy education aims to fulfill this growing need while undertaking a momentous amount of responsibility. Training skilled play therapists is a complex endeavor requiring a combination of foundational knowledge, advanced clinical and conceptual skills, and supervision that surpasses classroom coursework requirements. The authors describe the evolution of Georgia State University's Center of Play Therapy Education and Play Therapy Training Institute to provide readers with a comprehensive model for play therapy training and supervision.

DOI: 10.4018/978-1-5225-8226-7.ch003

INTRODUCTION

"In play a child is always above his average age, above his daily behaviour; in play it is as though he were a head taller than himself... play contains all developmental tendencies in a condensed form" (Vygotsky, 1966/2016, p. 18). From this 1933 lecture, Vygotsky emphasized the role of play within his larger cultural-historical approach, noting that "play is the leading source of development in preschool years" (as cited in Bodrova & Leong, 2015, p. 376). Children's need for play remains a constant factor in their development. Recent changes in child development have increased concerns among parents and professionals alike. Georgia State University's (GSU) Center for Play Therapy Education and Play Therapy Training Institute put child development at the forefront of instruction, practice, and supervision training experiences, allowing students and practicing professionals to address children's mental health concerns in a developmentally appropriate way: through play.

Parental responses to a national survey of children's health showed one in seven children (14%) aged two to eight years old had a diagnosed mental, behavioral, or developmental disorder (Bitko et al., 2016). Reviewing national data, Knopf, Park, and Paul Mulye (2008) similarly concluded that 20-25% of youth experience symptoms of emotional distress and about one in ten may have significant impairment from moderate to severe symptomatology. By 2030, the U.S. Department of Health and Human Services (2002) estimates there will be 83.2 million children under 18 years of age in the US, an increase from 72.0 million children in 2000, creating an arguably greater need for child mental health practitioners in the next decade.

Reporting on the state of children's mental health, U.S. Surgeon General, Admiral David Satcher, wrote, "growing numbers of children are suffering needlessly because their emotional, behavioral, and developmental needs are not being met by the very institutions and systems that were created to take care of them" (U.S. Public Health Service, PHS, 2000, Foreward, para. 1). Satcher called for including child- and family-centered mental health services in all systems that serve this population, engaging families, and integrating children's perspectives in mental healthcare planning (PHS, 2000). GSU's programs now involve parents and teachers, however, these and other child mental health training institutions face a number of program complexities; the changing and growing needs of the helping professions have created a training gap between the focus of education programs and the knowledge and skills needed for successful practice (Hoge, Huey, & O'Connell, 2004; Huang, Macbeth, Dodge, & Jacobstein, 2004).

Scarcity of Child Mental Health Professionals

Child-focused clinicians must develop both basic and advanced skills, navigate multiple systems, incorporate families into treatment, apply multiple systemic interventions in both schools and communities, and deliver services that are culturally competent (Huang et.al., 2004; Mellin & Pertuit, 2009). Factors such as insufficient funding, low priority placed on mental health in the public health agenda, and inadequate training of children's mental health providers contribute to the aforementioned training gap (Huang et al., 2004; Kieling et al., 2011; Saraceno et al., 2007; Saxena, Thornicroft, Knapp, & Whiteford, 2007; Tolan & Dodge, 2005).

The President's New Freedom Commission on Mental Health (2003) highlighted professionals' lack of education, training, and supervision as contributing factors to the shortage of well-trained child and adolescent mental health practitioners. This shortage has left providers without adequate training serving children and adolescents (Koppelman, 2004), and has created "poor working conditions in public mental health services, a lack of incentives to work in rural areas,... [and] in mental health specialists spending time providing care rather than training and supervising others" (Saraceno et al., 2007, p. 1171). GSU combats these challenges by encouraging community service and providing play therapy-specific supervision training to reinforce the strength and stability of the child and adolescent mental health provider workforce.

Traditionally, clinical mental health counseling programs focus on adults, and school counseling programs do not prepare school counselors to work with acute mental health concerns on a long-term basis (Mellin & Pertuit, 2009). Although the American School Counselor Association (ASCA, 2012) approves of school counselors providing individual and group counseling services, they list "providing therapy or long-term counseling in schools to address psychological disorders" under "inappropriate activities for school counselors" (ASCA, p. 3). In a review of the Council for Accreditation of Counseling and Educational Program's (CACREP) 2009 standards, Mellin and Pertuit (2009) found that *youth, children,* and, *adolescents* were not included in clinical mental health counseling and that *mental health* was not present within school counseling standards. Our review of the 2016 CACREP standards found the same. Although the Council on Rehabilitation Education (CORE) merged with CACREP in 2017 (CACREP, 2017), CORE's former standards did not include any specific requirements for rehabilitation counseling programs to provide coursework specific to children and adolescents (e.g., Mellin, Hunt, Lorenz, 2009).

Studies examining student access to graduate-level courses specializing in child and adolescent counseling are bleak. Mellin et al. (2009) surveyed 46 CORE- accredited rehabilitation counseling programs. Despite student interest, only eight programs (17%) offered a child and adolescent development-specific course; five programs (11%) offered a child, adolescent, and family helping relationships course. Only 4% of respondents reported receiving specialized instruction in youth psychiatric disabilities; only 2% indicated the availability of classroom instruction *and* clinical experience (Mellin et. al., 2009). Surprisingly, however, 73% of programs indicated that students could work with these populations during practicum and internship (Mellin et. al., 2009). Russ (2016) randomly sampled 2,000 American Mental Health Counselors Association members and found fewer than 60% of participants attended graduate programs that offered specific coursework on counseling children and adolescents and only 20% of these programs required these courses. Those who took childhood-specific courses or courses with childhood content reported feeling more prepared to work with children during internship, although only participants who took childhood-specific courses reported higher levels of expertise (Russ, 2016).

Recommendations for closing this educational gap include moving away from generic training models and offering specialized coursework and clinical experience to students working with children and adolescents (Hoge et. al., 2014; Mellin & Pertuit, 2009). Tolan and Dodge (2005) advised orienting programs to a developmental framework that includes epidemiology, prevention, and mental health promotion. Furthermore, utilizing licensed instructors and supervisors who currently practice (Hoge et. al., 2014) and creating opportunities for students to participate in multidisciplinary team treatment approaches (Huang et. al, 2004) helps students operate within an established professional network.

The American Academy of Pediatrics (AAP) urged pediatric providers to "write a prescription for play" (e.g., Yogman et al., 2018, p. 1), noting that cultural shifts in less parent engagement, more digital distractions, fewer safe spaces to play, and an increased focus on academic readiness, comes at the expense of the learning, skills, and social-emotional benefits developed through play. They eloquently stated:

Play is not frivolous; it is brain building. Play has been shown to have both direct and indirect effects on brain structure and functioning. Play leads to changes at the molecular (epigenetic), cellular (neuronal connectivity), and behavioral levels (socioemotional and executive functioning skills) that promote learning and adaptive and/or prosocial behavior. (Yogman et al., 2018, p. 5)

GSU meets child-specific mental health education recommendations and prescribes play by offering play therapy training to graduate-level students and practicing mental health professionals in university-based and continuing education formats. In turn, these students and professionals may provide developmentally appropriate services to children and families in different settings, such as community mental health agencies and public schools, so that mental health care access does not become a barrier to mental health treatment.

Play Therapy Credentialing and Effectiveness

The Association for Play Therapy (APT), a national organization established in 1982, exists "to promote the value of play, play therapy, and credentialed play therapists" (APT, 2018b). APT (2018c) defined play therapy as "the systematic use of a theoretical model to establish an interpersonal process wherein trained play therapists use the therapeutic powers of play to help clients prevent or resolve psychosocial difficulties and achieve optimal growth and development" (para. 1). Several different forms of play therapy were regarded as promising and evidence-based practices by the U.S. Substance Abuse and Mental Health Services Administration (SAMSHA), who listed them on their National Registry of Evidence-based Programs and Practices (NREPP) until SAMHSA ended their relationship with NREPP in 2018 (Ray, 2018). There are several forms of play therapy currently recognized as evidence-based by the California Evidence-Based Clearinghouse for Child Welfare (CEBC), an entity "highly regarded as a credible reviewer of mental health interventions for children... and a stable force in assessing evidence-based interventions" (Ray, 2018, p. 21).

Providing play therapy requires extensive specialized education, training, and experience. APT offers three credentials that licensed mental health professionals, certified school counselors, and school psychologists can earn after having demonstrated the depth and breadth of their specialized play therapy education, training, and experience. For twenty-five years, APT has offered the Registered Play Therapist (RPT) and Registered Play Therapist-Supervisor (RPT-S) credentials, and the School Based-Registered Play Therapist (SB-RPT) credential since 2016.

To meet the educational requirements necessary to obtain the RPT/S and SB-RPT credentials, training courses must be taken from an approved center of play therapy and/or an approved provider of continuing education. APT grants three-year approval status to approved centers at colleges and universities offering master's or doctoral degrees in a mental health field that satisfy requirements, such as (a) generating play therapy instruction, supervised clinical experience, and supervisor training, and employing faculty members with play therapy expertise and RPT/S credentials, (b) producing original play therapy-specific research, especially research advancing evidence-based play therapy practice, and publishing such research in professional peer-reviewed journals within and outside of the play therapy community, and (c) contributing to the advancement of play therapy and the growth of the play therapy community (APT, 2018a, para. 2).

APT also grants approval to approved providers who offer continuing education opportunities for professionals seeking licensure, continuing education, and play therapy credentials. APT-approved providers may be agencies, individuals, organizations, or businesses that award play therapy credit for continuing education purposes for a period of three years (Type I) or for one event of five days or less that offers up to 25 hours of play therapy credit (Type II; APT, 2018b). For both types, this coursework must satisfy specific approval criteria that aims to:

Improve client care, either directly or indirectly, by demonstrating evidence of either: (a) systematic use of a therapeutic model, the establishment of an interpersonal process using the therapeutic powers of play, and intent to prevent or resolve psychosocial difficulties and/or achieve optimal growth and development; or (b) content that enhances the specific professional proficiency of mental health practitioners who are engaged in the clinical practice of play therapy, the supervision of play therapists, or the instruction of play therapy. (APT, 2018b, p. 1) Meeting such stringent requirements helps "promote and protect the credibility and viability of the play therapy profession through strong academic rigor and ethical training standards" (Lebby, 2018b).

As public awareness of the effectiveness of play therapy grows, there is an increasing demand for professionals trained in this specialized modality. Beginning mental health graduate students and new professionals are increasingly challenged to meet the needs of their child and adolescent caseloads. As the flagship national professional play therapy association in the US, APT currently boasts more than 6,800 professional and student members, over 52% of whom have earned an RPT/S or SB-RPT credential (Lebby, 2018a). This growing trend of seeking professional recognition through credentialing validates the importance of play therapy and highlights the critical need for play therapy-specific training and research to demonstrate its effectiveness.

Several researchers have established play therapists' effectiveness through the publication of meta-analyses and other research. Lin and Bratton (2015) found small (d=.33) but statistically significant favorable outcomes for externalizing and internalizing behavior problems, caregiver-child relationship stress, and self-efficacy across 24 studies. Ray, Armstrong, Balkin, and Jayne (2015) found small (d=.21-.38) but statistically significant positive outcomes for externalizing and internalizing behavior problems, self-efficacy, academic, and other problems across 23 studies. Bratton, Ray, Rhine, and Jones (2005) found medium (d=.72) and statistically significant favorable outcomes for behavior problems, social adjustment, self-concept, anxiety, development, and relationship issues across 67 studies. LeBlanc and Ritchie (2001) also found medium (d=.66) and statistically significant positive outcomes for emotional and social adjustment, reaction to traumatic event(s), academic and behavior problems, and family adjustment across 42 studies. In addition, Ray and McCullough (2016) further detailed 25 randomized control trials, 25 observational studies, and 20 case reports and qualitative studies that have demonstrated play therapists' effectiveness in producing favorable outcomes on the aforementioned variables and others.

Play therapy education and training aims to fill the knowledge, awareness, and skills gaps inadequately trained child mental health clinicians demonstrate and to promote the growing need for child-specific mental health services. This responsibility is a momentous and complex endeavor, requiring a combination of teaching and training that integrates foundational knowledge and advanced clinical and critical thinking skills, such as case comprehension and conceptualization, personal awareness, and professional insight. Programs also must offer students support, encouragement, and supervision. GSU has a thirty-year history of providing post-graduate training in play therapy in the College of Education and Human Development's Department of Counseling and Psychological Services (CPS).

ORIGINS OF PLAY THERAPY AT GEORGIA STATE UNIVERSITY

In the late 1980s, Dr. JoAnna White, EdD, LPC, CPCS, RPT-S, offered the first Introduction to Play Therapy graduate course at GSU. She built a solid foundation upon which her successors could stand and continue to innovate and expand. This program obtained national recognition from APT as its second Approved Center of Play Therapy Education in July 2009 and as an Approved Provider of Continuing Education under the name "GSU Play Therapy Training Institute." Dr. White co-founded the Institute with Dr. Lauren Stern, PhD, LPC, NCC, RPT-S, a Clinical Professor and play therapy instructor at GSU during that time. Dr. White still serves the Institute as Director Emerita.

With her contributions, as well as those from Dr. Stern, Dr. Jeff Ashby, and current Director Dr. Tiffany McNary, both the Center of Play Therapy Education and the Play Therapy Training Institute have garnered renown in the Southeast for play therapy training. There are several key elements that make GSU's play therapy training approach effective and appreciated by students and practicing professionals. We enumerate these below to encourage readers to incorporate effective practices that meet children's developmental and mental health needs into their own play therapy centers and institutes for continuing education.

Building a Solid Training Foundation

In 1988, the first Introduction to Play Therapy course was offered at GSU to respond to a need for developmentally appropriate approaches to counseling young children within and outside of the school setting. This course was rooted in child-centered play therapy (e.g., Landreth, 2012) and integrated concepts from Adlerian play therapy (e.g., Kottman, 2011). Mental health and school counseling students received play therapy theory and were introduced to basic play therapy skills. The impact of this specialized course on students' clinical and child development conceptualization skills was remarkable.

With the success of the introduction course, coupled with the increased need for play therapists in and around Atlanta, a second play therapy graduate course was added to the CPS curriculum: Advanced Play Therapy. It served as a continuation and expansion of the introduction class for mental health and school counseling master's-level students, and specialist- and doctoral-level students in School Psychology and Counselor Education and Practice programs, adding advanced play therapy skills to their repertoire and extending their theoretical knowledge to other seminal play therapy theories (cf. O'Connor & Braverman, 2009) and filial therapy (e.g., Guerney, Guerney, & Andronico, 1966).

Both courses were offered each academic semester, though availability sometimes alternated based upon course registration numbers. Approximately six to fifteen students would enroll in each course. Small class sizes allowed the instructor to attend to individual student needs and encouraged group cohesiveness and sharing.

During these early years, Dr. White taught these classes using videos of her own play therapy sessions to demonstrate the use of play therapy theories and skills for students. In class, students would practice play therapy skills by role playing with each other using portable play kits. Recognizing the need for and the value of more experiential instruction with children in a live setting, though, she designed and built GSU's playroom in 1999 to provide a dedicated play therapy training space to facilitate skill development through direct practice and to provide teaching and supervision under optimal real-time learning conditions.

With the addition of the playroom, a graduate teaching assistant was hired to accompany children to and from the playroom and to film sessions. Although the graduate teaching assistant is not necessarily independently licensed, s/he is a doctoral student that must have successfully completed several classes before beginning in the position, such as the Introduction and Advanced Play Therapy courses and the doctoral-level Supervision of Counseling Services course. Additionally, s/he must be concurrently enrolled in the doctoral-level Applied Supervision Internship course, serving as a supervisor-in-training under a licensed and RPT-S credentialed professor while working in the graduate teaching assistant position.

Facilitating Practice and Teaching

The playroom design, based upon Dr. White's play therapy experience, follows Landreth's (2012) recommendations in terms of size, toy selection, and the installation of training equipment. It includes toys selected from Landreth's recommended categories, two sand trays (one wet and one dry), approximately 500 miniatures, a fully functioning sink, a bop bag, and a one-way observation mirror, behind which the teaching assistant can monitor the play session and operate the camera equipment. It is wired and equipped with state-of-the-art audio and video technology for real-time screen projection into the adjacent classroom, where the remaining students and course instructor can observe and discuss the session in progress.

From 1999 forward, requirements for both classes included practicing newly learned play therapy skills with children within and beyond the classroom setting. The in-class required practice invites children from GSU's Child Development Center to be play therapy participants. This center, located on campus, offers child care and a preschool learning environment for the children of GSU faculty, staff, and students. Nearly twenty-five years ago, Dr. White initiated a collaborative relationship with the Child Development Center, with both she and the CPS Department assuming ultimate responsibility for the children's care and wellbeing during this time. This partnership flourished under her leadership and the following procedures, implemented then, still exist today.

Through documented informed consent procedures, parents consent to their children participating in and being video-recorded during "special play times" under direct instructor supervision to help graduate-level play therapists-in-training apply their play therapy knowledge and skills in the playroom setting. Child assent to special play time is obtained verbally after parents have consented to participation in written form. Each academic semester, new informed consent forms are disseminated to parents through the Child Development Center, allowing them to decide how often their child participates in special play time and to withdraw their child from this experience at any time. Parents understand that video recordings of their children may be used for teaching, training, and research purposes. This 25-year collaboration has contributed greatly to the university's research efforts and continues to offer an ideal setting for play therapists-in-training to learn about young children's development while practicing and polishing their play therapy skills.

GSU's playroom is centrally located among the offices and classrooms within the CPS Department. For Introduction to Play Therapy students, the graduate teaching assistant accompanies each child on foot from the Child Development Center to and from the playroom for special play time. The child selected for that day's class rotates among all children with permission to attend, and the play therapist-in-training does not necessarily work exclusively with one child. For Advanced Play Therapy students, one of the first class sessions is dedicated to forming a student-child dyad at the Child Development Center so the relationship begins in a familiar space (the child's classroom) and near a familiar and presumably safe person for the child (the child's teacher); this dyad remains paired exclusively throughout the semester. The Advanced Play Therapy students have the privilege of accompanying their child from the Child Development Center directly to the playroom and back, further building their relationship during their walks before and after their play sessions together.

This in-class experience allows the play therapist-in-training thirty minutes with a child in the playroom while the teaching assistant records the session from behind the one-way mirror. The rest of the class remains in the adjacent classroom, viewing the session live, while the course instructor encourages the class to note what basic and advanced play therapy skills are being employed, and what strengths and areas for improvement they see in their colleague's approach. This feedback is captured on a play therapy evaluator's form that is shared orally and in writing with the play therapist-in-training after the session. The professor also comments on what the play therapist-in-training and/or the child is doing in the session, further enhancing students' understanding of play therapy theories and process dynamics in real time. Therefore, students learn by doing and by actively observing their peers while direct supervision and commentary is provided by their professor.

Other introductory and advanced course requirements include recruiting and obtaining consent and assent to practice play therapy in special play times outside of the classroom setting with one child on the students' personal time; transcribing recorded sessions to better understand one's personal process and the development of the therapeutic relationship through play therapy; and completing reports on how different theoretical orientations approach case conceptualization, practice, and parent feedback. Students learn to develop encouraging feedback and to deliver this information to their colleagues orally and in writing, which represents an active form of attendance and participation in class and a professional development skill that later serves them in working with future clients' parents/guardians, teachers, other professionals, and eventually their own supervisees.

PROGRAM EVOLUTIONS AND CURRENT PRACTICES

With a solid foundation from which to teach and practice, GSU's Center of Play Therapy Education carried on the mission initiated by Dr. White for twenty years with procedures that remained relatively unchanged during that time. The evolutions that have emerged in current procedures respond more to meeting societal and technological demands for security than changing the underlying play therapy teaching and practice philosophy. All of these differences have spurred enhancements that allow the program to operate to the highest possible ethical and legal standards while adding greater diversity and depth to class discussions.

Tracking the Evolution of Current Practices

Since 2010, the CPS Department and the Child Development Center have agreed to assume joint responsibility for accompanying child participants to and from the playroom. Child participants are now accompanied back and forth from sessions with one of their teachers in addition to either the CPS graduate teaching assistant (in Introduction to Play Therapy) or the play therapist-in-training (in Advanced Play Therapy). Beyond providing an extra layer of physical security to the children, this double accompaniment also promotes children's emotional security to have a person they already trust (their teacher) there to ensure their wellbeing, acting as a secure base for them (Verschueren & Koomen, 2012) while they develop a therapeutic relationship with the play therapist-in-training. This reflection for the child's safety also was extended to bathroom breaks requested by the child during play sessions; children are always accompanied to the restroom by their teacher and their play therapist-in-training.

To better include parents, the course instructor encourages them to sit in the observation room with their child's teacher and the graduate teaching assistant during the session. The parents may openly communicate their questions or concerns and receive immediate answers from the graduate assistant, who is well-trained in play therapy, child development, and supervision, or from the professor after the session. However, if the parent is not present, no feedback is offered after the session. Additionally, parents are better informed about data security procedures employed through updated informed consent forms.

Sessions are digitally recorded and stored on a server developed uniquely for the Center for Play Therapy Education. This server allows only the course instructor and teaching assistant to access files, though both may digitally send encrypted files to students through a password-protected account. The course instructor works closely with the College of Education and Human Development's lead technology staff person, participating in specialized technology trainings twice a year to comply with the highest levels of data security and ethical responsibility (e.g., American Counseling Association, 2014; American Psychological Association, 2018).

In addition to the technological changes within the Center of Play Therapy Education, the program has updated its original coursework to reflect current CACREP standards and APT objectives, and now includes three additional course offerings. This three-course expansion provides a more comprehensive and well-rounded perspective on child development and further play therapy-specific knowledge and skills in several crucial domains. Notably, professors put special populations and settings at the forefront of play therapy education, such as working with traumatized children and families through play and expressive arts and working "outside the box" of the four-walled classroom through adventure therapy facilitation and education.

Expanding Course Offerings

A total of five graduate-level courses are currently offered and taught by two different professors: Tiffany McNary, PhD, LPC, NCC, CPCS, RPT-S, Clinical Assistant Professor of Counseling, and Jeff Ashby, PhD, ABPP, RPT-S, Full Professor of Counseling Psychology. The difference in the play therapy professors' professional identities provides students with licensure, supervision, and play therapy credentialing advantages; students can seek education and training across disciplines or supervision from a professor within their discipline, as those disciplines may require.

Three of GSU's courses provide students with 67.5 hours each of the mandatory 150 education hours required for RPT/S certification through APT, and the remaining two courses offer 30 hours each towards RPT/S certification. A registration wait-list is necessary to account for the ever-increasing demand for these courses. Enrollment is intentionally limited to increase instructors' abilities to respond to students' specialized training and supervision needs. Additionally, students may benefit from play therapy-specific supervision groups that meet weekly on campus to focus on child and adolescent cases. Each semester, approximately 12-18 master's-level students in practicum and internship classes receive play therapy supervision by faculty members (including one part-time instructor) with doctoral degrees, a mental health license, certified supervisor credentials, and the RPT-S credential from APT.

The development of graduate-level course programming is an intricate task wherein professors are expected to reflect the values, mission, policy and procedures of multiple entities within their syllabi (e.g., university and department standards, accrediting agency guidelines, and specialty certification requirements). GSU play therapy syllabi specify all of these components and align course learning objectives with APT's requirements for RPT/S credentialing. We provide course descriptions in Table 1 as examples that may be useful to other approved centers or individual providers designing coursework for play therapy credit.

Since the inception of GSU's play therapy program thirty years ago, instructors have emphasized that providing an adequate training environment and promoting collaborative relationships among participants allows students to grow in their professional identity as play therapists and to flourish in their skill development. The specific concepts that are emphasized and employed in the GSU teaching approach are worth noting and incorporating in any center for play therapy education or continuing education setting. We describe them here to encourage readers to think globally about how their training programs will make a difference in the professional

Table 1. Georgia State University play therapy course offerings

Course	Course Objectives	Course Content	Course Format	Text(s)	Attendance hours offered toward RPT/S credential
Introduction to Play Therapy[a]	Acquire play therapy knowledge and skills. Utilize play therapy skills with children from GSU's Child Development Center and children recruited outside of class time.	Play therapy history, seminal play therapy theories, basic play therapy techniques, and issues related to counseling children.	Lecture, case studies, video presentations, and experiential activities. Limited to 15 students.	Landreth (2012) Kottman (2011)	67.5
Advanced Play Therapy[a]	Develop and deepen play therapy knowledge and skills. Build a one-on-one therapeutic relationship with a child from GSU's Child Development Center. Review recorded sessions in individual play therapy-specific supervision. Participate in group supervision activities outside of class time.	Play therapy history, additional play therapy theories, play therapy research, and recent innovations in play therapy. Guest speakers present on special topics of interest, directly linking theories and special issues to real-world practice.	Lecture, case studies, video and oral presentations, and experiential activities. Limited to 13 students.	Ray (2011)	67.5
Treating the Traumatized Child: Integrating Play Therapy and the Expressive Arts[a]	Acquire traumatology and traumatic play dynamics knowledge. Gain exposure to working with traumatized children through play and expressive art therapies and the neurosequential model of therapeutics.	Discussion and delineation of common concerns, research bases, and practice guidelines among traumatology, play therapy, and expressive art therapy theories and practices.	Lecture, discussion, video and oral presentations, and experiential activities. Limited to 30 students.	Findling, Bratton, & Henson (2006) Gaskill & Perry (2017) Herman (1992/2015) Malchiodi (2014) Steele & Malchiodi (2011)	30
Family Systems, Theory and Interventions: Integrating Play Therapy and the Expressive Arts[a]	Acquire knowledge of family systems theories and working with families in play therapy. Integrate play and expressive arts techniques into family therapy sessions using art, puppets, sand tray, storytelling, and drama.	Family therapy history, major family therapy theoretical orientations, family therapy research and ethics, and family play therapy techniques.	Lecture, discussion, video and oral presentations, and experiential activities. Limited to 30 students.	Gil (2016) Gladding (2015) McGoldrick, Gerson, & Petry (2008)	30
Facilitating Adventure Therapy and Education[b]	Acquire knowledge about adventure/challenge therapy. Learn to facilitate adventure/challenge therapy.	Dynamics of adventure experiences, therapeutic application of adventure activities, and effective group facilitation and processing skills.	Lecture, video, class discussion, and participating in and leading a variety of experiential exercises in high-, low-, and no-ropes settings. Limited to 12 students.	Ashby, Kottman, & DeGraff (2008) Gass, Gillis, & Russel (2018)	30

Note. [a]Denotes courses taught by Dr. Tiffany McNary, PhD, LPC, NCC, CPCS, RPT-S, Clinical Assistant Professor of Counseling at Georgia State University. [b]Denotes courses taught by Dr. Jeff Ashby, PhD, ABPP, RPT-S, Full Professor of Counseling Psychology at Georgia State University.

lives of their students and those students' future or current clients as a result of having participated in readers' own play therapy education and training programs.

TEACHING APPROACH AND THEORETICAL CONSIDERATIONS

Attending to the logistics, details, and setup of a training institute are paramount to its establishment and success. Equally as important are the relationships and connections we have with one another. Developing a sense of community among students aids in fostering a sense of belonging to the course, the program, and the profession as a whole, and helps them build a professional network with their colleagues. While integrating psychological and developmental theories and models, clinical experience, and experiential practice into each class, course instructors underscore connection to the play therapy material, to each other, and to the professor. Several practices are key to GSU's teaching approach to experiential education. For example, instructors emphasize creating a learning community, incorporating supervision directly into the teaching model, and discussing the importance of trauma-informed instruction and care, multiculturalism, and social justice during class sessions.

The program incorporates tiered teaching and supervision experiences to develop a cadre of play therapy professors/trainers and supervisors, addressing Saraceno et al.'s (2007) concerns for developing more practicing supervisors. Furthermore, professors encourage students to use their play therapy skills on a volunteer basis to help others and further promote the play therapy profession. Finally, offering courses in a continuing education format to practicing clinicians allows the GSU Play Therapy Training Institute to have a greater community impact on child clients, answering Satcher's call to expand child mental health services (PHS, 2000). We discuss each of these components in turn to inspire readers to build a solid training foundation for students and simultaneously perform community outreach and strengthening through their own programs.

Creating a Learning Community

This part of GSU's teaching style is multifaceted and includes didactic learning, experiential components, and creativity. Instructors integrate clinical skills into the classroom environment and highlight attunement, intentionality, student strengths, and the use of encouragement, thereby creating a safe and nurturing environment in which to learn and develop personally and professionally. This approach recognizes the developmental processes involved in becoming both a helping professional and a play therapist. Instructional style and depth are informed by the students' developmental levels, as instructors aim to support students' transition from novice learners to competent clinicians. In accordance with Vygotsky's (1978) teachings on the zone of proximal development, instructors are mindful of the level of scaffolding, assistance, support, and encouragement needed for students to complete the various tasks required of them.

This multi-layered approach to teaching, which captures students' unique and varied learning styles, may begin, for example, with a Power Point presentation and lecture embedded in a thought-provoking discussion, followed by a case study from the instructor's clinical practice. Then, students transition to viewing a video of the professor facilitating a play therapy session, cued to highlight the skill taught in the Power Point. Finally, students work experientially using play and expressive activities designed to increase students' awareness of the class topic.

Incorporating Supervision Into the Teaching Model

Supervision is an important component to require within a didactic and experiential training program, for students initially learning play therapy skills and for licensed mental health professionals that supervise others. GSU's Center for Play Therapy offers supervision experiences and training to accommodate different students' needs: requiring supervision of play therapists-in-training and offering tiered teaching and supervision opportunities to doctoral students learning to supervise others in play therapy practice.

Offering Supervision as a Part of Initial Play Therapy Training

Instructor awareness of clinical supervision models (e.g., Bernard & Goodyear, 2018; McNeill, Stoltenberg, & Romans, 1992; Stoltenberg, 1997) offers greater conceptualization of student development. Understanding students' individual professional development stage (i.e., length of time in graduate program and previous courses taken) provides instructors with a roadmap of how to enhance clinical understanding and skills for each class member. For instance, a first semester student will approach and comprehend course material vastly differently than a student entering his or her final semester who has completed basic skills, counseling theories, and practicum.

When these two types of students are in the same class, the instructor can make use of each of their skill levels to create connections and further skill development for all students simultaneously. For example, the instructor can invite more advanced students to describe their experiences to the class, thereby activating case conceptualization and presentation skills, to engage less advanced students in observation through active listening, discussion, and connecting to others and the course material through asking questions and giving feedback. The integrated developmental model (e.g., Stoltenberg, 1997; McNeill et al., 1992) also recognizes that student development may vary within the same cohort year, with some students integrating material and skills more quickly than others.

Meeting students at their developmental level is central to helping them integrate new knowledge and increasing their willingness to examine and reflect upon their practice. Accordingly, professors must balance their roles of educator, supervisor, model, mentor, and consultant. Instructors must be keenly aware of their responsibility to the clients that these students serve (currently or eventually). The discrimination model (e.g., Bernard & Goodyear, 2018) highlights three main skill areas for supervisees that can translate directly to play therapy-specific courses: intervention skills, conceptualization skills, and personalization skills. Intervention skills address counseling interventions and skills; conceptualization skills attend to understanding patterns and choosing interventions; and personalization skills focus on personal counseling style (Bernard & Goodyear, 2018). When addressing each of these skill areas, supervisors will utilize and shift between teacher, counselor, and consultant roles (Bernard & Goodyear, 2018). In the teacher role, the supervisor provides structure, instruction, feedback and modeling; in the counselor role, s/he increases a supervisees' reflection and awareness of their inner world; and in the consultant role, the supervisor challenges the supervisee to trust his or her own insights and to choose his or her own actions (Bernard & Goodyear, 2018).

However, Allen, Folger, and Pehrsson (2007) posited that standard supervision training falls short in recognizing the unique adult-child relationship, non-verbal communication, and projective approaches inherent to play therapy. They emphasized the need for play therapy supervisors to be grounded in play therapy education, theory, and techniques. Muro, Holliman, Blanco, and Stickley (2015) found significant improvements following play therapy training on students' attitudes, knowledge, and skills following in vivo-experiences of providing play sessions under weekly supervision. They explained that students may experience increased doubt in their skill set when first working with children, and they argued that skill practice is critical to student and skill development.

Allen et al. (2007) provided a three-step model for supervising novice play therapists that focuses on developing content, feeling (at a distance), and interpersonal reflection skills. Following a developmental model, Ray (2004) highlighted how play therapy supervisors often provide structure and specific skills feedback to novice supervisees and peer consultation to those with more advanced training. She asserted that play therapy supervisors aid in developing a supervisee's basic skills, such as nonverbal behaviors and verbal responses, and advanced skill sets, such as limit-setting, identifying themes, and interpreting play behaviors. She further advised that supervisors remain aware of their supervisee's personal and professional limitations and how these may affect the clients with whom they work. She suggested using supervision to process the supervisee's feelings that arise when working with a child who is rejecting or hurtful within the therapeutic relationship.

Teaching How to Supervise Through Tiered Supervision Experiences

Training and supervising students in play therapy requires a different skill set than practicing as a clinician. As such, the GSU Center of Play Therapy Education takes a first-hand role in developing the next generation of play therapy educators and supervisors. Doctoral-level counselor educator/supervisor and counseling psychology students may serve as teaching assistants and supervisors-in-training (SIT) in play therapy courses and supervision groups through tiered teaching and supervision experiences.

Current CPS doctoral students may engage in a full-year SIT experience. These students partner with a CPS faculty member and assist with a variety of teaching and supervision responsibilities. SITs co-facilitate weekly group supervision classes with their assigned faculty member. In addition to co-facilitating weekly master's-level practicum supervision groups, SITs are required to meet for one hour a week individually with one or two master's-level students who are also members of the larger weekly group. Each year, one or two doctoral students who manifest an interest in learning to supervise play therapy interns are permitted to do so as SITs.

In a tiered format, SITs from all different supervisory disciplines (e.g., clinical mental health, school counseling, and play therapy) also meet once a week in an advanced supervision class with a different faculty member to take supervision on their supervisory experiences. This class allows SITs to focus on their roles as instructional and supervisory managers (of master's-level individuals and groups), advocates for multicultural competency, and gatekeepers. All of these skills are paramount to furthering child mental health practice in general and the play therapy profession more specifically.

Incorporating Trauma-Informed Practices

Play therapy courses offered through GSU's Center of Play Therapy Education are designed and facilitated in ways that are consistent with trauma-informed practices. SAMHSA's (2014) 4R trauma-informed approach includes *realizing* the widespread impact of trauma and understanding potential paths to recovery; *recognizing* the signs and symptoms of trauma; *responding* by integrating knowledge about trauma into policies, procedures and practices; and *resisting re-traumatization*. SAMHSA (2014) further highlighted the importance of several principles of trauma-informed care, such as promoting safety, trustworthiness, transparency, collaboration, and empowerment; giving voice; and recognizing cultural, historical, and gender issues present within the trauma and more globally within the person's life.

Trauma-sensitive counseling is taught and modeled in parallel structure to trauma-informed practice. Each semester-long course begins with an overview, purpose statement, and opportunity for the instructor and students to share about themselves and their relation to the course. In the beginning phase, instructors are intentional in establishing safety and connection to allow students a space to fully engage in play therapy. In the middle phase, "the work" is accomplished: the learning, experiencing, challenging, and growing that occurs within the course. Finally, each semester ends with a dedicated space to reflect on their work and transition to other professional and personal endeavors with a sense of closure. The instructors highlight the prevalence and effects of trauma in both a specialized course and throughout all courses with the realization that students will encounter various forms of trauma while working with children, adolescents, and families.

Emphasizing Multiculturalism and Social Justice Advocacy

Multicultural competency encompasses an awareness and ownership of one's own biases, assumptions, and values (Sue, Arredondo, McDavis, 1992). Personal identities influence assumptions, values, and attitudes that can manifest in counseling (Bernard & Goodyear, 2018). As such, multiculturalism needs to be addressed within classrooms, and multicultural competencies must be developed within students. Ratts, Singh, Nassar-McMillan, Butler, and McCullough (2016) emphasized that competence begins with self-awareness that "extends to clients, to the counseling relationship, and to counseling and advocacy interventions and strategies" (p. 35). Multicultural and social justice counseling researchers and advocates have repeatedly highlighted the importance of understanding the effects of power, privilege, and marginalized identities within the counseling relationship (e.g., Constantine, Hage, Kindaichi, & Bryant, 2007; Hays, Dean, & Chang, 2007; Ratts et al., 2016). Ratts et al. (2016) further underscored the importance of understanding the impact oppression has on mental health.

To further facilitate multicultural competency, Hays et al. (2007) suggested holding open discussions involving students' reactions and biases towards clients and highlighting contextual and systemic factors that impact clients during case conceptualization. They posited that multicultural competency is linked with knowledge of privilege and oppression and argued that educators can increase students' awareness through "discussing invisible minority status" (p. 323). To meet these recommendations, GSU's Center of Play Therapy Education incorporates multicultural conversations into each course, attending to systemic and individual client factors, differences and similarities within the counseling relationship, and student self-exploration and reflection in relation to diverse clientele.

We argue that part of being multiculturally competent play therapists is to recognize and understand the multiple systemic factors impacting the lives of children. As with all clients, race, religion, socioeconomic status (SES), sexuality, gender identity, and ability status are variables that must be considered when working with children. Children, however, are also faced with additional systemic factors over which they have limited control and minimal voice to initiate change. Understanding a child's family dynamics, school life, and the state laws governing their rights and freedoms are central factors to understanding a child's world. Additionally, child mental health professionals need to be equipped to navigate and, when possible, integrate multiple systems while keeping the child's interests at the forefront of all treatment. As such, we make every effort to ensure that case vignettes, videos of play therapy sessions viewed in class, and children brought from the Child Development Center for sessions include diverse characteristics along many lines, such as nationality, race, and SES. Professors acknowledge and process different dynamics that arise in session pertaining to the client's world, his or her potential lived experiences, as well as students' reactions and assumptions that may affect the therapeutic relationship.

Understanding the role of social justice advocacy is crucial to providing multiculturally competent counseling. Social justice advocacy allows individuals to have a voice, gain information, understand their rights, and make more informed choices (Stewart & MacIntyre, 2013) by focusing on issues of oppression, privilege, and social inequity and promoting equitable treatment and allocation of resources (Chang, Barrio Minton, Dixon, Myers, & Sweeney, 2012). Furthermore, social justice advocacy within the counseling profession involves identifying needs and taking action to change inequity and systemic barriers (Ratts et al., 2016; Trusty & Brown, 2005).

Children are a vulnerable population and most often a voiceless population. Students must learn to recognize the power dynamic that exists in most child-adult relationships and that, within many systems, children are entirely powerless. Therefore, play therapists work to dismantle this power differential from their first interactions with children and parents through gathering assent and consent for services, promoting autonomy, and returning responsibility to children in play. GSU's Center and Institute helps play therapists-in-training develop these skills through discussion, modeling, and direct practice.

ADDITIONAL PROFESSIONAL DEVELOPMENT OPPORTUNITIES

Part of teaching play therapy is modeling how we advocate for children's inherent rights to protection, to express an opinion and to be heard, to be silent, and to play (United Nations, 1989, art. 15). As educators and play therapists, we are well positioned to advocate for the changes that will directly impact and assist our youngest clients in their communities. The GSU Play Therapy Training Institute offers opportunities for students to impact children in the community through philanthropic and continuing education opportunities, and awards some with a scholarship for demonstrating their commitment to the play therapy profession.

Encouraging Play Therapy Philanthropic Opportunities

Dr. McNary created "Play Therapy Serves," the Play Therapy Training Institute's service component, in 2016. The mission is to promote play therapy, advocacy, volunteerism, and to provide community service to children and families. Over 120 volunteer hours have been provided by GSU play therapy graduate students above their coursework with Child Development Center participants. This community outreach has served children and their families in Atlanta-area schools, hospitals, community-based mental health centers, and homeless shelters, and could be replicated in other communities.

Providing Play Therapy Scholarship Opportunities

Awarding play therapy students with graduate funding opportunities recognizes their commitment to the profession. Since 2015, the GSU Play Therapy Training Institute has offered the JoAnna White Play Therapy Scholarship, a $1,000 scholarship awarded to a current play therapy graduate student in good standing who has exhibited a strong interest and commitment to the play therapy profession through research, practice, and service.

Offering Continuing Education Through the Play Therapy Training Institute

Recognized by APT as an approved Provider of Continuing Education since 2009, GSU's Play Therapy Training Institute has had four different directors since its establishment. This Institute is the state of Georgia's only college or university that trains professionals in play therapy through university-based courses or continuing education trainings. Approximately ten trainings are offered each year to current students, alumni, and community mental health professionals through GSU's Institute. Twice per year, the Institute invites nationally recognized play therapists to give a full day of training, providing continuing education to 100 attendees or more.

FUTURE PLAY THERAPY PERSPECTIVES AT GEORGIA STATE UNIVERSITY

Play therapy faculty are mindful of the developmental processes involved in becoming a play therapist and their intricate roles as educators, supervisors, models, mentors, and consultants. As GSU's Center for Play Therapy Education and Play Therapy Training Institute both look ahead into the future, there are several common themes in their goals that revolve around offering more training opportunities and continuing to provide cutting-edge teaching methods and materials.

Offer More Training Opportunities

One goal is to continue to offer five play therapy courses to graduate students in mental health professions. Additionally, we wish to expand the current course offerings, allowing additional sections to open on the academic calendar to reduce wait-lists and to promote the therapeutic powers of play (e.g., Schaefer & Drewes, 2014) more widely.

Another possibility is to connect with community agencies or directly with families by keeping GSU's website updated and placing brochures in pediatricians' offices, for example, to market free play therapy services to children in nearby communities. Students would benefit from real-world skill development, and families would benefit from increased access to mental health care through GSU's services.

Provide Cutting-Edge Teaching Methods and Materials

A strength of GSU's teaching method is that we use recorded sessions for teaching and supervision purposes. Connecting a livestream from the playroom to the adjacent classroom or utilizing a one-way mirror allows students to learn and reflect on practice issues and to observe and give feedback to others in real time. Following class sessions with group supervision encourages, strengthens, and provides specific feedback for students' skill improvement.

Structuring class times with didactic and experiential learning opportunities and processing encourages students to engage in, grapple with, and dialogue about the material. Creating an environment that demonstrates safety, honesty, transparency, and openness provides students with the support they need to take risks, explore ideas, self-reflect, and self-evaluate.

Intentionally integrating teaching strategies that promote creativity, play, and expressive arts-based approaches fosters clinicians' ability to move from an adult-client mindset to a child mental health perspective in engaging ways. This can be accomplished by emphasizing the importance of the child-therapist relationship and the therapeutic powers of play, promoting attunement to children's nonverbal and verbal communication, understanding the child's world, and training play therapists to enter the child's world and learn about their experiences from the child's perspective.

We will further model this mindset shift by stimulating students' thinking about individual, family, cultural, and systemic factors that may impact children, highlighting advocacy competencies and ethical considerations in each course. Providing detailed clinical examples that span race, religion, SES, disability, sexuality, and gender identity and encourage open discussion on students' responses to clients with various and intersecting cultural backgrounds helps students craft appropriate treatment responses in their practice sessions within and outside of the classroom.

CONCLUSION

As play therapists, we know that children are not little adults, that their problems are unique, and that their viewpoints are worthwhile. Play therapy courses offer many students their first in-depth exposure to considering child development in context, to counseling children, and to choosing developmentally appropriate interventions and modalities that promote children's self-expression and healing. GSU's play therapy program has embraced this responsibility for over thirty years. Because graduate students and professionals are the foundation of our future profession, when trained in the art of play therapy, they weave threads of trauma-informed practice, multicultural, and social justice competencies into the fabric of our next generation with their impact on the children they serve. We hope that our training models encourage other play therapists to establish or enhance their own programs to help current and future clinicians use the therapeutic powers of play in more creative ways in their own work.

REFERENCES

Allen, V. B., Folger, W. A., & Pehrsson, D. E. (2007). Reflective process in play therapy: A practical model for supervising counseling students. *Education, 127*, 472–479.

American Counseling Association. (2014). *ACA code of ethics*. Alexandria, VA: Author.

American Psychological Association. (2018). *Ethical principles of psychologists and code of conduct*. Washington, DC: Author.

American School Counselor Association. (2012). *ASCA national model: A framework for school counseling programs. Executive summary*. Alexandria, VA: Author.

Ashby, J. S., Kottman, T., & DeGraff, D. (2008). *Active interventions for kids and teens: Adding adventures and fun to counseling*. Alexandria, VA: American Counseling Association.

Association for Play Therapy. (2018a). *Approved center of play therapy education*. Retrieved from https://www.a4pt.org/page/ApprovedCenter

Association for Play Therapy. (2018b). *Approved provider guide*. Retrieved from https://www.a4pt.org/resource/resmgr/education_&_training/approved_provider_guide_-_au.pdf

Association for Play Therapy. (2018c). *Why play therapy?* Retrieved from https://www.a4pt.org/page/WhyPlayTherapy

Bernard, J. M., & Goodyear, R. K. (2018). *Fundamentals of clinical supervision* (6th ed.). Upper Saddle River, NJ: Pearson Education.

Bitko, R. H., Holbrook, J. R., Robinson, L. R., Kaminski, J. W., Ghandour, R., Smith, C., & Peacock, G. (2016). Health care, family, and community factors associated with mental, behavioral, and developmental disorders in early childhood: United States, 2011-2012. *MMWR. Morbidity and Mortality Weekly Report*, *65*(9), 221–226. doi:10.15585/mmwr.mm6509a1 PMID:26963052

Bodrova, E., & Leong, D. J. (2015). Vygotskian and post-Vygotskian views on children's play. *American Journal of Play*, *7*, 371–388.

Bratton, S. C., Ray, D., Rhine, T., & Jones, L. (2005). The efficacy of play therapy with children: A meta-analytic review of the outcome research. *Professional Psychology, Research and Practice*, *36*(4), 376–390. doi:10.1037/0735-7028.36.4.376

Chang, C. Y., Barrio Minton, C. A., Dixon, A. L., Myers, J. E., & Sweeney, T. J. (2012). *Professional counseling excellence through leadership and advocacy*. New York, NY: Routledge. doi:10.4324/9780203829165

Constantine, M. G., Hage, S. M., Kindaichi, M. M., & Bryant, R. M. (2007). Social justice and multicultural issues: Implications for the practice and training of counselors and counseling psychologists. *Journal of Counseling and Development, 85*(1), 24–29. doi:10.1002/j.1556-6678.2007.tb00440.x

Council for Accreditation of Counseling and Related Educational Programs. (2017). *CACREP/CORE merger: July 2017 announcement.* Retrieved from https://www.cacrep.org/news-and-events/cacrepcore-updates/

Findling, J. H., Bratton, S. C., & Henson, R. K. (2006). Development of the Trauma Play Scale: An observation-based assessment of the impact of trauma on the play therapy behaviors of young children. *International Journal of Play Therapy, 15*(1), 7–36. doi:10.1037/h0088906

Gaskill, R. L., & Perry, B. D. (2017). The neurobiological power of play: Using the neurosequential model of therapeutics to guide play in the healing process. In C. A. Malchiodi & D. A. Crenshaw (Eds.), *Creative arts and play therapy for attachment problems* (pp. 178–196). New York, NY: Guilford Press.

Gass, M. A., Gillis, H. L., & Russel, K. C. (2018). *Adventure therapy: Theory, research, and practice.* New York, NY: Routledge.

Gil, E. (2016). *Play in family therapy.* New York, NY: Guilford Press.

Gladding, S. T. (2015). *Family therapy: History, theory, and practice* (6th ed.). Upper Saddle River, NJ: Pearson.

Guerney, B. G. Jr, Guerney, L., & Andronico, M. (1966, March). Filial therapy. *Yale Scientific Magazine, 40*(6), 14, 20.

Hays, D. G., Dean, J. K., & Chang, C. Y. (2007). Addressing privilege and oppression in counselor training and practice: A qualitative analysis. *Journal of Counseling and Development, 85*(3), 317–324. doi:10.1002/j.1556-6678.2007.tb00480.x

Herman, J. L. (2015). *Trauma and recovery: The aftermath of violence from domestic violence to political terror.* New York, NY: Basic Books. (Original work published 1997)

Hoge, M. A., Huey, L. Y., & O'Connell, M. J. (2004). Best practices in behavioral health workforce education and training. *Administration and Policy in Mental Health, 32*(2), 91–106. doi:10.1023/B:APIH.0000042742.45076.66 PMID:15586846

Huang, L., Macbeth, G., Dodge, J., & Jacobstein, D. (2004). Transforming the workforce in children's mental health. *Administration and Policy in Mental Health, 32*(2), 167–187. doi:10.1023/B:APIH.0000042745.64582.72 PMID:15586849

Kieling, C., Baker-Henningham, H., Belfer, M., Conti, G., Ertem, I., Omigbodun, O., & Rahman, A. (2011). Child and adolescent mental health worldwide: Evidence for action. *Lancet, 378*(9801), 1515–1525. doi:10.1016/S0140-6736(11)60827-1 PMID:22008427

Knopf, D., Park, M. J., & Paul Mulye, T. (2008). *The mental health of adolescents: A national profile, 2008*. San Francisco, CA: University of California, National Adolescent Health Information Center.

Koppelman, J. (2004). *The provider system for children's mental health: Workforce capacity and effective treatment* (NHPF Issue Brief No. 801). Washington, DC: National Health Policy Forum.

Kottman, T. (2011). *Play therapy: Basics and beyond*. Alexandria, VA: American Counseling Association.

Landreth, G. L. (2012). *Play therapy: The art of the relationship* (3rd ed.). New York, NY: Brunner-Routledge. doi:10.4324/9780203835159

Lebby, K. (2018a, October). *Year in review*. CEO keynote presented at the Annual Association for Play Therapy International Conference, Phoenix, AZ.

Lebby, K. (2018b, December). From the CEO [Editorial]. *Play Therapy, 13*(4), 2.

LeBlanc, M., & Ritchie, M. (2001). A meta-analysis of play therapy outcomes. *Counselling Psychology Quarterly, 14*(2), 149–163. doi:10.1080/09515070110059142

Lin, D., & Bratton, S. (2015). A meta-analytic review of child-centered play therapy approaches. *Journal of Counseling and Development, 93*(1), 45–58. doi:10.1002/j.1556-6676.2015.00180.x

Malchiodi, C. A. (2014). *Creative interventions with traumatized children*. New York, NY: Guilford Press.

McGoldrick, M., Gerson, R., & Petry, S. (2008). *Genograms: Assessment and intervention* (3rd ed.). New York, NY: W. W. Norton.

McNeill, B. W., Stoltenberg, C. D., & Romans, J. C. S. (1992). The integrated developmental model of supervision: Scale development and validation procedures. *Professional Psychology, Research and Practice, 23*(6), 504–508. doi:10.1037/0735-7028.23.6.504

Mellin, E. A., Hunt, B., & Lorenz, D. C. (2009). Rehabilitation counselor preparation for working with youth with psychiatric disabilities. *Rehabilitation Education, 23*(1), 33–42. doi:10.1891/088970109805059191

Mellin, E. A., & Pertuit, T. L. (2009). Research priorities for mental health counseling with youth: Implications for counselor preparation, professional development, and research. *Counselor Education and Supervision*, *49*(2), 137–155. doi:10.1002/j.1556-6978.2009.tb00093.x

Muro, J. H., Holliman, R. P., Blanco, P. J., & Stickley, V. K. (2015). Exploring play therapy training: An investigation on the impact of practice on attitudes, knowledge, and skills with master's level students. *International Journal of Play Therapy*, *24*(4), 234–247. doi:10.1037/a0039811

O'Connor, K. J., & Braverman, L. D. (Eds.). (2009). *Play therapy theory and practice: Comparing theories and techniques* (2nd ed.). Hoboken, NJ: John Wiley & Sons.

President's New Freedom Commission on Mental Health. (2003). *Achieving the promise: Transforming mental health care in America* (DHHS Publication No. SMA-03-3832). Retrieved from https://govinfo.library.unt.edu/mentalhealthcommission/reports/FinalReport/downloads/FinalReport.pdf

Ratts, M. J., Singh, A. A., Nassar-McMillan, S., Butler, S. K., & McCullough, J. R. (2016). Multicultural and social justice counseling competencies: Guidelines for the counseling profession. *Journal of Multicultural Counseling and Development*, *44*(1), 28–48. doi:10.1002/jmcd.12035

Ray, D. (2004). Supervision of basic and advanced skills in play therapy. *Journal of Professional Counseling, Practice, Theory, & Research*, *32*(2), 28–41. doi:10.1080/15566382.2004.12033805

Ray, D. C. (2011). *Advanced play therapy: Essential conditions, knowledge, and skills for child practice*. New York, NY: Routledge. doi:10.4324/9780203837269

Ray, D. C. (2018, March). The evidence-based determination: A moving target. *Play Therapy*, *13*(1), 21.

Ray, D. C., Armstrong, S. A., Balkin, R. S., & Jayne, K. M. (2015). Child centered play therapy in the schools: Review and meta-analysis. *Psychology in the Schools*, *52*(2), 107–123. doi:10.1002/pits.21798

Ray, D. C., & McCullough, R. (2016). *Evidence-based practice statement: Play therapy* [Research report]. Retrieved from http://www.a4pt.org/?page=EvidenceBased

Russ, B. R. (2016). *Counselor preparation and adolescent youth: A study of clinical mental health counselors* (Doctoral dissertation). Western Michigan University. Retrieved from http://scholarworks.wmich.edu/dissertations/2463

Saraceno, B., van Ommeren, M., Batniji, R., Cohen, A., Gureje, O., Mahoney, J., & Underhill, C. (2007). Barriers to improvement of mental health services in low-income and middle-income countries. *Lancet*, *370*(9593), 1164–1174. doi:10.1016/S0140-6736(07)61263-X PMID:17804061

Saxena, S., Thornicroft, G., Knapp, M., & Whiteford, H. (2007). Resources for mental health: Scarcity, inequity, and inefficiency. *Lancet*, *370*(9590), 878–889. doi:10.1016/S0140-6736(07)61239-2 PMID:17804062

Schaefer, C. E., & Drewes, A. A. (Eds.). (2014). *The therapeutic powers of play: 20 core agents of change* (2nd ed.). Hoboken, NJ: Wiley.

Steele, W., & Malchiodi, C. A. (2011). *Trauma-informed practices with children and adolescents*. New York, NY: Routledge.

Stewart, A., & MacIntyre, G. (2013, April). Advocacy: Models and effectiveness. *Insights, 20*. Retrieved from https://www.iriss.org.uk/sites/default/files/iriss-insight-20.pdf

Stoltenberg, C. D. (1997). The integrated developmental model of supervision. *Psychotherapy in Private Practice*, *16*(2), 59–69. doi:10.1300/J294v16n02_07

Substance Abuse and Mental Health Services Administration. (2014). *SAMHSA's concept of trauma and guidance for a trauma-informed approach* (HHS Publication No. SMA 14-4884). Retrieved from https://store.samhsa.gov/system/files/sma14-4884.pdf

Sue, D. W., Arredondo, P., & McDavis, R. J. (1992). Multicultural counseling competencies and standards: A call to the profession. *Journal of Counseling and Development*, *70*(4), 477–486. doi:10.1002/j.1556-6676.1992.tb01642.x

Tolan, P. H., & Dodge, K. A. (2005). Children's mental health as a primary care and concern: A system for comprehensive support and service. *The American Psychologist*, *60*(6), 601–614. doi:10.1037/0003-066X.60.6.601 PMID:16173893

Trusty, J., & Brown, D. (2005). Advocacy competencies for professional school counselors. *Professional School Counseling*, *8*(3), 259–265.

United Nations. (1989). Convention on the Rights of the Child. *Treaty Series*, *1577*, 3.

U.S. Department of Health and Human Services. (2002). *Trends in the well-being of America's children and youth. Section 1. Population, family, and neighborhood*. Retrieved from https://aspe.hhs.gov/report/trends-well-being-americas-children-and-youth-2002

U.S. Public Health Service. (2000). *Report of the surgeon general's conference on children's mental health: A national action agenda*. Washington, DC: Department of Health and Human Services.

Verschueren, K., & Koomen, H. M. Y. (2012). Teacher-child relationships from an attachment perspective. *Attachment and Human Development*, *14*(3), 205–211. doi:10.1080/14616734.2012.672260 PMID:22537520

Vygotsky, L. S. (1978). Interaction between learning and development. In M. Cole, V. John-Steiner, S. Scribner, & E. Souberman (Eds.), *Mind in society: The development of higher psychological processes* (pp. 79–91). Cambridge, MA: Harvard University Press.

Vygotsky, L. S. (2016). Play and its role in the mental development of the child (N. Veresov & M. Barr, Trans.). *International Research in Early Childhood Education, 7*(2), 3-25.

Yogman, M., Garner, A., Hutchinson, J., Michnick Golinkoff, R., & Committee on Psychosocial Aspects of Child and Family Health, Council on Communications and Media. (2018). The power of play: A pediatric role in enhancing development in young children. *Pediatrics, 142*(3), e20182058. Retrieved from http://pediatrics.aappublications.org/content/pediatrics/142/3/e20182058.full.pdf

Chapter 4
The Clinic as the Classroom:
Blending Educational and Clinical Preparation in Play Therapy

Dee C. Ray
University of North Texas, USA

Hannah Robinson
University of North Texas, USA

ABSTRACT

Play therapy training clinics are vital to the success of the field of play therapy, as they serve as the foundation for play therapists' education and clinical training. Furthermore, play therapy training differs depending on the developmental level of the play therapist. In this chapter, the authors present a clinical educational program for graduate level students designed to prepare play therapists through practicum experiences based in a play therapy training clinic. The authors address the structure of beginning and advanced play therapy trainings as well as practicum and internship courses, and provide detailed information regarding supervisors, potential course assignments, scheduling, play therapy skills, play therapy rooms, and supervision.

INTRODUCTION

Due to the growing recognition of play therapy as an evidence-based intervention supported by research on its effectiveness (Lin & Bratton, 2015; Ray, Armstrong, Balkin, & Jayne, 2015), counselors and therapists benefit from thorough attention to the preparation of play therapists through integration of knowledge and skills

DOI: 10.4018/978-1-5225-8226-7.ch004

in play therapy training programs. Play therapy training clinics are tasked with preparing students to provide play therapy for a wide range of child clients. In university settings, the integration of play therapy training within counseling clinics involves addressing the developmental needs of student counselors while providing ethical and therapeutic services to clients. Because play therapy supervision and training are ideally structured depending on students' developmental levels, training for novice and advanced play therapists differ (Ray, 2011). The education of play therapy students requires that students are exposed to knowledge through scholarly literature but also necessitates learning through graduated clinical experiences. Hence, progressive clinical experiences within a counseling clinic are essential components of play therapy courses. Blending practice and real clinical experiences throughout the play therapy curriculum fosters readiness of the play therapist to effectively serve child clients in the real world.

In order to integrate clinical experiences with educational curriculum, a training clinic requires procedures, resources, materials, and structure that effectively supports the education and facilitation of play therapy. Intake, scheduling, and file procedures contribute to successful training practices through appropriate matching of educational level and training experience. Video recording equipment and maintenance of equipment is essential to the immediate observation and consistent supervision of play therapy experiences. Play therapy training rooms have two-way mirrors, with observation rooms attached to the play therapy rooms equipped with audio devices that supervisors and group members can use during session to observe the sessions live. People resources, such as on-site supervisors, waiting room staff, and babysitters are necessary to provide delivery of services to clients while play therapists are in training. Perhaps most importantly, the clinical setting includes a therapeutically-equipped playroom that meets the needs of child clients, as well as play therapists in training. According to Landreth (2012), the structure, location, size, and contents of the playroom are imperative in facilitating the child's ability to feel comfortable and free. Materials for the playroom are carefully selected to meet the emotional and play needs of children, providing an experience that allows for full emotional expression. The play therapy student not only practices play therapy skills within the clinic setting, but observes and experiences the structure and procedures of play therapy through working within the functional clinic.

This chapter includes recommended structures and course requirements for introduction to play therapy, advanced skills in play therapy, and practicum and internship courses. Within each section the authors will address rationale, content, potential course requirements, and structure of play therapy clinical experiences within the play therapy clinic. Additionally, the authors will include materials that may be used for supervised practice of the clinical experiences, including sample clinical training schedules and *The Play Therapy Skills Checklist* (PTSC).

PLAY THERAPY SKILLS CHECKLIST

The Center for Play Therapy created the PTSC, which is intended to be used as a clinical form to facilitate skills and ways of being for students learning play therapy (see Appendix 1). Initially created by the Center for Play Therapy for use during both beginning and advanced play therapy trainings, the PTSC has undergone several revisions during the many years of its' use. The PTSC closely follows the play therapy skills outlined by Landreth (2012) and Ray (2011) in their foundational play therapy books. Additionally, the PTSC has been included as a component of supervision for play therapists in research studies in order to ensure the play therapists follow child-centered play therapy (CCPT) protocol (Ray, Purswell, Haas, & Aldrete, 2017). The PTSC is used developmentally across the clinical play therapy curriculum and in play therapy clinics. While basic descriptions of the PTSC and its' components are included below, readers are encouraged to reference Ray (2004) and Ray and colleagues (2017) for more information regarding the PTSC and its' use in research and supervision.

Initially, the PTSC is provided to students in the introductory course to teach the basic non-verbal and verbal skills. The *PTSC* is used by supervisors in initial practice times to provide feedback to students on their play therapy sessions, helping students to become aware of the concepts put into action during sessions with children. The PTSC is beneficial to beginning play therapy students because it provides students with concrete examples and feedback regarding the skills used in their play therapy sessions. Additionally, this checklist provides a specific structure for feedback sessions which includes ample opportunity for encouragement, leaving room for supervisors to discuss both strengths and areas of growth during the feedback time. As students practice and have more advanced play therapy experiences, the PTSC is a tool for clinics to help students review their own sessions and assess their progress. Supervisors may use the PTSC to provide feedback directly to supervisees or they may ask supervisees to rate themselves for further exploration during supervision sessions. Alternately, supervisors and supervisees may want to use the PTSC while observing the same segment of a session to explore their similar or alternate perceptions of a play therapist's skills.

The PTSC begins with a section for "be with" attitudes are included at the top of the PTSC. On the checklist nonverbal and verbal skills are included, as well as areas designated for therapist responses and alternative responses for each skill. Nonverbal skills include posture, expression, and interest level of the therapist; verbal skills include tracking, reflecting content and feeling, esteem building, facilitating decision making and creativity, facilitating relationship, reflecting meaning, limit setting, and rate of responses. Brief descriptions of each section are included below. For further explanations of skills included, other sources may be referenced as needed (Landreth, 2012; Ray, 2004; Ray, 2011)

"Be With" Attitudes

The "be with" attitudes, initially discussed by Landreth (2012) as healing messages and later by Landreth and Bratton (2006) in the Child-Parent Relationship Training model, includes four messages that are essential to convey to children in play therapy. The messages include "I am here.", "I hear you.", "I understand.", and "I care." "I am here" conveys to the child that the therapist is physically, mentally, and emotionally present in the playroom with the child. "I hear you" is the therapist's desire to fully engage and listen to the child's verbal and nonverbal behaviors in the room. "I understand" includes all of the therapist's responses that aid the child in feeling heard and seen in the room. Lastly, the final healing message, "I care", is sufficiently conveyed if the first three healing messages are successfully conveyed and experienced by the child. The "be with" attitudes on the PTSC are used to provide feedback to the play therapy student about moments of connectedness and relationship between play therapist and child.

Nonverbal Communication

The degree to which therapists communicate nonverbally in the play therapy session can be indicated on the PTSC. Nonverbal communication is an essential component to successful play therapy (Landreth, 2012; Ray, 2011). Firstly, the therapist has an open posture and leans forward in his or her chair. The therapist appears interested in and focused on the child and his or her play throughout the duration of the play therapy session. Furthermore, the therapist seeks to feel relaxed in session, indicated through both verbal and nonverbal expressions. The play therapist also pursues a state and expression of congruence, both to match the child's affect and to match the therapist's own responses. For example, if the child is angrily hitting the bop bag with strong punches and furrowed eyebrows, the therapist who excitedly and brightly exclaims, "You're angry!" in a high-pitched voice would not be reflecting in a manner consistent with the child's affect. Similarly, a therapist who states, "You figured that out" in a dull, uninterested and matter-of-fact tone of voice would not be demonstrating a tone and expression congruent with the response made.

Verbal Communication

All verbal responses should ideally consist of 10 words or less, as including more than 10 words may make it difficult for the child to hear or understand what the therapist is communicating (Landreth, 2012). Therefore, succinct responses are favorable to wordy responses and are noted on the PTSC. Additionally, the rate of responses ideally match the child's activity level and manner of play. Descriptions and examples of each skill in this section serve only as reminders of their use in clinical supervision, and readers are encouraged to review more thorough rationale, descriptions and examples of each skill in Landreth (2012), Ray (2004), Ray (2011), and Ray and colleagues (2017) as needed.

The PTSC includes nine verbal response categories that guide the verbal facilitation of play therapy by the therapist. *Tracking responses* are verbal responses to the child's nonverbal behavior by stating what is observed. Examples of tracking include "you put that over there" and "you are moving that one all around". *Reflecting content* occurs when the therapist paraphrases the verbal content provided by the child. For example, if the child says, "I went to a birthday party last week and had cake and played with all of my friends," a reflecting content response would be, "You did a lot of fun things at the birthday party." *Reflecting feeling responses* include labeling the child or object's emotion or responding to emotional content in session, such as "You're angry." and "You seem disappointed that our session is almost over." *Facilitating decision making and responsibility responses should* encourage and empower the child to make their own decisions and take responsibility. Examples of decision-making and responsibility responses include "You decided to make a new one." and "That looks like something you can do." *Facilitating creativity and spontaneity responses* encourage children to be free and creative, and include responses such as, "In here, that can be whatever you want it to be." *Esteem building and encouraging responses* foster the child's experience of stronger and capable sense of self. Esteem building and encouraging responses include "You worked really hard on that.", "You made it just the way you like.", and "You're proud of yourself." *Facilitating relationship responses* focus on the relationship between the therapist and child client and include "you" and "me" in the response. Examples of facilitating relationship responses are "You wanted to tell me about that." and "You want to take care of me." *Reflecting larger meaning* is an advanced play therapy skill that focuses on the child's theme or pattern of play. For example, a reflecting larger meaning response for a child high in power and control may be "You like to be in charge when we play." *Limit-setting responses* follow Landreth's (2012) ACT limit setting model, in which the therapist acknowledges the child's feeling (A), communicates the limit (C), and targets alternative choices (T). An example of a limit-setting response is "You're excited to shoot me, but I'm not for shooting. You can choose to shoot the bop bag and pretend it's me."

The PTSC is a clinical form that brings together the building blocks of play therapy skills and clinical experiences by highlighting the therapeutic relationship, the non-verbal communication between therapist and child, and the verbal communication of therapist. Additionally, the PTSC allows the supervisor and/or play therapy student to focus on areas of strengths and growth while learning effective practice of play therapy. The PTSC is available as a standard form in a play therapy clinic and used throughout the play therapy educational curriculum.

INTRODUCTION TO PLAY THERAPY

In the first play therapy course typically referred to as introduction to play therapy or play therapy basics, students are learning the basic tenets of play therapy for the very first time. Some students may have prior experience working with adults and children, but the first play therapy course is most often an introduction to students' first experiences working with children in a therapeutic setting. Thus, training of beginning play therapists focuses on child-centered play therapy principles (Axline, 1947; Landreth, 2012). Ray (2011) stated that it is beneficial if novice play therapy supervisors focus on concrete and definitive skills in supervision and provide ample encouragement throughout the process. Hence, the structure of beginning play therapy trainings are organized to match the developmental stage of novice play therapists. The introductory play therapy course instructor collaborates with the play therapy clinic to structure a beginning level clinical practice experience. Table 1 presents each of the clinical assignments that may be involved in an introductory course and responsibilities of both the instructor and clinic director to ensure a favorable learning experience in the clinic.

Observations

Clinical experiences in an introductory course begin with observation of play therapy, the opportunity to view the reality of play therapy with child clients. Observations are the initial collaboration between the clinic and educational curriculum. Students are required to observe at least two play therapy sessions with clients in the first few weeks of the initial play therapy course. In order to prepare students for observations, they become familiar with clinic rules regarding confidentiality and professionalism. Frequently, students at this level may not have experience being in a clinic setting. Preparation for observation may include informing the students to use soft voices when checking in with clinic staff so as not to announce the observation to clients who may be present, quickly and unobtrusively taking their places for observations, not sharing any material they see or learn during the observation outside of the class setting, as well as other considerations. Additionally, the instructor and clinic administration work together to carefully select play therapy sessions conducive to beneficial observation. Instructors and clinic administrators consider the experience and skill level of the play therapist to be observed, the nature of the case being observed, and schedule availability. When students observe, they are asked to notify the play therapist of the observation and to plan to spend brief time with the play therapist following the session to ask questions. Students are also encouraged to help the play therapist clean the room following a session which serves several purposes including making effective use of process time, helping the play therapist, and learning more about playroom structure. Additionally, students are asked to write a reflective paper of the observation including their feelings and reactions, as well as specific skills they observed.

Initial play therapy observations impact the processes and procedures of a counseling clinic and deserve careful preparation. In a given semester of one introductory course, the clinic may need to accommodate up to 40 or more observations depending on the number of enrolled students. The play therapy instructor is sensitive to potential for disruption of clinic services to offer this learning experience and works closely with the clinic director to ensure that clients remain a priority. In turn, the clinic director is aware of the essential nature of observations as learning experiences and works to help students feel comfortable while learning professionalism in the clinic setting.

Practice Sessions

In a second possible assignment for an introductory play therapy course, students are asked to practice two play sessions with a child who is not an identified client. The purpose of these sessions is help students become comfortable with children and to practice skills with a child who is not experiencing emotional or behavioral problems. The instructor provides an informed consent to students to give to the volunteer parent in which the nature of the assignment is explained including that the session is not a play therapy session but a practice time. Typically, this assignment is completed outside of the clinic setting as students use friends and family members. However, occasionally the student does not have access to an appropriate setting. In these cases, the instructor might involve the counseling clinic to serve as a site for the assignment. When using the clinic as a practice setting, the student provides the volunteer parent with an informed consent that specifies the time of the session as well as a statement that the practice session will be held within the clinic but not part of clinical services. The student works with clinic staff to identify a room and time for the practice session and follows clinic procedures for checking in. Because this particular assignment involves video recording to submit to the instructor, the student works with the clinic to set up recording. Practice sessions are monitored by clinic staff to ensure limited crossover between the student who is not considered trained yet to be a play therapist and perception of the practice time being an authentic play therapy session. Due to the need for monitoring, clinic staff typically is responsible for scheduling the room and recording in order to ensure that the practicing student does not have access to client information or sessions. Practice sessions within an operating counseling clinic require considerable clinic efforts and therefore should be scheduled sparingly.

Micropracticums

For the introduction to play therapy course, two to five micropracticums are scheduled throughout the semester, in which students participate to gain experience working directly with volunteer children utilizing play therapy. Micropracticums are a structured experience for practice held within the last half of an introductory play course and within the clinic, and serve as mini-practice experiences in which students are provided the opportunity to work with volunteer children in short, intensive, and highly supervised experiences. Micropracticums, therefore, differ from practicum and internship experiences in that they serve as introductory clinical experiences for students who are just beginning clinical coursework in counseling.

A micropracticum is typically held within one class period and provides the opportunity for each student to practice play therapy skills with a child while under supervision of an experienced play therapist. The micropracticum experience is directly supervised and monitored by the course instructor with the approval of the clinic director. Because of the experiential nature, the assignment is considered the cornerstone of learning for play therapy students and essential to the introduction course. Micropracticums involve the participation of volunteer children, students in the course, play therapist supervisors, course instructor, and clinic staff.

Children who participate in micropracticums are children who are volunteered by parents, typically developing, and do not present with concerning clinical issues. Optimal ages for beginning level practice are four to seven years old, although older ages up to nine are appropriate. The authors identify volunteer children mostly through personal contacts of students, faculty, or clinic staff. Because children are often unknown to the instructor, screening of children is a crucial component to a successful experience. Instructors are encouraged to confirm with referral source about how the person knows the child, whether the person has any concerns about the child, whether the child has shown any behavioral or emotional problems beyond the expected, and to discover how well the child separates from primary caregivers. Children who are referred because the contact has concerns about the child are not scheduled for micropracticum. Along these same lines, children who are seeking or participating in clinic services are not scheduled for inclusion. The number of children needed for micropracticum is based on the number of play therapy students but typically the authors suggest one child for every three play therapy students.

Supervisors are a necessary and significant component of micropracticum experiences. The Association for Play Therapy *Best Practices* (2016) states, "play therapists offering clinical supervision services are adequately trained in supervision methods and supervisory skills" (p. 14). Supervisors have experience with facilitating play therapy with their own child clients in order to integrate their own experiences into their supervision with beginning play therapists. Ideally, the supervisors chosen for these play therapy trainings have completed training in supervision and have also completed advanced coursework in play therapy; additionally, it is preferable if supervisors have completed a master's degree in a professional mental health field. However, some play therapy training programs are limited in their access to experienced play therapists and supervisors. In these cases, the authors recommend that instructors and clinic directors select supervisors who have demonstrated knowledge and basic skills in play therapy to help facilitate the growth of students new to play therapy. The authors further recommend that the instructor conduct special training with supervisors on identification of skills in new play therapists and how to provide effective feedback for growth.

Regarding micropracticum structure, there are numerous options to choose from when scheduling students with volunteer children: scheduling all students in a group with the same child, scheduling each student in a group with a different child but keeping the dyads consistent among all micropracticums, or assigning each student a new child during each micropracticum. The authors believe there are benefits to all options discussed above. For example, scheduling each student with the same child for each micropracticum allows the student to practice specific areas of growth discussed during feedback in the next session with the child and allows the student the opportunity to continue developing a stronger relationship with the child throughout the numerous sessions. On the contrary, scheduling students with a new child for each micropracticum experience allows students the opportunity to develop their basic skills with different children with varied presenting behaviors and personalities. Therefore, it is up to the instructor and practice clinic to decide how they would like to schedule their own experiences.

Structure across micropracticums includes the assignment of one supervisor to work with a total of three to four students. The day begins with 30-minute focus sessions, in which the supervisor meets the group members and describes the overall structure of micropracticum. During this time supervisors often ask group members if they have any questions, introduce the students to the playrooms, and briefly describe the feedback process. This focus session time allows the supervisor the opportunity to learn more about each of the students and begin developing relationships with the group members. When the focus group is completed, the sessions begin. Each student works with a child client for 30 minutes while the rest of the group observes the session from the observation room attached to the playroom behind the one-way mirror. Directly following the session, the group has supervision to process the session for 30 minutes. The micropracticum structure involves the rotation of one student facilitating play therapy while the small group and supervisor observes, small group processes session, and then the next student facilitates play therapy, and so on. In order to accommodate a large play therapy course, another group is put into rotation in which that group is using the playroom while the first group is in process time allowing alternative use of playroom and process room to efficiently allow for more play sessions. Appendix 2 includes a sample micropracticum schedule in order to further clarify the structure. Bratton, Landreth, and Homeyer (1993) discussed a similar structure for an intensive three-day play therapy training that may be reviewed for an alternative structure for training.

The micropracticum component of the introductory course is dependent upon the use of the clinic and clinic procedures. Because micropracticum is time- and resource-intensive, the experience can be disruptive to clinic processes and must be carefully planned. Dates for micropracticum are set as a collaborative effort between the instructor and clinic director months prior to implementation. The clinic director works with the instructor on best times for micropracticum (e.g., holding micropracticums on Thursday afternoons because the clinic has less clients that day). Clinic staff informs clients about upcoming micropracticums by having counselors report to clients that the clinic might be busy with more children than usual on the week of the micropracticum. Clinic staff may prefer that micropracticums be set off schedule from usual client times (e.g., starting on the hour if client times are usually at the half hour). At times, the clinic may have to cancel, reschedule, or change rooms for clients if micropracticums are using the playrooms. Although up to five micropracticums is optimal, the disruption to clinic procedures may not be worth the ideal number; hence, the instructor limits micropracticums to three per semester. Additionally, because of the number of children involved in micropracticum and frequent coming and going to playrooms, the experience requires babysitters for children which is an added consideration to cost, person resources, and space. For a class of twelve students, micropracticum frequently involves having two babysitters, a separate waiting room for children to play, and two play therapy rooms. These considerations are often in addition to normal resources provided by clinics for serving clients on a daily basis. Necessary clinic resources for micropracticum may seem daunting or discouraging but our experience is that many people involved in play therapy are eager to volunteer their time and energy in order to help others learn play therapy. The authors believe that the learning outcomes of micropracticum far outweigh the organizational and resource obstacles.

Table 1. Introductory play therapy course clinical assignments

Assignment	Assignment Description	Instructor Responsibilities	Clinic Responsibilities
Play Therapy Observation	Student is required to observe and write reflection on two play therapy sessions.	• Informs clinic director of assignment due dates. • Works with clinic director on putting together observation schedule. • Prepares students to engage in confidential and unobtrusive clinic observation.	• Provides instructor with observation schedule based on collaborative discussion on potential for beneficial experiences. • Provides instructor rules and preferences for student observation conduct within clinic. • Prepares clinic staff for facilitating observation procedures.
Play Therapy Practice Session	Students who are unable to access an appropriate space for play and recording may be required to conduct practice times in the clinic setting. These sessions are typically 30 minutes in length and required to be recorded.	• Works with student to find an appropriate site outside of clinic. • If clinic is only appropriate setting, instructor works with clinic director to arrange for student practice sessions. • Provides student with appropriate informed consent that limits the nature of holding session in clinic setting.	• Works with instructor on setting up student to practice in clinic setting. • Prepares and organizes clinic staff to schedule, monitor, and record student practice session in clinic.
Micropracticum	Three to five classes of the introductory course structured to provide a practice experience to each play therapy student.	• Set dates with clinic director for micropracticum at least two months prior to first assignment. • Identify supervisors for micropracticum and prepare for supervision and feedback. • Identify volunteer children for participation. • Set up schedule for micropracticum days and disseminate to clinic and students. • Set up babysitting for children during micropracticum experience. • Communicate with clinic director following each micropracticum to evaluate for changes to procedures.	• Collaborate with instructor regarding micropracticum dates. • Identify playrooms to use for micropracticum. • Inform counselors of micropracticum dates and work with counselors on rescheduling or rearranging if needed. • Identify space and preferences for waiting area for micropracticum children. • Ensure that micropracticum is not therapeutically disruptive to clinic services to clients. • Communicate with instructor regarding any possible disruptions that can be avoided.

INTERMEDIATE PLAY THERAPY TRAINING AND COURSES

After completion of introduction to play therapy, students progress to advanced skills in play therapy. Therefore, students taking advanced skills in play therapy have completed some training in play therapy, know basic child-centered play therapy skills, and have worked with child practice clients in the micropracticum trainings. Hence, the structure of advanced play therapy training differs from beginning play therapy training. Students are now ready to engage with child clients under supervision. In advanced play therapy training, students often work with one child client weekly and meet with a supervisor in triadic supervision weekly. The supervision is tailored to meet the developmental needs and skill set of advanced play therapy students. Child clients are children who present with minimal clinical symptoms and have been screened through the clinic intake system as being appropriate for a novice play therapist under supervision. Table 2 presents clinical experiences involved in advanced educational training and responsibilities of both the instructor and clinic director to help with continued professional growth of the new play therapist.

When students begin to see clients in play therapy, clinics and course instructors ensure substantial monitoring and supervision to address client care. The responsibility of clinic staff is to help match clients with new play therapists and provide monitoring of sessions on-site. The responsibility of course instructors is to confirm that play therapists receive appropriate knowledge for serving clients as well as consistent and effective supervision. Identification of clients for newly practicing play therapists involves detailed intake procedures in which clients who need more experienced therapists are routed to those therapists and away from new play therapists. Clinic directors ensure that child clients matched to new play therapists are not reported to be highly aggressive toward adults or demonstrate highly dysregulated or impulsive behaviors (e.g., running away, serious self-harm). Other presenting issues may be concerning for play therapists but may provide valuable learning experiences when under close supervision. Once play therapists are matched to clients, clinic staff provide on-site monitoring by having an experienced clinic staff member available when the new play therapist sees clients. Such procedures safeguard client welfare as the play therapist is learning. On-site supervision helps to address the play therapist's anxiety regarding unexpected events which allows the play therapist to be more fully present with child clients.

The instructors of advanced courses are responsible for reviewing processes and procedures for difficult client situations. Weekly classes involve addressing the current experiences of the play therapists who are now serving child clients with emotional and behavioral issues. The instructor provides solutions and facilitation of therapeutic decision-making for students at this level. Most importantly, the instructor selects supervisors who are well-trained and effective in supervision of students at the intermediate learning level. Ideally, supervisors have a master's degree in a mental health profession, completed advanced coursework in play therapy, have training in supervision and currently see child clients. In supervision, supervisors focus on advanced skills of identifying themes, connecting with children, working with parents, and limit setting (Ray, 2004; Ray, 2011), while simultaneously ensuring that the basic nonverbal and verbal skills are present and sufficient. The PTSC is used regularly to raise the student's awareness of skill facilitation and provide concrete feedback on improvement.

Supervisors at this level facilitate effectively through role-play of situations taking place in play therapy sessions. Encouraging play therapists to practice skills aloud in role-play helps them to find words and ways of being that are natural yet therapeutic for their clients. Although not always possible, live supervision of sessions is helpful to the process of clinical supervision. When viable, supervisors observe sessions at the clinic and then engage in short process/feedback times following the session. Immediate feedback is often appreciated by the supervisees due to the relevance in the moment as they end a session. Effective play therapy supervision entails the use of video recording of sessions. Clinical supervisors observe their supervisees' facilitation of play therapy on a weekly basis without exception. Because self-report is known to be an inaccurate description of events in counseling (Ellis, 2010; Reichelt & Skjerve, 2002), supervisors are ethically responsible to observe the play therapist's work in play therapy in order to evaluate effectively.

Video recording is yet another blended component of play therapy training between curriculum and clinic. Clinics need to have working recording capabilities while supervisors persist in using recordings in supervision. Video recording may present difficulties in play therapy training for multiple reasons from multiple sides, including equipment problems, supervisee resistance to showing recordings, or limited time allotted for supervision. The clinic's role in maintaining recording equipment is primary to the supervision process. Yet, maintaining equipment can be expensive and time-intensive. Clinics benefit from having alternate plans for recording when equipment is not functioning such as having ready-to-go cameras that can be placed in the room. These types of alternative procedures require attention to confidentiality through use of encrypted and password-coded equipment. Regarding other obstacles to review of recordings, instructors confirm with supervisors that supervisees are sharing recordings during supervision and processing through solutions when supervisees are resistant. Instructors are also responsible for ensuring that supervisors are provided enough time for supervision to meet the needs of each supervisee. There may be times when the instructor modifies supervision schedules or configurations of supervisees to provide enough time for viewing of recordings.

Table 2. Advanced experiences in clinical play therapy experiences

Experiences	Assignment Description	Instructor Responsibilities	Clinic Responsibilities
Play therapy with one client	• Student is expected to facilitate play therapy at least once per week with one client under supervision.	• Collaborate with clinic director on number of students that need to see clients. • Work with clinic director on matching play therapy student with appropriate client. • Address relevant play therapy situations from the week in class. Follow-up on any concerning therapeutic issues.	• Prepare clinic staff for number of new play therapy students seeing clients. • Orient new play therapists to clinic procedures. • Work with instructor and students on scheduling clients. • Review intake procedures to ensure that new play therapists are matched with appropriate clients. • Maintain play therapy materials and rooms. • Maintain recording equipment. • Assign an experienced play therapy staff to be on-site when new play therapists are seeing clients.
Supervision	Student is expected to engage in supervision one hour per week.	• Identify supervisors to engage in supervision. • Meet weekly with supervisors to ensure that supervision involves observation and effective feedback/processing. • Engage in live supervision when possible. • Communicate with clinic director regarding any client or play therapist concerns.	• Work with supervisors to schedule live supervision. • Provide spaces and equipment for supervision. • Communicate with instructor regarding any client or play therapist concerns.

PLAY THERAPY PRACTICUM AND INTERNSHIP CLINICAL EXPERIENCES

Following successful completion of introduction of play therapy and advanced skills in play therapy, students progress to practicum and internship experiences. According to Ronnestad and Skovholt (2013), students at this stage have moved into a new developmental level, thus requiring different supervisory experiences. Therefore, supervision and coursework for play therapy practicum and internship experiences should be structured according to the students' level of development and imminent transition out of graduate school and into the field of play therapy. Table 3 presents clinical experiences involved in practicum and internship courses, as well as responsibilities of both the instructor and clinic director to help with continued professional growth of the student play therapists.

Having completed prior coursework and supervision, students at this stage are well-equipped to see child clients who may have more significant presenting concerns, including child clients who have difficulties with impulsivity such as running away or self-harm behaviors, and those child clients who are reportedly highly aggressive toward adults. Additionally, consideration must be given to the length of time that the practicum or internship student will be seeing clients at the training clinic, as child clients who require more long-term care may not be appropriate for placement with a student who will only be at the clinic for one semester.

Client load is also necessary to consider when assigning play therapists new clients. In many clinical training settings, students at the practicum and internship level are required to see adult clients, and potentially adolescent clients, in addition to play therapy clients. Therefore, it is recommended that course instructors communicate with the clinical staff to determine the needs of the clinic and also assess the capacity of the student when determining the ideal number of clients. Client load should be determined on an individualized basis because some students are better equipped to be assigned more clients when compared to others.

In practicum courses, it is recommended that students focus on holding a small caseload of approximately 1-2 play therapy clients per week. Because students in practicum are just beginning to see clients on a consistent basis, additional time should be allotted for session preparation, file maintenance, client conceptualization, peer consultation, and supervision. Therefore, practicum students spend approximately 10 hours per week on these additional factors per client. As students become more comfortable in their new counseling roles and progress to internship experiences, they are encouraged to take on more clients. Therefore, students in internship are recommended to see at least 8-10 play therapy clients weekly across a semester, totaling approximately 20 hours of clinical work a week when supervision, preparation, file maintenance, and additional factors are included.

The practicum and internship course instructor should regularly communicate with clinic staff to ascertain whether play therapy practicum and internship students are successfully meeting clinical policies, including starting and ending sessions on time, providing ethical services to clients, keeping playrooms maintained, and more. Failure to meet responsibilities set forth by clinical staff should result in repercussions including potential lowering of course grade, remedial training or supervision, and in the most severe cases, failure to successfully complete the practicum or internship course. Therefore, it behooves the course instructor and clinical staff to maintain close relationships with one another, as it benefits all parties involved to do so.

Supervision of the Advanced Play Therapy Student

Novel, exciting, and anxiety-provoking experiences are the nature of the practicum/internship structure, requiring broad and deeper levels of supervision. Similar to advanced play therapy educational experiences, the play therapy clinic provides an on-site supervisor available to the practicum/internship play therapist at all times when clients are present. As the play therapist begins to see child clients who exhibit more behavioral and emotional challenges, an experienced play therapist is needed on-site to walk the novice play therapist through effective practices when problems occur. On-site, immediate supervision also allows the play therapist to process through emotionally challenging sessions while the play therapist is engaged in the emotionality. During the practicum/internship phase of training, the play therapist is engaged in consistent, weekly supervision with an experienced play therapist supervisor. Again, because the novice play therapist is now serving clients with more demanding needs, close supervision is necessary in which the supervisee is provided time and focus to develop effective responses and treatment plans, while also processing through personal reflections and awareness. The supervisor may assign the PTSC as a self-reflection tool to the supervisee to notice ways-of-being and use of skills in individual sessions and with specific clients.

In addition to focus on processing clinical sessions, supervision at this stage should also be focused on file maintenance. According to The Association for Play Therapy's *Best Practices* (2016), it is mandatory to maintain up to date and accurate clinical files for all clients. Supervisors are tasked with not only providing weekly supervision for practicum and internship students, but also ensuring that students' progress notes and files are maintained in a timely and appropriate manner. This means that supervisors should initially read through session summaries weekly to verify that summaries are complete and provide accurate depictions of the clinical sessions; over time, supervisors may choose to review session summaries less frequently depending on the quality of the students' summaries.

Upon completion of clinical services, supervisors should ensure that supervisees complete treatment summaries for all clients seen during the course. Treatment summaries should include a brief yet comprehensive summary of the client's presenting concern, diagnosis, counseling procedures utilized in sessions, client progress and therapeutic outcomes, and recommendations (Bernard & Goodyear, 2018; Ray, 2011). It is ideal if the treatment summary is limited to one to two pages in length and attached as the leading file document. Lastly, treatment summaries should include basic demographic information of client, in addition to the total number of sessions, and date of initial and final clinical sessions.

Gatekeeping

According to the Association for Play Therapy *Best Practices* (2016), "play therapist supervisors do not recommend unqualified students or supervisees for certification, licensure, employment, or completion of an academic or training program." Hence, supervisors of practicum and internship students should regularly assess play therapy students' progress and clinical skills. The supervisor and course instructor are responsible for ensuring students have adequate clinical skills and demonstrate professional and ethical behavior before completing the course. The Play Therapy Skills Checklist (PTSC) may be used to assess students' clinical skills in a variety of ways, including as documentation for students who demonstrate limited progress.

Case Conceptualization

One of the course requirements for the play therapy practicum and internship course includes a case conceptualization, in which the student presents a recording of a clinical play therapy sessions to the class and provides a conceptualization of the client before receiving feedback from the course instructor and fellow students. The purpose of this assignment is twofold: the student is required to intensely focus on one of their clients and conceptualize the client according to their chosen theoretical orientation, and the instructor is able to see the student's clinical skills. The instructor may choose whether they allow the students to choose their own client to use for the case conceptualization, or whether they would prefer to assign the client they would like to be presented to the course.

CONCLUSION

Play therapists serve an essential role providing children with developmentally appropriate treatment, and as research supporting effectiveness of play therapy as well as awareness of play therapy continue to grow the demand for well-trained play therapists will continue to increase. The play therapy training clinic provides the setting for the development and implementation of clinical education for play therapists and is responsive to the play therapist's developmental level, need for clinical training and supervision, and course structure while doing so. In this chapter, we provided the essential components and potential course structures for clinical

Table 3. Practicum and internship in clinical play therapy experiences

Experiences	Assignment Description	Instructor Responsibilities	Clinic Responsibilities
Play therapy with 1-2 clients for practicum and 8-10 clients for internship.	Student is expected to facilitate play therapy at least once per week with 1-2 clients for practicum and 8-10 clients for internship while under supervision.	• Collaborate with clinic director on number of students that need to see clients. • Work with clinic director on matching play therapy student with appropriate client(s) and number of client(s). • Address relevant play therapy situations from the week in class. Follow-up on any concerning therapeutic issues. • Ensure students are following clinic procedures.	• Prepare clinic staff for number of Practicum/Internship students seeing clients. • Reorient/introduce play therapists to clinic procedures. • Work with instructor and students on scheduling clients. • Ensure that play therapists are matched with appropriate clients. • Ensure that play therapists are given appropriate number of clients in caseload. • Maintain play therapy materials and rooms. • Maintain recording equipment. • Ensure play therapist students are informed of clinic crisis procedures.
Supervision	Student is expected to engage in supervision one hour per week.	• Identify supervisors to engage in supervision. • Meet weekly with supervisors to ensure that supervision involves observation and effective feedback/processing. • Engage in live supervision when possible. • Communicate with clinic director regarding any client or play therapist concerns.	• Provide spaces and equipment for supervision. • Regularly communicate with course instructor regarding any student therapist concerns.
Record maintenance	Student is expected to write weekly progress notes for all clients and write treatment summaries upon termination.	• Ensure supervisors are regularly checking clinical files for completion and accuracy. • Work with students to revise treatment summaries. • Review all files at end of semester for completion.	• Monitor and audit files on a routine basis. • Communicate with instructor regarding lapse in a student's clients' files. • Maintain file storage that is secure and HIPPA compliant.
Case Conceptualization	Student is expected to present at least one clinical session of choice to class.	• Ensure student is providing ethical and clinically competent counseling services. • Provide feedback to student on counseling skills and conceptualization of client.	

components of introduction to play therapy, advanced skills in play therapy, and play therapy practicum and internship courses. Integration of clinical experiences as formal learning assignments require collaboration and organization between clinic administration and course instructors. It is our hope that the information included in this chapter facilitates the creation and development of additional play therapy training clinics.

REFERENCES

Association for Play Therapy. (2016). *Play Therapy Best Practices*. Clovis, CA: Author.

Axline, V. (1947). *Play Therapy*. New York: Ballantine.

Bernard, J. M., & Goodyear, R. K. (2018). *Fundamentals of clinical supervision* (6th ed.). Boston, MA: Allyn & Bacon.

Bratton, S., Landreth, G., & Homeyer, L. (1993). An intensive three day play therapy supervision/training model. *International Journal of Play Therapy*, *2*(2), 61–78. doi:10.1037/h0089366

Ellis, M. V. (2010). Bridging the science and practice of clinical supervision: Some discoveries, some misconceptions. *The Clinical Supervisor*, *29*(1), 95–116. doi:10.1080/07325221003741910

Landreth, G., & Bratton, S. (2006). *Child parent relationship therapy (CPRT): A 10-session filial therapy model*. New York, NY: Routledge.

Landreth, G. L. (2012). *Play therapy: The art of the relationship* (2nd ed.). New York, NY: Routledge. doi:10.4324/9780203835159

Lin, Y., & Bratton, S. C. (2015). A meta-analytic review of child-centered play therapy approaches. *Journal of Counseling and Development*, *93*(1), 45–58. doi:10.1002/j.1556-6676.2015.00180.x

Ray, D. (2004). Supervision of basic and advanced skills in play therapy. *Journal of Professional Counseling, Practice, Theory, & Research*, *32*(2), 28–40. doi:10.1080/15566382.2004.12033805

Ray, D., Armstrong, S., Balkin, R., & Jayne, K. (2015). Child centered play therapy in the schools: Review and meta-analysis. *Psychology in the Schools*, *52*(2), 107–123. doi:10.1002/pits.21798

Ray, D. C. (2011). *Advanced play therapy: Essential conditions, knowledge, and skills for child practice*. New York, NY: Routledge. doi:10.4324/9780203837269

Ray, D. C., Purswell, K., Haas, S., & Aldrete, C. (2017). Child-centered play therapy-research integrity checklist: Development, reliability, and use. *International Journal of Play Therapy*, *26*(4), 207–217. doi:10.1037/pla0000046

Reichelt, S., & Skjerve, J. (2002). Correspondence between supervisors and trainees in their perception of supervision events. *Journal of Clinical Psychology*, *57*(7), 759–772. doi:10.1002/jclp.2003 PMID:12205716

Ronnestad, M. H., & Skovholt, T. M. (2013). *The developing practitioner: Growth and stagnation of therapists and counselors*. New York, NY: Routledge.

APPENDIX 1

Table 4. Play Therapy Skills Checklist – Micropracticum Feedback Form

Therapist:________________ Child/Age: ___________________ Date: ___________ Observer: ______________________		
Demonstrated "Be With" Attitudes (I am here, I hear you, I understand, I care):		
Therapist Non-Verbal Communication:	**Feedback**	
Lean Forward/Open		
Appeared Interested		
Relaxed/Comfortable		
Tone/Expression Congruent with Child's Affect		
Tone/Expression Congruent with Therapist's Responses		
Therapist Responses:	Therapist Responses/ Examples	Other Possible Responses
Tracking Behavior		
Reflecting Content		
Reflecting Feelings		
Facilitating Decision Making/ Responsibility		
Facilitating Creativity/ Spontaneity		
Esteem Building/Encouraging		
Facilitating Relationship		
Reflecting Larger Meaning		
Limit-Setting		
Rate of Responses		
Succinct/Interactive		
Areas of Strength:		
Areas for Growth:		

APPENDIX 2

Table 5. Sample Micropracticum Schedule

Playroom #	114; Supervision large conference room	110; supervision small conference room	114; supervision large conference room	110 supervision small conference room
Time	**Counselor**	**Counselor**	**Counselor**	**Counselor**
1:00-1:30	Focus Group	Focus Group		
1:30-2:00PM	Student 1 (Child Name)	Student 4 (Child Name)	Focus Group	Focus Group
2:00-2:05 PM	Transition	Transition	Transition	Transition
2:05-2:35 PM	***Supervision***	***Supervision***	Student 7 (Child Name)	Student 10 (Child Name)
2:35-2:40 PM	Transition	Transition	Transition	Transition
2:40-3:10 PM	Student 2 (Child Name)	Student 5 (Child Name)	***Supervision***	***Supervision***
3:10-3:15 PM	Transition	Transition	Transition	Transition
3:15-3:45 PM	***Supervision***	***Supervision***	Student 8 (Child Name)	Student 11 (Child Name)
3:45-3:50 PM	Transition	Transition	Transition	Transition
3:50-4:20 PM	Student 3 (Child Name)	Student 6 (Child Name)	***Supervision***	***Supervision***
4:20-4:25 PM	Transition	Transition	Transition	Transition
4:25-4:55 PM	***Supervision***	***Supervision***	Student 9 (Child Name)	Student 12 (Child Name)
4:55-5:25 PM			***Supervision***	***Supervision***

Chapter 5
Role of University-Based Training Clinics:
Facilitating the Advancement and Growth of Play Therapy

Latifey B. LaFleur
University of Louisiana at Lafayette, USA

Irvin G. Esters
University of Louisiana at Lafayette, USA

ABSTRACT

This chapter will focus on the formation and operation of a university-based play therapy clinic. Attention to the role of the clinic in experiential training, which is an important part of counselor and play therapy preparation will be addressed as well. The mission, functions, and benefits of a university-based play therapy training clinic will be explored in depth and suggestions for forming and administering the clinic will be made. Further, the authors will discuss the effect of a play therapy clinic on training, credentialing, and the promotion of play therapy along with the influence of accrediting entities such as CACREP. Finally, to assist interested programs in the development of a play therapy training clinic, components such as funding, space, design, equipment/materials, administration, and ethical considerations are discussed.

DOI: 10.4018/978-1-5225-8226-7.ch005

INTRODUCTION

The purpose of this chapter is to explore the role and advantages of a university-based play therapy training clinic. The authors will examine current policies, procedures, and clinical training programs, and comment on their efficacy in facilitating instruction and research. The chapter will expand on the concepts related to operating a university-based mental health training clinic, including effective policies and procedures which can be implemented in play therapy training clinics.

It would appear from a review of the extant literature and the most recent two editions of the CACREP standards (2009 and 2016), that the importance of campus-based training clinics for counselor training has been de-emphasized. Language in the 1994 CACREP standards was clear and unequivocal regarding university-based clinics as a requirement for accreditation. Much has changed. The sparse language related to the clinical learning environment and university-based clinic in the 2009 standards foreshadowed what would become a virtual elimination of such language in the 2016 standards (CACREP, 2009, CACREP, 2016). Mobley and Myers (2010) cite advances in technology which have made supervision possible in various formats as a primary force influencing this de-emphasis. Additionally, one would need only to look at the current list of CACREP accredited programs to see the proliferation of online universities among those accredited. For those programs, a campus-based clinic is not a possibility. It might be accurate to say that if university-based clinical learning environments were the only way to meet the standard, online programs would not be eligible for accreditation. Mobley and Myers (2010) go on to note that a review of the standards is called for, and perhaps two sets of standards should be considered which include online programs as well as university-based clinics.

While the CACREP standards have de-emphasized the necessity of university-based clinical learning environments through the years, it is the present authors' assertion that the experiences students gain in such settings are representative of best practices and are exceptionally valuable in preparing the next generations of counselors, including play therapists. Our students have identified their internship or practicum assignment in our university-based play therapy clinic as the most formative experience in their program of study. University-based clinics provide for modeling skills and strategies and for live and recorded supervision. The service aspect is also an important facet of the model, as is providing an ideal for conducting a practice of play therapy. We hope to provide, in the following chapter, some of the details of operating a university-based training clinic with the emphasis on preparing play therapists.

Threefold Mission: Training, Research, Service

University-based clinics have a trifold mission. The most often cited primary reasons to have a university-based clinic is for training and supervising developing practitioners and to provide a service to the community. The present authors are faculty in a program that operates a university-based clinic. The emphasis at our clinic is on training and supervision but we are acutely aware of the dearth of mental health services in our community and we take our service mission seriously. Research is, for us, a tertiary mission of the clinic and any research conducted therein must conform to and co-exist without disrupting in any way, the training and service missions.

Training in our campus-based clinic has three "levels." Pre-practicum instruction in skills and strategies is the first level. Here, students enrolled in the beginning play therapy class, the advanced play therapy class, the beginning helping skills class, and the advanced helping skills class, demonstrate the skills and techniques taught in the classroom setting. In these classes, students utilize the clinic as a lab in which to develop, practice and demonstrate skills and techniques. Their capstone experience in the two general helping skills courses is a video portfolio recorded in the clinic. In the play therapy class, the clinic is used to demonstrate play therapy interventions which are critiqued by the instructor and classmates. All first-level clinical experiences involve classmates serving in the role of clients. The second level of training is practicum. All students in the Clinical Mental Health Track, including those in play therapy, must complete their practicum in the university-based clinic. The requirements for practicum include 100 hours on-site with 40 hours being in direct client service. Practicum students also run a psychoeducational group for undergraduates at this level. The third level is internship where students complete 600 hours with 240 in direct service to clients. In both practicum and internship, program students see "real" clients and record their sessions for supervision. This tiered protocol allows for a more natural progression of skill and professional development throughout training.

It is during the second and third level of clinical training that the service part of the mission is enacted. Practicum and Internship students see clients from the university and surrounding community. Intakes are conducted by internship students and cases are staffed at a weekly meeting. The suitability of the client for treatment at our clinic is discussed with the faculty clinic director, with the intent being that practicum students will be assigned lower risk clients. Interns are assigned clients considered to be higher risk or those presenting with more complicated issues. The two main problems we encounter are waiting lists and dealing with semester breaks and other "timeouts" imposed by the academic calendar. Also of note is that some clients will require treatment beyond an intern's tenure in the clinic. For that reason, care is taken to transfer clients in the most facilitative ways possible. We will address this more completely in a section of this chapter dealing with ethical challenges.

University-based play therapy training clinics substantially improve and facilitate the efficiency of teaching and evaluating the play therapy skills of mental health professionals-in-training. Trainees receive supervision from experienced play therapists, while gaining the necessary training and experience required for credentialing. Providing supervision and instruction to students as they acquire the specific play therapy knowledge and skills can help students strengthen these skills, better understand the nuances of the techniques, and build their confidence.

The Clinic as a Research Site: Promoting the Value of Play Therapy

The Association for Play Therapy (APT) aims to promote the value of play, play therapy, and credentialed play therapists (a4pt.org). As previously noted, we believe the university-based play therapy training clinic can support this mission through training, service and research. In addition to teaching and supervision of skills development, training clinics offer a myriad of research opportunities for faculty and students alike. The data collected in studies utilizing the university-based clinic have the potential to contribute to the ongoing advancement of play therapy. Engagement of trainees in research enriches growth and learning, while strengthening confidence and appreciation for outcome research and evidence-based play therapy practices.

A university-based play therapy training clinic is in alignment with the mission of the Association for Play Therapy (APT). Institutions of higher education offering Master's or Doctoral degrees in the mental health field can apply for the designation of Approved Center of Play Therapy Education (AC) through the Association for Play Therapy. These Centers are selected to generate play therapy research, peer-reviewed publications, instruction, and supervised clinical experiences at universities (a4pt.org). This collaboration between universities and the Association for Play Therapy (APT) greatly increases opportunities to enhance the credibility, advancement and growth of play therapy. The development of a play therapy training clinic improves the program's capabilities while offering a valuable service to the university and the community.

While it is certainly true that the university-based play therapy clinic can be a rich source of data to support research. Care must be taken to assure that policies and procedures that address the ethical treatment of participants are firmly in place. Federal law regarding behavioral research conducted in any institution that receives federal funding dictates that participants must be protected according to strict guidelines (Office of Human Research Protections, 2018). Universities will have Institutional Review Boards (IRB) in place to assure compliance. Any faculty member, student, or clinician conducting research in the play therapy clinic must seek and receive IRB approval before beginning a research project. There are 3 levels of IRB approval which may apply to research conducted in play therapy clinics located on university campuses. A complete review of the criteria can be found in 45 CF 46 but we will provide a brief synopsis in the following paragraphs.

All research conducted at the university, which includes the play therapy clinic, must be approved by the IRB. A category of "Exempt" exists for research which meets certain criteria where risk to the participants is non-existent. Even though the term "exempt" is used, the researcher will be required to present evidence to the IRB that the research meets the criteria. In all likelihood, the participants in most, if not all, research conducted in the play therapy clinic will be minors. Minors are considered to be a vulnerable population and as such, any research conducted with them as participants must undergo at least an "Expedited" review. No research conducted with minor participants will be "Exempt." Much of the type of research conducted in a play therapy clinic would involve minimal risk to the participants and would receive an "Expedited" review. However, if greater than minimal risk, as defined in 45 CF 46, is present the study must go through a "Full" review in order to be approved. Each institution has a research review process which must be followed to assure compliance. An additional consideration for research conducted with human subjects and involving mental health issues must be HIPPA compliant.

Association for Play Therapy Credentialing

The Association for Play Therapy (APT) is a national professional society leading the advancement of the play therapy modality and expanding the knowledge and expertise of mental health professionals. This is accomplished through developing and enriching the training and credentialing processes for those interested in play therapy practice, instruction and supervision (a4pt.org). APT offers several pathways to engage in the required specialized education, training and experience for credentialing purposes. The current avenues include approved Centers of Play Therapy, Universities offering Play Therapy, Approved Providers of Play Therapy Continuing Education and the Annual Association Play Therapy Conference. To be certified, mental health professionals or trainees engage in 150 hours of play therapy specific instruction from institutions of higher education or APT approved providers, acquire 500 supervised direct client contact hours and 50 hours of simultaneous play therapy supervision (a4pt.org).

A University-based play therapy training clinic could apply to become an approved Center of Play Therapy Education or could be a component in the offering of a play therapy graduate program or internship. Approved centers are designated by the APT to generate research specific to play therapy and to be the genesis of publications germane to the field. Such in a professional peer-reviewed source while advancing evidenced-based play therapy practice (a4pt.org). Centers offer play therapy instruction, supervised clinical experience, and host faculty members with play therapy expertise and RPT/S credentials (a4pt.org). The Association for Play therapy (APT) endorses "well-rounded" play therapy education (i.e. incorporating various theories and models), and supervised experience, attained in a manner that is conductive to the assimilation of content and the demonstration of proficient play therapy skills (a4pt.org). Play therapy training clinics can provide the means to facilitate this curriculum/training in the recommended manner offering a method to illustrate, deliver and refine learned skills under play therapy specific instruction and supervision.

APT has recently updated credentialing requirements specific to supervision that become effective January 1, 2020. Changes stipulate that all supervision and play therapy experience hours earned for the RPT and RPT-S credentialing process are to be under the supervision of an RPT-S only, in contrast to any licensed mental health professional board approved supervisor. Play therapy training clinics are positioned well to meet this change in requirement, hosting RPT-S credentialed faculty to deliver supervision, increasing the amount of potential applicants for the prestigious RPT and RPT-S credentials.

Pragmatic Considerations for Operating a University-Based Clinic

Facilities for a university-based or graduate program operated play therapy clinic would be similar to any clinic or private practice setting for the delivery of play therapy. Several exceptions exist. The first exception is, the play therapy clinic will often be integrated into the broader clinic which might consist of group therapy, family therapy and individual therapy settings. As such, the play therapy clinic may be one or more rooms set up exclusively for play therapy (see section below regarding setting up a play therapy room), or a room which can double as a facility for play therapy, group meetings, or family meetings. The former, of course, would be the preferred situation as it would provide a dedicated space for play therapy with permanent furniture and equipment unique to play therapy. This would be especially true if more than one room can be dedicated to play therapy as clients often require overlapping time slots. The authors have observed, in their own clinic that play therapy clients tend to seek sessions after school so multiple spaces within the clinic dedicated for play therapy allows for more children and counselors to utilize a play room. The latter facility layout would likely require that play therapy equipment and materials be transported into the multi-purpose room when it is to be used as a play therapy room. In the author's own program clinic which is campus-based and serves individuals, groups and families in addition to play therapy clients, a larger room is established exclusively as a play therapy room complete with the requisite equipment and materials. Other rooms in the clinic, less specific in their utility also serve as secondary sites for play therapy. This is accomplished by using a pre-equipped cart (or tote bag) which can move materials and equipment from storage into the room efficiently, thus making the room a play therapy friendly space, if only temporarily. The cart can be set up according to age or specific needs of the client and can be "loaded" in preparation for the meeting. A second consideration in any training clinic is supervision. In earlier times, direct observation via one-way mirrors was the standard practice. These type opportunities for observation have increasingly given way to, first making video tapes and more recently to the use of digital audio-visual technology by which to capture the session. This method is far less time constraining than direct, real-time observation, and far less cumbersome than videotaping sessions. Video tapes present security problems and are bulky and more of a management problem. Digital video recording of sessions requires specific equipment which can get expensive. While "low-tech" devices such as portable digital cameras and "GoPros" are capable of making perfectly usable recordings of sessions, they can be viewed as intrusive and, in part because the recording resides on the device until it can be downloaded and erased. The downloaded copy must now reside on a flash drive or similar device present problems with security of the taped session. The better solution, in the authors' experience is a system designed specifically for clinical applications of which several are commercially available. The authors' clinic utilizes the Viso software from Noldus coupled with a dedicated server and network which provides for HIPPA compliant recording. Live viewing from faculty offices or a viewing room and recordings made and stored digitally on the secure server are accessed through the network for supervision. All data is stored on the server and accessible by the maker and the supervisor without the necessary step of downloading the data on a portable format. This contributes to security. We have found that two cameras work best in the play therapy room to provide multiple angle access to the often active participants in play therapy sessions.

Playroom Location, Design and Materials

Playroom location should be chosen in order to minimize potential problems inherent in the practice of play therapy. Children at play can, naturally, become noisy, which can be distracting or disturbing to others within earshot. Playrooms should, therefore, be located in an area identified as least likely to interfere with daily functions within the setting. Confidentiality can also be an issue if the location is not conducive to privacy, including unintentional disclosures though the actions of the child or the often, if not mandatory, presence of the parent or guardian in the waiting area.

Children may feel uncomfortable or concerned with parents or others hearing the happenings within the playroom. Being located within a campus building, often shared with other departments and programs, increases the level of traffic near and through the clinic at times. Door liners and white-noise machines are a helpful means to reduce the noise level and protect privacy. An established waiting area for parents and children before the session will decrease the likelihood of disturbances within and around the clinic. The present authors have experienced said challenges due to the lack of an established waiting area, other than dedicated benches along the wall across from the therapy rooms. The use of white-noise machines and establishment of clear rules such as "no cell phone use" posted around the clinic help us to avoid disruption of ongoing sessions.

The size of a playroom has specific implications for the play therapy process. Due to the nature of play itself, the ability to move around easily and safely are important considerations which require an adequate amount of space. However, while space for movement is essential, the ability for the play therapist to observe a child's play is equally fundamental. A properly sized playroom assures a child is never too far away (Landreth, 2012). Landreth (2012) recommends a room approximately 12 feet by 15 feet with an area around 150 to 200 square feet to achieve this balance within the space. Special considerations should be made for play therapy groups with more than two to three children. Activity level, personal space boundaries and the opportunity to create individualized space for group members, if needed, would require a larger playroom of approximately 300 square feet to accommodate groups of up to five children (Landreth, 2012).

Other Considerations for the Playroom

Safety, privacy, and durability are key in the design of a playroom. Flooring such as vinyl tiles offer ease of cleaning and can be replaced easily if damaged. If carpet is used, select types designed for high traffic areas and regarded as extremely durable (i.e. consider fiber, twist and density). A washable, easy to clean paint finish will stand up to sticky fingers and colorful materials and is more practical for a playroom. The authors used a neutral color to balance out with the colorful toys that fill the playroom. Child sized furniture made from sturdy wood or similar hard-surface material is necessary in the playroom. Furniture height should be considered in order for smaller children to reach toys and materials without assistance or engaging in unsafe climbing. Landreth (2012) recommends that the top shelf be no higher than

38 inches in height for the abovementioned reasons. The playroom in the authors' clinic is furnished with a table and chairs, six in total, including two adult-sized for the play therapist, co-therapist or parent when applicable. Additionally, two large wooden shelves are placed along the walls to display toys and materials, and a custom built miniature shelf of the recommended height (see shelf height above), depth and design (less depth of shelf and space between shelves is recommended to maximize space and avoid over filling shelves) compliments the furnishings for ease and functionality. The table provides an accessible, easily cleaned surface for painting or other art activities, use of play dough, clay or similar materials, and other structured directive activities that require table work space. When designing or remodeling a new playroom, the inclusion of a small bathroom with a cold water sink (hot water poses a danger) would minimize challenges with bathroom breaks outside of the playroom. Landreth (2012) points out the therapeutic benefits of a bathroom as an extension of the playroom, creating opportunities to utilize the space for staging bathroom-related scenes, as a hiding or retreating space, or to clearly shut out and ignore an adult.

Therapeutic Toys and Materials

Playroom toys and materials are selected based on guidelines that align with the reasoning for play therapy and are conducive to the achievement of play therapy goals and objectives (Landreth, 2012). Simply put, toys and materials should offer a variety of choices for self-expression and self-awareness. Selected toys and materials should facilitate the exploration and expression of a wide range of feelings and real-life experiences. Additionally, the variety of mediums should offer opportunities to develop self-understanding, self-control, and a positive self-image while establishing a safe relationship within the play therapy process (Landreth, 2012).

The selection of materials should be intentional, with a therapeutic rationale, while taking into account developmental level, interests, and diversity. Lastly, as with other features of a playroom, toys and materials should be safe and of well-made construction for active use. An example would be a wall mounted shatter resistant mirror in which children can act out play scenes while offering an opportunity to create a measure of self-awareness (i.e. facial expressions, body posture, etc.). A few examples of other furnishings from the present authors' clinic include: A wooden play kitchen, a large doll house and a stage for puppet shows.

Landreth (2012) categorized toys and materials into three categories: real-life toys, aggressive-release toys, and creative expression and emotional release toys. Examples of real-life toys which can represent parts of the child's life, aiding in the direct expression of thoughts, feelings and experiences includes a play kitchen, a doll house, or a puppet stage (Landreth, 2012). Landreth (2012) recognizes that particular toy construction and design can elicit certain behaviors and emotions (such as a bop bag) and the expression of anger, hostility or frustration. The bop bag is a durable, child-sized punching bag, which is an example of the aggressive-release toy category. Authors have found foam bats, foam swords and small tabletop punching bag as other helpful options within this category. Finally, sand and water are examples of mediums for unstructured creative expression and emotional release. While the potential exists for unwanted "messiness" with the inclusion of sand and water, we have had good experiences with these tools and regard them as manageable assets to the play therapy process.

Scheduling and Other Administrative Considerations

Scheduling is occasionally an issue with the play therapy room for two primary reasons: 1. More play therapy clients need the same time-slot and there is no play therapy room available to them, and 2. Time outside of the session is necessary to set up the room or to clean up after the session has ended. We have addressed the first issue, as noted previously, by converting a group or family counseling room to a temporary play therapy room by bringing in play therapy materials on a cart. While this is not an ideal solution, it does provide for more than one play therapy client to be seen in the same time slot. The second issue is solved by adhering to a strict 50 minute session which allows for 10 minute set up between sessions and eliminates the need to schedule the room for a longer period than the traditional hour. Alternatively, it has proven useful to schedule the play therapy room on one and one-half hour intervals, as occasionally the therapist becomes a post-session custodian when water or sand finds its way onto and into every aspect of the therapy space or when miniatures end up strewn about the room. This assures that the space is orderly for the next counselor and client.

If the training clinic accepts fees for services, a mechanism consistent with the host institution's policy must be devised to handle money. The authors' clinic focuses on training so fees for services are limited and designed to be as nonrestrictive as possible while still providing some funding for incidentals such as paper, copying costs, crayons, sand, and other consumables as needed. A nominal one-time fee, currently $25, is assessed as an "intake fee" payable by money order or cashier's check only. No charge is levied for subsequent sessions, regardless of the frequency of meetings or duration of treatment. This fee is far below the standard rate for play therapy sessions but it, along with intake fees from individual, group, and family counseling, provides adequately for those aforementioned expenses. The low fee enables parents and children without financial means to engage in play therapy which would be unaffordable otherwise. We have limited payment to cashier's checks and money orders to simplify our collection process. Fees are collected by the clinician and handled by the department administrative assistant. No cash is ever "on hand" and no personal checks ever come back NSF. We have even speculated that the extra step of going through the process of obtaining a cashier's check or money order might serve to strengthen the commitment to counseling. With no cash exchanging hands or personal checks having to clear often strained bank accounts, the money trail from the student-clinician to the clinic account at the university cashier's office is simple and secure. Other possible funding sources for a training clinic could include university or department budgets, grants, endowments, contributions, lab fees from students, or as mentioned to some degree above, fees for services from clients.

Administration of the clinic is supervised by a faculty director of clinical experiences. Day-to-day operations are the responsibility of a senior-level graduate assistant who has been appointed as Clinic Manager. This person acts somewhat similarly as would a Chief Resident in a hospital, assigning clients, assisting with scheduling, acting as liaison between the student clinicians and the faculty, and generally managing the daily operations of the clinic. The Clinic Manager earns indirect internship hours in addition to Graduate Assistantship compensation and a tuition waiver. The clinic, including the play therapy component is staffed by counseling graduate students enrolled in practicum or internship.

Ethical/Legal Considerations

University-based training clinics should develop policies and procedures appropriate to the resources of the program (i.e. faculty experience/credentials, specific instruction/training, etc.). Types of services offered and clients served are delineated in the clinic policy manual (i.e. age range, potential referral sources, level of need). Authors have found that these boundaries around services help to screen potential referrals to the appropriate providers. For example, referrals from an inpatient hospital, with a high level of need, would not be suitable for a training clinic that may potentially have a waiting list and will have semester breaks and regular counselor transfers due to graduating clinicians. When a situation does occur where a client's level of need exceeds the ability of the clinic to accommodate, we have a developed referral protocol and referral list. This provides for a smooth transition to a more appropriate service that best meets the client's identified needs. This type of consideration can help to preclude ethical or legal issues related professional responsibility. Guidelines for handling unsafe or potentially suicidal clients and the commitment to providing adequate support and supervision are also necessary as the authors have found that no screening regimen can completely circumvent suicidality.

Student-Clinicians are constantly supervised, usually via recorded sessions, but occasionally by live observation. In the author's experience, the in-person availability, in the clinic of a licensed professional (i.e. a core faculty member) has proven useful on multiple occasions. One example of this is when, due to a client disclosing a high risk for suicide, the clinician is required to break confidence. Admittedly, this is not usually a problem in play therapy because we require parents or guardians to wait while the child is in session. The requirement to have a faculty member present in the building, available for emergency consultation, can mean that faculty make themselves available outside of classes or regular office hours, especially when the clinic is open during extended hours.

Another issue involves maintaining client records within the training clinic. Authors have a well-established protocol for storing, accessing and securing all clinic records. Client documentation such as intake paperwork, treatment plans, progress notes and other related documents that constitute the client's official record are stored in a locked filing cabinet in a locked room only accessible to students and faculty working in the clinic in a given semester. As noted, our students record all sessions for supervision. Video recording is a condition for being a client with only one exception. Clients who refuse recording of their sessions can be seen only if a mutually agreeable schedule can be established so that live supervision of all sessions can be done by a faculty member. The recordings are intended for supervision and we classify them in the same category as "personal therapy notes" that do not become part of the client's record. As such, all recordings are erased from the secure server after the session has been reviewed by a faculty member and after the student-clinician has received constructive feedback on their performance.

Site Evaluation

Feedback is an integral part of a training clinic, helping to advance the growth and development of trainees and ensure quality of services. Evaluation of services in the form of feedback-informed treatment (FIT) compliments the intentional culture of feedback within a counseling training clinic. FIT empowers clients to provide helpful feedback to inform treatment and services through a systematic assessment and offers many potential benefits. FIT enhances the collaborative, client-as-expert dynamic within the counselor/client relationship while illustrating client responsibility within the treatment process. This inclusion of FIT can help to lower drop-out rates, increase client satisfaction of services, and improve client outcomes. Miller's (2018) Outcome Rating Scale (ORS) and Session Rating Scale (SRS) are the FIT performance metrics utilized by the Authors. The ORS and SRS are easy to incorporate into the session and are designed to be administered repeatedly. This particular performance metric (ORS, SRS) offers age specific modification of materials (adult, child, and younger child-defined as age 5 or younger) making it ideal for a play therapy training clinic that might provide services to all the mentioned populations.

CONCLUSION

With the modernization of training, particularly as emerging technologies are incorporated into service delivery, evaluation of services, and supervision, play therapy training clinics can serve as a hub for education, training, and research, providing opportunities for faculty and students to conduct investigations into the play therapy and supervision processes. The Association for Play Therapy (APT) encourages play therapy research that "demonstrates the value and effectiveness of play and play therapy, increases play therapy knowledge or improves play therapy techniques, and supports evidence-based play therapy practices" (a4pt.org). The development of a play therapy training clinic with up-to-date technology enables programs to collect data originating at the facility for research projects and would expand the capabilities of programs to achieve the aforementioned objectives. Service to individuals and families with financial insufficiencies can be provided to those for whom play-therapy would be excluded as a form of intervention. Finally, a campus-based play therapy clinic can provide exemplary training and supervision opportunities to the next generation of play therapists.

REFERENCES

Association for Play Therapy. (n.d.a). Retrieved from http://www.a4pt.org/page/educationtraining

Association for Play Therapy. (n.d.b). Retrieved from http://www.a4pt.org/page/CredentialsHomepage

Council for Accreditation of Counseling and Related Educational Programs (CACREP). (n.d.). *2009 Standards*. Available: www.cacrep.org/wp-content/uploads/2017/07/2009-Standards.pdf

Council for Accreditation of Counseling and Related Educational Programs (CACREP). (n.d.). *2016 Standards*. Available: https://www.cacrep.org/for-programs/2016-cacrep-standards/

Hittner, J., & Fawcett, M. (2012). *Developing a Counselor Education Training Clinic: The First Year*. Retrieved from https://www.counseling.org/knowledge-center/vistas/by-subject2/vistas-education-and-supervision/docs/default-source/vistas/vistas_2012_article_22

Landreth, G. L. (2012). *Play Therapy: The Art of the Relationship* (3rd ed.). New York, NY: Routledge Taylor & Francis Group. doi:10.4324/9780203835159

Miller, S. D. (2018). *Performance Metrics-Licenses for the ORS & SRS.* Available: https://scott-d-miller-ph-d.myshopify.com/collections/performance-metrics/products/performance-metrics-licenses-for-the-ors-and-srs

Mobley, A. K., & Myers, J. E. (2010). *Developing and Maintaining Counselor Education Laboratories* (2nd ed.). Retrieved from https://www.acesonline.net/resources/developing-and-maintaining-counselor-education-laboratories

Office of Human Research Protections. (2018). *45 CF 46*. Available: https://www.hhs.gov/ohrp/regulations-and-policy/regulations/45-cfr-46/index.html

Chapter 6
University/District Collaboration Play Therapy Clinics

Ryan P. Holliman
Dallas Counseling and Treatment Center, USA

Pedro Blanco
Tarleton State University, USA

ABSTRACT

Many elementary schools must make due with a single school counselor, leaving many children in need of services. The authors of this chapter propose a unique partnership to create sustainable school-based play therapy clinics. The proposed clinics provide free services to children in schools and also allow for the collection of data by university professors hoping to examine and advocate for effectiveness of play therapy. The chapter will discuss how to select appropriate partners, how to build relationships with school professionals, how to establish research and clinics in the schools, training concerns, and ethical issues.

INTRODUCTION

The American Association of School Counseling Association (ASCA) recommends a ratio of one counselor to every 250 students (2017). However, a recent study of trends in student to counselor ratios indicates that in some states the ratio is as low as 200:1 and as high as 924:1 (ASCA, 2014). It is obvious that with ratios this high, a school counselor can only provide limited counseling to the highest need

DOI: 10.4018/978-1-5225-8226-7.ch006

children. The challenges that elementary schools deal with are legion, and the school counselor is often overwhelmed at the prospect of being the sole individual trained and responsible for the mental health concerns for all students in the school. Our hope is that by developing and operating a school based play therapy clinic in collaboration between a university and a local school district will not only aid in the school counselor stress but also better meet the social emotional needs of the children attending the school.

Building Relationships

For a collaborative clinic to exist, relationships must be forged. This relationship is often one of give and take, in which both the school and the clinic have to have mutual benefits. It is often the case that for this to be a reciprocal value both parties must have a foundation of trust. One of the eternal truths about public education is that time and space will always be sought after commodities.

Establishing a Relationship With the Principal

The principal of a school can be a great asset to a collaborative clinic. However, one must understand that the tasks that a principal has been entrusted with vary greatly from those that a therapist holds dear. Principals are entrusted with the efficient and successful administrations of public schools (Ruff & Shoho, 2016), and at the elementary level a principal is often tasked with not only the academic minutiae that may seem insignificant to the counselor, but also with handling problematic behaviors and discipline. This by no means indicates that the principal and the counselor must be natural enemies. Rather, it indicates that the counselor must approach the relationship in such a way to establish the collaboration clinic as a win-win situation. First and foremost, when the collaborator approaches a principal they must be able to identify how they can help the school. In our experience principals are initially hesitant to bring in outside projects to their campus. The authors have found that sharing how a play therapy clinic in their school would not only aid in providing additional support to the school counseling, but that there is indeed a wealth of research demonstrating the effectiveness of play therapy increasing academic achievement. By providing this evidence and demonstrating that a collaborative play therapy clinic will free up some of the school counselors time school administrators/principals have been more willing to establish such a project.

Being conversant in play therapy literature and the ways in which it may help the principal and their school will be an important part of the process. A key part of engaging with non-mental health professionals is being somewhat of a salesperson.

When you're in sales, you have to sell things that other people want to buy, as opposed to simply selling things that you want to sell. What principals in general want to buy are things to will help their children learn better with a minimal impact on the daily operations of their school.

Dollarhide, Smith, and Lemberger (2007) conducted a study of critical incidents which impacted relationships between school based counselors and principals. One finding from the study was that when principals were confronted with evidence of a school-base counselors influence on the students, teachers, parents, and system of the school it led to shift in how they were perceived. It was found that these types of interactions led to the school-based counselor's skills defining their role in the school, as opposed to the principal being the one to delineate their role (Dollarhid et al., 2007). As such, school-based counselors may be best served when they consider how to serve the entire school as opposed to just a student. Another important issue is how to present evidence to advocate for the importance of one's presence in the school and to illuminate the value that has been added to the school system by the work of the counselor. One suggestion that the authors have to facilitate these kinds of counselor-principal experiences is to collect data on students on both the individual and group level, specifically using outcome variables of use to the principal. For example, a counselor that is seeing a child might gather data about referrals to the principal's office before play therapy and after 10 sessions. Providing a concrete impact on the child can help the principal see in a concrete way how a school-based clinic is helping the school reduce behavioral issues which impact academic achievement.

A second theme in the critical incidents identified by Dollarhide et al. (2007) was the ability of school-based counselors to see the "big picture" of the school. Specifically, this means school-based counselors who understand and appreciate the mission of the school, see students holistically, work for systemic change in the school, and collaborate with all partners in a school system. These are a few concrete practices that may help counselors see the "big picture" of the school. First of all, when talking with the principal a school-based counselor should be able to easily connect the work they are doing with the mission of the school and make that connection explicit in their conversations with the principal. Secondly, the counselor should talk not solely about mental health outcomes but how their work has improved the physical health, social skills, academic status, and mental health of children. Finally, a school-based counselor should view the entire school as their client and work on developing interventions and programs that have links to impacting students at a school-wide level, as well as how to systematically work with other partners in the school.

Establishing a Relationship With the School Counselor

A positive relationship with the school counselor can make all the difference in a collaboration clinic. A good school counselor has their finger on the pulse of the school, and knows children who are struggling, and what their home lives are like. A collaboration clinic can be very appealing to a school counselor, because it can provide an influx of counseling services that they would not likely be able to provide on their own. One possible issue of conflict for the school counselor and the collaboration clinic is that the school counselor could possibly feel threatened. In most of the elementary schools where the authors of this chapter have developed collaboration clinics, the elementary school counselor is the *only* counselor in the building. As such they are accustomed to being the only mental health professional, aside from perhaps a school psychologist that may be shared by multiple campuses. As such in building the relationship with the school counselor, it will be important for the representatives of the collaborative clinic to clearly state that their intention is not to *take over* or *replace* the school counselor rather that the goal is to help the school counselor in cooperative way. Delineating what exactly the clinic will do, and making regular contact with the school counselor will be helpful. As well, frequent planned communication is typically the best way to maintain such a relationship. School counselors in the experience of the authors of this chapter take a great deal of responsibility for the school and how the mental health services are conducted, and staying in touch is a way to honor the seriousness with which they approach their job.

One strategy that the authors have used is to look for potential collaborations with school counselors in which we have already developed sort of relationship. Because the collaboration is often between a university and a specific school it possible that previous alumni are already working in the schools as school counselors. The authors have benefited from reaching out to school counseling alumni when looking at establishing partnerships as the often are familiar with what our potential needs are, and can provide a familiarity of the program to their administrators. If you are in the position where you are new to the area or do not have any past relationships with any of the school counselors in potential collaborative districts, we encourage you to attempt to see if any school counselors describe themselves as play therapists or report that the conduct play therapy in the bio page from the school websites is available. Another strategy may be by checking in with a random school counselor within the district and seeing if he/she is aware of any campus that may be in need of additional support.

Establishing Relationships With the Teachers

While the school counselor and the principal are both very important, the person who spends the most time with children are usually their teachers. It has been the experience of the authors that teachers have perhaps the most voluminous knowledge of a child's family situation as well as their day-to-day functioning in the classroom. However, teachers and clinical counselors do not always see things the same. The authors of this chapter believe that one of the principle reasons for this may be that in general most disciplines believe that they have the market cornered on the *truth* and how to address the real problems of the day. Many clinical counselors believe that if people would simply listen and apply their perspective on working with children, then the world would be a better place. However, such a view speaks to a lack of understanding and empathy for the position that others take. So to build a relationship with teachers, the clinicians and faculty must admit that teachers have a unique and valid perspective. Secondly, while they may have a different viewpoint on how to best help children, we should not view them as adversaries, but rather as helpful allies in our attempts to improve the lives of children and therefore our communities. This section has addressed some of the philosophical elements of building relationships with teachers but what about the practical elements? First, make time to introduce yourself to the teacher at the beginning of the year, if you are going to be seeing a child who is a member of their class. When you introduce yourself you should ask questions about how to best retrieve a child for therapy, while not disrupting the classroom. You also want to gauge the teacher's level of excitement (or chagrin) about the prospect of their child participating in the program. You also want to check in with them during a planning period to see how things are going. It does seem that teachers are frequently under-appreciated in our current social climate, and treating them as well-trained professionals to whom respect is due is well worth the investment. In the past we have met with teachers during staff development days or during their teaming period to go over the plan of the collaboration, basic information of play therapy, and expectations.

When developing relationships with teachers we have found that it is of the utmost importance to validate the teachers experience and training. Never offer advice or strategies when working with teachers unless the teacher has requested aid. Many teachers are continually overburdened by not only their task of educating and building working relationships with large numbers of students, but they are often charged with the undertaking of additional administrative tasks that take them away from the actual class instruction. When working with teachers as collaborators we have found that demonstrating understanding and attempting to find ways to alleviate any of their stress is your best chance in forging a partnership.

Establishing Relationships With the Parents

Finally, one must learn how to develop a relationship with the parents of the child. This can be a rather significant challenge in school-based collaboration clinics because parents do not accompany their child to sessions as they might at a community clinic. The experience of the authors has been primarily in Title I elementary schools where there is a high proportion of families that qualify as economically disadvantaged. It has been our experience that parents who have economic difficulties are under a large degree of stress and that they often can be difficult to contact (Velsor & Orozco, 2007). In the experience of the authors, some of the Title I school districts that the authors have worked in have had a higher proportion of parents who did not speak English than non-Title I school districts. When such barriers to communication occur, the authors have found it imperative to find translators or recruit student counselors who are bilingual so that the counselors can fully communicate with the parents. However, it should be noted that this may be a feature of the schools with which the authors have worked in the southern United States, where there is a high population of Spanish only speakers.

The authors have found that making connections with parents in crucial to the success of any program within the school setting. Without parental consent, children cannot be seen. Sometimes parents are reluctant to have their child enrolled in services within the school setting. In the past we have made attempts to inform parents about school based play therapy collaborations by providing workshops on parenting and various other topics on child mental health at the local parent teacher association. Having a presence in the school and being visible is also a way to demonstrate to parents that you are there to help. When children are in services it is essential to provide parents with updates/consults either by phone or in person.

Velsor and Orozco (2007) have outlined a few important ways to establish relationships with parents. One of the first major principles in establishing a positive relationship with a parent is to contact them with opportunities or good news. It is not uncommon for parents to hear from schools only when problems are occurring. A counselor at a collaboration clinic may reach out to parents when there are groups, classes, or other programs that they think will specifically benefit the family. It can also be helpful to call parents with good news about the child. For example, if a child has shown marked improvement in therapy, a phone call about how well the child is doing can help establish phone calls from the clinic or school as a positive event rather than a disciplinary event.

A second suggestion that Velsor and Orozco (2007) suggested is making home visits. This is a suggestion that requires a significant shift in how the counselor approaches work with families. Typically a therapist that works in a private practice or an agency expects families to come to the counselor. Making home visits can overcome barriers that prevent the parents from coming to the school to speak to the counselor. As well, it provides a less formal relationship which can minimize power differentials.

Another suggestion is to take time as a collaboration clinic to help families address issues that are not necessarily centered specifically on the child (Velsor & Orozco, 2007). It is easy for a play therapist to view the child as the client. However, it is the view of the authors that in play therapy the entire family system is the client. To that end, addressing issues which cause stress to the family unit may allow for the family to have more energy to engage in the play therapy of their child. Some of the issues which may cause stress are difficulty accessing medical services, nutritional needs, housing challenges, and employment issues. By providing the family with referrals to agencies that can help address these needs, the school-based clinic can help establish itself as not another entity that wishes to make demands of parents but one that solves real life problems that are pressing for the family.

A final suggestion is one that comes from the medical field. For many families, especially those who have immigrated to the United States, navigating the public education system can be difficult (Hill & Torres, 2010). Knowing how to advocate for a child, how to become involved in their education, and how to access special services is difficult for parents not familiar with the workings of a public school district. One method that has been used by hospitals is a peer navigator system. A peer navigator is someone who is an individual who is a para-professional and helps the individual navigate things in the medical community such as making appointments, understanding diagnoses, and accessing the medical care they need (Jandorf, Gutierrez, Lopez, Christie, & Ikzkowitz, 2005). The authors propose that an educational peer navigator that helps parents become aware of programming at the school, facilitating appointments with school professionals, and helping advocate for parents needs would be a helpful addition to help parents become more engaged.

EVALUATING SCHOOL DISTRICTS

Developing a school-based play therapy clinic is no small undertaking as this chapter has discussed. While this chapter has addressed all the ways in which one might develop a school-based play therapy clinic. It is also important to evaluate the schools in which such a clinic might be most suited. As such, the authors have identified several ways in which one might evaluate a school for establishing a clinic.

Evaluating the district tends to focus more on policies and attitudes that the district may have regarding the establishment of a school-based play therapy clinic. You will note that at the district level, most of the questions will be focused on conducting research, while the questions that will be important for the campus are more of a mixture of research and clinical. One of the first set of policies that will be important to evaluate will be the institutional review board (IRB) requirements of the school district.

Is Outside Research Allowed?

This is an important first question. Many districts are understandably cautious when it comes to allowing outsiders into the school district to work with their children. In the current climate of violence in schools, a district wants to have tight control over those who enter the school on a regular basis. A search of the website for the school district should provide some preliminary information about the school and it's openness to research.

What Are Requirements/Limitations Regarding Research?

Even if a school does in fact allow research, it does not mean that you will be allowed unfettered access to conduct your research. Are there requirements/limitations regarding how often and for what duration of time a child may be pulled from class as part of the research study and/or clinic? Another important topic for consideration is the limitations that may surround the idea of session recording. Some schools make the caveat that sessions may be recorded, but that the camera should focus on the clinician and the child should not be visible in the frame. Others may have requirements regarding what sort of recording media is used for sessions (e.g. audio, video, etc…). Some school districts have a policy against recording of any kind. If faculty members intend to use students for this work, an understanding of limitations of recording will help determine the feasibility of conducting it in a specific district.

Limitations Regarding Time

For some districts, the amount of time required for both students and staff will be a deciding factor not only in whether your request to conduct research is even approved but also how successful the venture may be. It has been the authors' experience that time in the schools if very different from time in the clinical world. It is not uncommon for sessions in the play therapy clinics to be 45 minutes of actual play therapy with the final 10-15 minutes reserved for parent/family consultation and restoring order to the playroom for the next session. However, to remove a child from a classroom for 45 minutes at least once a week would be a considerable hardship not only for the individual teacher, but it would pose a considerable amount of concern in regard to district approval. Another issue that will be important to discuss is what efforts you will need on the part of the school staff to help make the clinic run smoothly. Some common issues that faculty and clinicians will need help with in the schools include: identifying appropriate children, sending home informed consent documentation and retrieving it, consultation regarding Child Protective Services cases, and managing scheduling issues. A successful collaboration clinic will minimize the amount of time required from staff.

Who Are the Decision Makers?

The informed consent document for the district Institutional Review Board will identify some of the persons that will be responsible for making decisions on campus-based research. It would behoove the faculty involved in creating the collaborative clinic to be aware of those persons and their backgrounds. Establishing professional relationships to ensure that both members of the school district can see the direct benefits of the program, while also making certain the expectations of the university administration are being met.

DEVELOPING RESEARCH

One of the essential parts of a collaborative clinic for the academic is developing a research agenda that can be met through one's work at the school. While certainly providing counseling services at a school can be rewarding in and of itself, collecting data for research helps provide an evidence based rationale for maintaining the clinic. When conducting research at schools, it is important to gain consent from parents, schools, and university institutional research boards (IRB). Usually the first step to gaining consent involves completing a school district IRB request and gaining consent of campus principals. Secondly, one must gain the university IRB's approval. Finally, once both the school district and university have agreed to the research plan, the parents of individual children must provide consent for their child to participate.

In the authors' experience, one of the consistent problems in developing a collaborative clinic is the availability of consistent and well-trained personnel. A collaborative clinic relies on the use of counseling students to provide services. The benefit to such an arrangement is that students working in a collaborative clinic as part of their internship usually do not draw a salary, which means it can be done with little or no budget. However, one of many challenges is that they are not fully trained professionals and as such will need extended training and supervision. As well, students graduate as a general rule, so you will have a high degree of staff turnover. Finally, students are a finite resource, and the more students you recruit the more management and supervision will have to take place. With this in mind, we are presenting a variety of research models which can be effectively accomplished with a small base of personnel.

Single Case Design

One of the models of research that is perhaps best suited to the unique position of a collaboration clinic is the single-case design study. A single-case design study is one in which the unit of analysis is the individual case (Ray, Minton, Schottelkorb, & Brown, 2010). The APA has identified large single-case design studies (e.g. 6-9 cases) as sufficient for one of the criteria for providing evidence to contribute to an intervention being recognized as a well-established treatments. The essence behind a single-case design study is the idea of continuous assessment, meaning that an individual serving as one of the cases in such a study should be administered an assessment instrument at least once a week, and possibly multiple times a week.

The classic model of single-case design is A-B-A where A=No treatment and B=Treatment. However, it should be noted that there are many models of single-case design, ABA is the simplest model. During the initial phase of no-treatment, the individual is provided assessments, for at least 3 measurement points. General guidance in the literature suggests that while 3 is the minimum, the true goal for single case design is to reach a relatively stable measurement. This phase serves as the baseline. The next phase introduces treatment and the continuous assessment continues. This may prove to be logistically challenging, because the child will need both play therapy and assessment which may need to occur at different times by different counselors. Finally, the last phase in the classic model is a no-treatment phase. During this portion of the research data is gathered which may help determine if gains are retained after treatment is withdrawn.

Single case design is a beneficial method in collaboration clinics for several reasons. First and foremost, it can be done with a minimum of personnel. Aside from student counselors, there are typically only two personnel positions which need to be filled. First, a faculty director that oversees reserach, training, and clinical supervision. Second, a clinic assistant, who may be an advanced student, whose duties include maintaining playrooms, developing schedules for the counselors, and communicating with the school counselor or principal about needs or concerns regarding the program. Secondly, you do not have to have a large sample size. Between groups research studies can be analyzed with parametric tests using samples sizes of n=30 (Pallant, 2016). Furthermore, if one wants to conduct single case design research, then the sample size can range from three to nine participants (Ray & Schottelkorb, 2010). To find large samples of children with a particular disorder can be difficult in some schools. For example, finding 40 children in one school who are diagnosed with depression or anxiety, can be a challenge. However, to find between three to nine children with those characteristics will be much easier. One major challenge to this approach however is timing. With at least six weeks needed for an initial baseline and non-treatment follow up stage, the researcher in the school is left with little time to provide the intervention stage in a typical school semester. If a typically university semester is comprised of sixteen weeks, then a researcher will have three weeks for baseline, ten weeks for intervention, and three weeks for the non-treatment follow-up stage. This will require researchers to work with school staff before the beginning of school to identify potential participants (if the research is done in the fall semester) or plan on starting research in spring semesters, using the fall semester to identify participants.

Instrument Studies

Another kind of research study which can be conducted in schools is investigation into validity and reliability properties of instruments. Establishing an instrument with sufficient reliability and validity can be a research agenda in and of itself (Kimberlin & Winterstein, 2008). One of the benefits to instrument studies is that they do not necessarily require intervention, and as such it may require much less work on the part of the faculty and collaboration clinic to conduct an instrument study. In terms of design, the most difficult part of an instrument study is actually getting individuals to return the instrument. Once it has been returned, the truly difficult part of conducting instrument study analyses occurs. The following are some different kinds of instrument studies that might be used in a collaboration clinic.

Population Validity Studies

Inferences about an assessment instrument are based on the population with which it was normed. One avenue for investigation is investigating the validity of an instrument with different populations, such as ethnic groups. Examining if the factor structure of an instrument holds for another population helps expand the usefulness of an instrument.

Reliability Studies

Researchers and use test-retest, split-half, or internal consistency approaches to reliability to ensure that an instruments performance is stable across time, users, and items. At most this requires administering the instrument at two different times points, and for certain designs it can be administered just once.

Small Between Groups Studies

This is the research design with which the authors have the most experience. In this type of study, the goal is typically to recruit at least 30 children and ideally 80. Each child is randomized to a condition, either experimental group (receiving play therapy) or the wait-list control group (who receives no treatment during the study, but receives it at the conclusion of post-testing). Then children are tested on the selected measurements and proceed in receiving whatever treatment they are assigned. After treatment concludes post testing is conducted. The analyses conducted may either be a mixed design split-plot ANOVA or a MANOVA depending upon how many analyses and variables are being examined.

Research studies using official assessment can be tricky in the school system. Self-report instruments tend to work well in the environment; however young children can be poor raters on presenting problems and it can be challenging to find appropriate instruments. Teacher-report instruments can work well depending on your relationship with the teacher and the frequency in which you are asking them to respond. Providing time or incentives for teachers can be helpful, for example providing a substitute teacher and snacks in the teacher's lounge for the teacher so they then complete the instruments. Gathering data from parents is often most challenging, as you have limited contact with them and often have to rely on sending assessments instruments home in a weekly folder. Incentives tend to help, but the response rate from parents tends to be lower than self-report or parent-report in our experience.

When conducting any type of research in the school system it is imperative to begin the process as early as possible to ensure success. Focusing on beginning the study during the Fall semester have proven to be imperative as it allows the summer to be a period of preparation and training, and also helps avoid the academic state testing that typically occurs in the Spring semester. One resource which may help in providing a timeline and to do list is the School Research Project Checklist initially developed by Blanco and Tsai and later published by Muro, Stickley, Muro, Blanco & Tsai (2015).

INITIAL DEVELOPMENT

One of the major differences that students and counselors working in a collaborative clinic might experience revolves around security. In collaborative clinics the members of the university do not function as employees of the school and in many ways they will have the experience of being an outsider on the school campus. In light of recent tragic events at schools, security measures are meant to scrutinize visitors. The following is list of concerns in regards to security for collaborative clinics.

Background Checks

Many schools require any visitors or volunteers to submit to a district background check. This can raise multiple issues for developing the clinic. First and foremost it may limit the counseling students that are allowed to participate. If a student has a history of criminal offenses in their past, even for charges such as drug possession, it may be within the districts purview to deny their request to serve as a volunteer at the school. The directors of the collaborative clinic will also have to gather the appropriate paperwork from the students, submit them before the start of the school year, and follow-up to make sure that all background checks have been received and approved.

School Entrance Security

The authors of this chapter have had a wide range of experience with different security protocols at school entrances. In one rural school in which we developed a collaborative clinic, the security procedure was writing your name on a sign in sheet at the front desk. Other campuses require a scan of a photo ID and have mag-locked doors that prevent access. It is important not only for clinic directors to be aware of these procedures but to communicate them to the counselors that will be serving the school. Nothing is more disappointing than being turned away at the door of a school due to poor preparation.

Room Access

Clinic directors will also have to arrange for access to the room in which they are planning to conduct play therapy. Sometimes your room will be in a portable building, which may be locked all the time, as it may be used for storage, or only special classes/situations. Other times you might be provided a playroom inside the school building, which may or may not be locked on a regular basis. Not only is it necessary to have regular access to a room key, but you may need a pass-card to get back into the building in case you need to enter/exit the building from a portable building or to drop-off/return a child from recess or other outside activities. The following is the protocol that we have found to be most effective for managing access control. Require that all students serving as counselors at the clinic wear a lanyard that displays their university student ID. Arrange for a copy of the room key and passkey to the building be left with the secretary/receptionist at the front desk of the school. Then instruct students that as they sign in for security they may pick up the key and as they sign out they must return it.

Another important issue to address is who else might have access to the room and what you keep in your playroom. The authors have had many experiences in which it appears that other people have had access to our playroom and used it for a variety of purposes. If other people regularly use the room you will have to consider carefully how to identify materials as belonging to you as opposed to the school. When sharing space you should also consider how the room will be used and how to limit the amount of disruption to the actual playroom space/materials. In addition if you are sharing space with other programs within the school ensuring a schedule is posted outside the door and an agreement is made about the best way to share the space.

TRAINING COUNSELING STUDENTS

The success of a collaboration clinic greatly depends upon the students who serve as the backbone of the operation. Running a clinic in a school is wildly different than running a clinic anywhere else. Students who might be highly capable clinicians find that school-based play therapy clinics provide unique challenges that they may not be prepared to deal with as graduate students. Therefore the successful collaboration clinic makes training clinicians for this new setting a priority.

Training Students About School Culture

Understanding the Role of Mental Health in the School

In counseling clinics, therapists, administrators, and clients alike understand that the primary purpose is to provide quality mental health care as the desired outcome. However, at a school mental health is a means to an end, rather than an end unto itself. Mental health in a school serves the purpose of removing barriers from educational attainment (DeKruyf, Auger, & Trice-Black, 2013). This can be a serious adjustment for many clinical counselors. There are a few practical things that counselors should be made of aware of to help them honor the goal of the school. First and foremost, counselors should seek to minimize time outside of the classroom. A school-based play therapy clinic cannot hope to succeed if they supplant the schools' goal of education with its own goal of mental health. Counselors should also become aware of particular classroom time which may negatively affect the child. For example, if a child is struggling in math, it would be counterproductive to schedule a play therapy session during math education time. An important aspect of training is to remind therapists about the importance of standardized testing and to be prepared for canceling sessions during times when standardized testing occurs. As well, counselors must be aware of special holidays, assembly days, and other days at schools which may require scheduling changes for a play therapy session.

We Are Guests

When you create a collaboration clinic, the counseling students and even professors involved must understand that they are guests in the school. This can be a challenge for professors who are used to having carte blanch in how they run their classroom or students who are accustomed to higher degrees of autonomy at a mental health clinic. Therefore, training students about how to be respectful guests in a school is essential. One of the first things to educate students about is how to avoid becoming critical of teachers or administrators. It can be easy to take a negative view of teachers or administrators when their view of how to work with children is very different from that of therapists. However, remind the students who are working in the school-based clinic, that they would likely not appreciate a teacher coming into their session and criticizing their interventions. Another thing to consider is that each school has their own sets of rules and policies, as guests you would want to follow as many of these procedures while in the school. This could be things as simple as setting limits about running down the hall before or after sessions, a practice that may be common within an agency or private practice setting. Being observant or asking about policies in the school with the school staff is always a good idea.

Frequent communication is a must in many aspects of a school-based play therapy clinic. There are aspects of working with children that the professors and clinicians may be well aware of how to handle, but in a school based play program, it is essential to reach out to appropriate personnel, specifically the principal and the school counselor. These will also be important issues to outline in any informed consent documents that are provided to parents as well as the school district. A non-exhaustive list of potential incidences which require such communication follows:

1. When an outcry of sexual abuse occurs, the counselor may consider contacting the school counselor. Many school counselor has their finger on the pulse of the lives of the children. Ethical issues, confidentiality, and policy may need to be addressed here for those who have never worked in a school (Trice-Black, Riechel, & Shillingford, 2013). A first step for graduate students is to consult with the on-site school counselor and/or their faculty supervisor. By informing the school counselor the school based play therapist can then collaboratively

work on the next best course of action in reporting. This communication of informing the school counselor also allows he/she to aid in any follow up or investigation. There will be instances in which a school is reluctant to file a report, and in such a situation, a graduate student should consult with their faculty supervisor about how to proceed.

2. When a child becomes hurt. Even if it is a minor injury, the clinician should at minimum inform the students teacher about the injury and inform the school counselor, so that the clinician is not linked to allegations of physical abuse. Accidents happen sometimes, and by letting the teacher and school counselor know about the injury less alarm may occur if a parent calls questioning how his/her child got hurt. It is also important that if the injury is small in the playroom, for instance small cut on figure, or a knee bang on a table, that the play therapist help calm the child before leaving. Having a child leave the room yelping in pain could disrupt the school and cause alarm when not needed. Furthermore, in more serious cases, the play therapist should consult the school nurse or follow any emergency procedures set by the school.
3. When scheduling becomes an issue. Some teachers are absolutely delighted for one of their students to be receiving therapy and they see the value that it produces for the child and their educational experience. Others are less excited, and may have very strict boundaries about when students are to be taken out. Therefore, it is important to communicate to the school counselor and the teacher about any proposed change in schedule. Sometimes demonstrating a little flexibly and understanding can go a long way. One trick that we have used in the past to alleviate this concern is if it the teacher has multiple children in his/her classroom. In these case, the play therapist could switch each individuals session time on a rotation, in this way the child does not miss this same course of study each week. Attempting to find creative solutions to get both the teacher's needs met while also ensuring the child gets their opportunity attend play therapy.
4. When the counselor must cancel the appointment. Counselors are people too and as such they will inevitably have personal issues which may prevent them from attending sessions. However, it is important to communicate with school staff that the counselor will not be able to attend sessions. If a therapist unexpectedly no-shows, it can lead to a child being upset, and sometimes, disruptive to the classroom. Therapist must be trained to be in frequent communication with not only their supervisor but also school staff to make sure that everyone is on the same page. Typically, this communication takes the form of an email to the teacher and the school counselor, who can the relay the information to the child.

How for Students to Develop Healthy Relationships With School Professionals

It is not enough for the faculty members who are the leaders of the clinic to develop healthy relationships with school professionals, they must also teach the students how to engage in healthy relationship building. The authors will here outline a few ways in which this may be accomplished. First and foremost, a culture of communication must be established. A culture of communication means that it is encouraged and required for student counselors to communicate with their faculty members, the school counselor, and relevant personnel about issues effecting the school. This starts with the faculty members introducing the counselors in training to the school counselor and teachers from whom they will be picking children up for therapy. This communicates that the clinic is one that needs to communicate with school personnel and that they do not operate in isolation. A culture of communication is also established through requiring student counselors to communicate with counselors and teachers about routine issues such as scheduling problems, when they will not be at the clinic due to sickness or vacation, and regularly asking for feedback from pertinent personnel.

Another way in which faculty members can help counselors in training to establish healthy relationships is through emphasizing the importance role of teachers and other educational staff in clinical supervision. It can be easy for a student counselor to view the teacher as someone whom the counselor needs to relay information to, and not someone that they can learn from. Discussing teacher consultations in supervision and highlighting their importance helps establish a relationship in which they value the feedback of others.

A final way which the authors think that healthy relationships can be maintained is by providing mechanisms by which the school and its staff can address concerns or problems with a student counselor. The authors suggest a few different ways in which the faculty can safeguard against such problems and respond to school concerns. The first safeguard is being selective about the students that work at the clinic. Having individual interviews much like a student would have at any other internship site can be helpful in determining if they are a good fit for working in a school environment as well as aiding in the early detection of any behavior problems.Another safeguard would be extensive training about how to conduct ones self in a school. The authors have utilized a four week training regimen in which students are provided guidance on how to relate to school staff, how to address common problems in a school, and the basics of school-based play therapy. The final safeguard that the authors have found helpful is regular evaluation in weekly clinical supervision. There are several forms that this may take. One is through the use of formal skills evaluations. The

Play Therapy Attitudes Knowledge and Skills Survey (Kao & Landreth, 1997) is a formal assessment of play therapy skills that may be used to measure the abilities of a therapist. As well, by watching regular recordings of play therapy sessions a supervisor may gain a sense of any problems that may occur. Finally, it would be helpful for a supervisor to seek regular feedback from school personnel that might have interactions with the student counselors. The faculty members should also work collaboratively with school professionals to develop a process by which the student counselor can receive feedback about both acceptable and unacceptable performance in the school-based clinic and be given a chance to be re-mediated, as well as clear actions that should occur if the student is unable to change their performance. Giving the school and the student counselor both a sense of agency and due process is an essential element to make sure that both the graduate students and the students of the school are being given a quality experience.

Documentation

When establishing a clinic in a school one very important and often forgotten practical piece of the clinician's work is documentation. In schools space is often a scarce commodity. So having a space that where only members of the play therapy team have access, is fairly uncommon. This creates several potential dilemmas. The first is where will client files of the children being seen in the school will be held. Second what will be included in the child's files? Third who will have access to the files? Lastly, what procedures will be put into place to meet HIPPA and/or FERPA guidelines?

Because our past collaborations have been in conjunction with our place of employment, a state university, we have chosen to keep all client files in a locked filling cabinet, within a locked office, within a locked suite on the university campus. The authors have found that there are several benefits to having all of the client records held off site. However, this means that the play therapist must complete their session notes at the university setting, and they often do not have the caregiver's contact numbers directly with them at the school. The authors consider the child's file part of our records and they are not directly provided to the school and are not considered part of the child's academic records. The authors do release records to the school when the parent has signed a release of information. In addition, we do submit summary documentation about the program, indicating how many sessions were provided, how many children have been served and other demographic information but in these reports no identifying client information is shared.

Requirements for Counselors-In-Training

The authors have identified several requirements which will be important for student counselors to meet before participating in the school-based clinic. These requirements fall into three major domains: (1) Academic requirements, (2) School-based requirements, (3) Commitments to the clinic.

Students participating in the school-based clinic should have completed all of the course work necessary for them to engage in supervised counseling practice. The authors have had a variety of students at the very beginning of their academic careers show interest in participating in the clinic. However, it is important to limit participation as a counselor to those who are ready to start their academic practicum in counseling (CACREP, 2016). Students not at this point in their training can find other ways to participate in the clinic, such as providing administrative support. The students will need to have completed formal or informal training in play therapy, with a focus on basic skills of play therapy, child development, and consultation with parents and teachers.

There are also a variety of requirements that are necessary for participating in the clinic that the school district would likely require. First, the student must be able to pass a background check conducted by the school. Students with prior convictions regarding drug use, violent offenses, and offenses regarding children will typically not be allowed to participate due to school district requirements, however this may vary, depending upon state laws and school district policies.. The school district may also require further paperwork to be allowed on campus as a volunteer (which in the experience of the authors is what most school-based counselors will be identified as. This may vary from school to school based on district policies).

Finally, there are some continuing requirements that it is recommended students adhere to. First the counselor must agree to attend initial training for the school-based clinic so that the faculty can assure a level of competence in working in schools. Weekly supervision is also requirement for students in programs accredited by the Council for Accreditation for Counseling and Related Educational Programs (. They must commit to a weekly schedule during school hours. Many students are interested in such programs, but they have full time jobs and as such may not be able to participate in the clinic, the availability of the elementary school students may conflict with a job schedule. It has been the experience of the authors that most schools operation from 8:00am to 3:00pm, which will conflict with a graduate students schedule if they work from 8:00am to 5:00pm.as it will need clinicians available from 8:00am to 3:00pm in most circumstances. Finally, students must be willing to commit to regular communication with school staff and submitting to the authority of school professionals.

ETHICAL ISSUES

Like with any clinical practice, one must be cautious of potential ethical violations, the same is true when developing a play therapy clinic within a school setting. One of the first couple of things to consider is ensuring that your policies and procedures are HIPPA and FERPA compliant. Several other specific areas of concern in our experience is confidentiality, the informed consent process, and the nature of mandatory reporting. Our hope is to highlight several of the essential problem areas we have experience when working in the school setting.

Confidentiality

The understanding and use of confidentiality from the school perspective can look quite different that the way mental health provider (Trice-Black, Riechel, & Shillingford, 2013). Therefore being very clear with the all school personal about the importance of confidentiality is imperative. Because the process of establishing a play therapy clinic in the school requires multiple school personal (teachers, school counselors, administrative staff, teachers aids, and staff) providing them with the necessary information to aid in the clinic Information in the school in essential. However, being provided with the details of a child's session or even knowing the child is attending services could be a breach of confidentiality. One must ensure that only the necessary information is shared in in conjunction with the coordination of services and the safely of the child.

In order for a play based therapy clinic to survive in a school, several individuals may play a role in the coordination of care. In order to have the clinic running, a point person leading the project should be established. This person should serve as the go between for the clinic to the school. It also helps to establish a contact person at the school that can ensure that the needs of the clinic are served. In the past we have found that the school counselor can server this role or an administrator at the school. This go to person usually serves as a liaison between you and the other school staff. They often help with the creation of schedules, the forwarding of consent forms, and the coordination of sending home and collection of information packets/assessments. In an attempt to keep things confidential packets are labeled as such with a return address to the liaison.

To further describe the importance of confidentiality, the play therapist will not discuss individual child clients with any school staff unless explicitly asked. To do so, the therapist would need a documented release of information. This can be frustrating to the school staff as they are often wanting information to aid in that child's academic success. With those releases we frequently will obtain information from teachers about how the child is doing in the classroom, and even discuss potential strategies to help the child in the room. But the child's activity in the playroom is never discussed to anyone with the exception of the child's legal guardians, the play therapist's supervisor, and the school counselor.

Informed Consent

One cannot stress enough the importance of obtaining informed consent. This sometimes can be a little tricky when working in the school setting. In the school setting the play therapy clinic may or may not have access to the students' academic records and consent forms are often sent home for a caregiver to sign. However, there are times when the caregiver at home may or may not be the custodial guardian who is able to grant the permission for the child to receive psychological services. This is why it is vital to have a member on your team or have a partnership with the school counselor or other school official who can obtain access to the school records to verify if the caregiver who signed the consent form is in fact listed in the school documents as the legal guardian.

One aspect of informed consent that is essential to the school based clinic is the approval for recordings. In the collaborations in which we have set up play therapy clinics in schools we have mandated the recording of all play sessions, it is not only helpful as it serves as a document of what occurred in session in but is also as it has aided our students in the process of supervision, and has helped the supervisors have a better picture of what was happening in session. Having direct statements about the requirement of sessions being recorded along with outlining the use of the recordings in not only necessary but ethically sound practice, here is what such a statement might look like. "The play sessions will be videotaped. The research team will observe the videotapes to ensure the quality of the study and to aid in the quality of services. All recordings will be destroyed at the end of this study. Student therapists will only have access to the recording initially at the school in which the recording took place. They will then turn in recording to the investigators, who will store them in a locked cabinet. These recordings are to be destroyed by shredding disks and the reformatting of flash drives at the end of the study."

Mandatory Reporting

When working with children as a professional counselor one must report to the appropriate authorities is an allegation is made (Barrett, Lester, & Durham, 2011). Being a collaborator at a school based clinic is no different. However, we mentioned earlier that we are a guest in the school. So finding out their policies and procedures as to how they handle contacting the appropriate authorities is recommended. Each school has unique policies and procedures when it comes to mandated reporting.

When a child makes an allegation in the playroom after the session, we require the play therapist to immediately contact the director of the clinic. There is then a meeting to observe the recording. After this consultation meeting, a report will be made in 48 hrs (which may vary depending upon state laws).. Some schools request that the report be made in conjunction with the school counselor; others have preferred that the clinic make the report independently. The key here is to make the report while also meeting the preferences of the school.

On-Site Supervision

Another issue to address for a school-based collaboration clinic is how to handle the issue of on-site supervision. Sometimes emergent issues present themselves and the student counselor may not be able to address without help form a supervisor. Two major issues for the collaboration clinic must be addressed: (1) Under what circumstances a supervisor should be consulted and (2) Who will serve as the on-site supervisor.

One of the challenges for a beginning counselor is that they may lack awareness about what they can and cannot handle on their own. What follows is a discussion about situations which commonly might call for an on-site supervisor consultation. However, it is important to note that schools tend to dynamic environments in which new and challenging circumstances occur and as such no list of events that would trigger the need for on-site supervision will ever be comprehensive.

The general principle of what constitutes the need for consultation with the on-site supervisor are situations which involve a time-sensitive response and those which directly impact the emotional and physical health of the child. The first and foremost example would include interactions with a child that raise the suspicion of physical or sexual abuse. Other situations which might be a cause for on-site supervision would be when a child is dysregulated to a degree to which the child is either disruptive or unable to engage in academic work.

The second issue, who serves as the on-site supervisor has a variety of answers and which solution is the best will depend on the personnel resources you have available. One option is for the school counselor to serve as the on-site supervisor. The advantage to this is that it requires no extra personnel to be assigned to the clinic. The down-side is that it creates more work for the school counselor. As well, school counselors might not always be reachable, as they may be in meetings, sessions, or guidance sessions.

Another option is to have a faculty-member who is associated with the collaborative clinic always available by phone. Faculty members associated with the clinic would block time during which they know they would always be available by phone and be able to help address any issues the clinician might have. The benefits to this arrangement are that it does not require the faculty to be physically present all the time and frees them up for other duties. As well, the counselor will be able to contact them without changing locations, which can be helpful. The downsides would be that if physical presence is required, it would be minimally helpful and it requires vigilance regarding making sure that one's phone is always charged, turned on, and answered.

A final solution would be using doctoral students to engage in block supervision. This would require the presence of a doctoral counseling program in which the students are being trained in clinical supervision. In this particular, model, the supervisors are provided graduate level education in supervision and then sign up for blocks of time to be physically present to address any concerns the student counselors may have. The positive aspect of this model is that it provides a mutual benefit to the student counselor and the supervisor. The challenge is that it requires a doctoral program and buy-in from the program to require students to engage in supervision practice.

CONCLUSION

In conclusion, while the development of a collaborative university/school district play therapy clinic can be tricky, it is also extremely valuable. A clinic of this nature can meet the needs of under-served at-risk children while also diminishing the stress placed on the shoulders of the school counselor. The process of developing such a clinic involves several factors such as finding the right school, developing a collaborative relationship with the school, developing a research agenda that is favorable to both the university and the school district, maintaining a program, and avoiding ethical pitfalls.

REFERENCES

American School Counseling Association. (2014). *State-by-state student-to-counselor ratio report 10 year trends.* Retrieved from https://www.schoolcounselor.org/asca/media/asca/Publications/ratioreport.pdf

American School Counseling Association. (2017). *The school counseling and comprehensive school counseling programs position statement.* Retrieved from https://www.schoolcounselor.org/asca/media/asca/PositionStatements/PS_ComprehensivePrograms.pdf

Barrett, K. M., Lester, S. V., & Durham, J. C. (2011). Child maltreatment and the advocacy role of professional school counselors. *Journal for Social Action in Counseling and Psychology*, *3*(2), 86–103.

Council for Accreditation of Counseling and Related Educational Programs. (2016). *2016 CACREP standards*. Retrieved from CACREP website: http://www.cacrep.org/wp-content/uploads/2017/08/2016-Standards-with-citations.pdf

DeKruyf, L., Auger, R., & Trice-Black, S. (2013). The role of school counselors in meeting students' mental health needs: Examining issues of professional identity. *Professional School Counseling*, *16*(5), 271–282. doi:10.1177/2156759X0001600502

Dollarhide, C. T., Smith, A. T., & Lemberger, M. E. (2007). Critical incidents in the development of supportive principals: Facilitating school counselor-principal relationships. *Professional School Counseling, 10*(4).

Hill, N. E., & Torres, K. (2010). Negotiating the American dream: The paradox of aspirations and achievement among Latino students and engagement between their families and schools. *The Journal of Social Issues*, *66*(1), 95–112. doi:10.1111/j.1540-4560.2009.01635.x

Jandorf, L., Gutierrez, Y., Lopez, J., Christie, J., & Itzkowitz, S. H. (2005). Use of a patient navigator to increase colorectal cancer screening in an urban neighborhood health clinic. *Journal of Urban Health*, *82*(2), 216–224. doi:10.1093/jurban/jti046 PMID:15888638

Kao, S. C., & Landreth, G. L. (1997). Evaluating the impact of child-centered play therapy training. *International Journal of Play Therapy*, *6*(2), 1–20. doi:10.1037/h0089405

Kimberlin, C. L., & Winterstein, A. G. (2008). Validity and reliability of measurement instruments used in research. *American Journal of Health-System Pharmacy*, *65*(23), 2276–2284. doi:10.2146/ajhp070364 PMID:19020196

Muro, J., Stickely, V., Muro, L., Blanco, P., & Tsai, M. (2015). Considerations for elementary schools and university collaborations: A guide to implementing counseling research. *The Journal of Research Administration*, *46*(1), 102–117.

Pallant, J. (2016). *SPSS Survival Manual*. London, UK: Open University Press.

Ray, D. C., Minton, C. A. B., Schottelkorb, A. A., & Brown, A. G. (2010). Single-case design in child counseling research: Implications for counselor education. *Counselor Education and Supervision*, *49*(3), 193–208. doi:10.1002/j.1556-6978.2010.tb00098.x

Ray, D. C., & Schottelkorb, A. A. (2010). Single-case design: A primer for play therapists. *International Journal of Play Therapy, 19*(1), 39–53. doi:10.1037/a0017725

Ruff, W. G., & Shoho, A. R. (2005). Understanding instructional leadership through the mental models of three elementary school principals. *Educational Administration Quarterly, 41*(3), 554–577. doi:10.1177/0013161X04269621

Trice-Black, S., Riechel, M. E. K., & Shillingford, M. (2013). School Counselors' Constructions of Student Confidentiality. *Journal of School Counseling, 11*(12), n12.

Van Velsor, P., & Orozco, G. L. (2007). Involving low-income parents in the schools: Community centric strategies for school counselors. *Professional School Counseling, 11*(1).

Chapter 7
Social Justice and Advocacy in University-Based Play Therapy Training Clinics

Emily C. Brown
University of Missouri – St. Louis, USA

Emily Oliveira
University of Missouri – St. Louis, USA

ABSTRACT

This chapter examines how university training programs and clinics can help play therapists develop social justice advocacy competency. Developing social justice advocacy can help play therapists understand social inequalities and oppressive systems, experience empathy with clients, and integrate advocacy action into their work. Training programs can help facilitate social justice advocacy for students through curriculum focus, service learning, and continuing education opportunities that promote awareness and empathy. Play therapy services offered in university clinics also offer opportunities for interns to increase understanding of social justice advocacy through client interactions and clinical supervision. Clinic directors promote social justice advocacy through managing just organization procedures and coordinating advocacy and outreach initiatives.

DOI: 10.4018/978-1-5225-8226-7.ch007

INTRODUCTION

According to the *Play Therapy Best Practices: Clinical, Professional, & Ethical Issues* published by the Association for Play Therapy (APT, 2016), training programs should include a focus on diversity issues. This is imperative as play therapists are serving increasingly diverse clients. Currently, almost half of children in the United States are racial and ethnic minorities, and it is estimated that more than 64% of children will be from racial and ethnic minorities by 2060 (Colby & Ortman, 2015). Mental health practitioners need cultural competence to respond to the needs of children and families in an increasingly diverse society, and the need for multicultural play therapy has been addressed in the play therapy literature (e.g., Davis & Pereira, 2014; O'Connor, 2005).

In addition to developing multicultural competence, mental health practitioners provide social justice advocacy to better serve clients. This is an intentional practice of seeking to meet the needs of disenfranchised clients based on an awareness of privilege, social inequality, and oppressive systems. Social justice advocacy can help clinicians understand and address the effects of social equalities and oppression on well-being. One framework for the integration of multiculturalism and social justice is provided in the Multicultural and Social Justice Counseling Competencies endorsed by the American Counseling Association (ACA; Ratts, Singh, Nassar-McMillan, Butler, & McCullough, 2015, 2016). To facilitate the development of these competencies, mental health training programs are tasked with providing education and supervision for mental health practitioners (Ratts et al., 2016). Play therapy training programs also need to provide multicultural training and awareness for play therapists on issues of diversity and social justice (Parikah, Ceballos & Post, 2013). Specifically, Parikah and colleagues (2013) recommended play therapists engage in "empathy training, activities that increase dialogue and immersion, the use of case studies, and role play . . . to increase their empathy and challenge their [belief in a just world], which may lead to an increase in their [social justice advocacy]" (p. 250). Parikh and colleagues (2013) suggested social justice advocacy attitudes could help play therapists enhance empathy in relationships with children and integrate advocacy into their work.

Despite recognition of the need for social justice advocacy training for play therapists, APT's (2016) guidelines have little to no information on advocacy, outreach, or social justice work. Therefore, this chapter provides university based play therapy training clinics with information on furthering social justice advocacy competencies in training programs with recommendations for training, clinical services, advocacy, and outreach efforts.

TRAINING PLAY THERAPISTS FOR SOCIAL JUSTICE ADVOCACY

Mental health practitioners recognize cultural competence and social justice as components of ethical practice (ACA, 2014; APA, 2017; NASW, 2017). Social justice includes understanding issues of oppression, privilege, and equality and taking social action for equity (Lee, 2012). Mental health practitioners use this understanding to provide social justice counseling considering "the impact of oppression, privilege, and discrimination on the mental health of the individual with the goal of establishing equitable distribution of power and resources through social advocacy" (Chang, Creather, & Ratts, 2010, p. 84). These principles and practices are rooted in a belief in a just world where all people have access to resources needed for physical and mental health. This professional call for social justice is embodied through advocacy actions with and for clients at various systemic levels.

To prepare mental health practitioners for multicultural and social justice counseling, training programs need to increase students' self-awareness, knowledge, and skills to take action (Ratts et al., 2016). Training that encourages advocacy action may be particularly salient given potential gaps between social justice advocacy perceptions and practice. Steele, Bischof, and Craig (2014) found many counselors believed social justice advocacy was important but fewer reported engaging in social justice advocacy action. Therefore, additional professional development and training may be needed to prepare mental health practitioners for advocacy action. Play therapy training programs can help address this through curriculum and continuing education. All of these training efforts help prepare students for clinical work in a university based play therapy training clinic and in future practice.

Graduate Coursework

Play therapists can develop social justice advocacy perceptions and practices when engaged in classroom instruction across the curriculum. Providing opportunities for reflection, experiential learning, and application helps students develop as social and advocacy-oriented practitioners (Hill, Harrawood, Vereen, & Doughty, 2012). To facilitate knowledge on counseling children in the training curriculum, instructors are encouraged to include case study examples of children. Instructors can also help play therapy students gain knowledge through a systems approach to client conceptualization and treatment planning. As students reflect on case examples, they should consider experiences of oppression, ecological factors, and therapeutic needs for children and families.

Even in classes that traditionally focus on adult clients, instructors could help play therapists develop social advocacy by incorporating examples of the impact of parental behaviors or mental illness on children and families. For example, discussing parental addiction and incarceration in an addictions course can help foster students' advocacy knowledge and skills when providing play therapy for families with these experiences. Case examples in psychopathology or diagnostic courses can include childhood examples of mental illness. Infusing discussions of childhood adversity and trauma across coursework can help play therapists gain perspective on systemic barriers and marginalization experiences connected to discrimination, poverty, homelessness, immigration, or mental illness. Also, students should develop an understanding of inequities in educational settings to more fully understand systemic barriers faced by school-age clients. Students should be encouraged to reflect on their developing awareness through class discussions and journaling for increased personal insight and growth.

Play therapy training programs offer play therapy specific coursework, such as Introduction to Play Therapy or Advanced Play Therapy courses. Assignments in these courses offer opportunities for experiential learning to develop multicultural and social justice counseling skills. APT (2010) provides a sample syllabus of an introductory play therapy course that recommends teaching practices in the course that help students "1) become and remain aware of their own cultural backgrounds, influences, and biases . . ., 2) acquire and continuously seek knowledge about how cultural backgrounds, influences, and biases operate in the lives of their clients, and 3) demonstrate culturally-appropriate therapeutic skills" (p. 3). These guidelines demonstrate the process of developing cultural competency. Within an introductory course, students can reflect on the influence of their culture on personal childhood play, cultural and diversity considerations when selecting materials for the playroom, and cultural implications when working with children experiencing adversity and oppression. Reflective practices in the course should help play therapy students explore biases and assumptions that can hinder empathy (Parikh et al., 2013). Students should also have opportunities for experiential learning, such as role play and providing practice play sessions with a "normal" child (APT, 2010). With this work, play therapy students could also reflect on cultural influences in the relationship established with the child and have opportunities to practice clinical conceptualizations from a systems perspective to prepare for social advocacy.

To help play therapists develop a systems perspective, graduate instructors can introduce Ecosystemic Play Therapy (O'Connor, 2016). Ecosystemic Play Therapy is a metatheory that requires play therapists to recognize and respond to the contextual systems of the child and family. This approach could help play therapists learn to consider how the child's presenting problems are linked to difficulties in various systemic levels (e.g., individual, caregiver, school, community, medical, judicial) and to develop treatment goals that meet client needs in these systems. Within this approach, students should be taught appropriate advocacy roles and personal and professional boundaries (O'Connor, 2016). Introducing this content and systems perspective can help play therapists understand the impact of various systems on children and learn to intervene for and with clients for social justice and advocacy work.

Graduate coursework in filial therapy is also recommended in university play therapy training to prepare play therapists for social justice advocacy work with families. Indeed, the preface for Landreth and Bratton's (2006) filial training text states mental health professionals must "empower parents to become therapeutic agents with their own children" (p. viii). Filial therapy has been implemented with families from diverse racial and cultural groups and with various presenting problems. For example, research supports filial therapy interventions with various trauma histories, including abuse (Costas & Landreth, 1999), family violence (Smith & Landreth, 2003), parental incarceration (Harris & Landreth, 1997), and foster care (Carnes-Holt & Bratton, 2014). These vulnerable children with trauma histories are often involved with child welfare and social service agencies, and play therapists need an understanding of these experiences and systems for social justice advocacy. Teaching filial therapy approaches to play therapists provides them with advocacy skills and knowledge that can be used to equip and empower caregivers with needed support and resources.

Service learning offers another opportunity to prepare play therapists for social justice counseling and advocacy through application of play therapy skills. Service learning should provide volunteer service opportunities in the community that are beneficial to participants and students (Baggerly, 2006). In addition, service learning activities include reflective practices for students to synthesize learning across contexts. Parikh et al. (2013) suggested activities that increase immersion could help play therapists develop empathy and gain new perspectives towards social justice advocacy. Several examples of play therapy service learning opportunities are found in the literature. These include play therapy at a federally funded preschool (Thanasiu, Rust, & Walter, 2018), play therapy at an elementary school with a play buddy program (Smith-Adcock et al., 2012), group play therapy services at an after-school care center (Baggerly, 2006), and an 8-week filial group for urban preschool parents (VanderGast, Post, & Kascsak-Miller, 2010). Graduate students provided play and filial services for high poverty children and families in each of these service learning examples. These examples highlight the mutually beneficial design of service learning activities that promote student learning and meet community needs. When designing service learning opportunities, course instructors and clinic directors should infuse social justice advocacy opportunities within communities where no cost play therapy services may be most needed.

Continuing Education

Universities can also provide play therapy training through continuing education opportunities. Since play therapists need continuing education in multicultural issues (APT, 2016), university based play therapy training clinics can offer training and help develop social justice competency for play therapists working in the community. For example, training clinics can host a summer play therapy conference. At the conference, affiliated program faculty can provide play therapy professional development for school counselors and community partners. Professional development with a social justice focus could include education on using play therapy to foster resilience for children and families from diverse cultural backgrounds or on advocacy approaches given disproportionate rates of adverse childhood experiences for children of color and children living in poverty (Sacks & Murphy, 2018). Clinic directors should use their awareness of community needs to inform topics of focus. For example, community needs assessments (such as those conducted by the United Way or other non-profit agencies) may highlight mental health or wellness needs of children and families. Clinic directors could connect professional development to this data to help mental health practitioners and play therapists respond to community needs. These efforts help integrate social justice and advocacy into professional development offered by the university based play therapy training clinic.

PROVIDING PLAY THERAPY SERVICES

Play therapy training clinic directors seek to provide exceptional clinical training experiences for students and play therapy services for clients. Promoting social justice advocacy in the play therapy training clinic involves careful reflection on organizational procedures and clinical supervision practices that affect the learning and experiences for students and clients.

Organizational Procedures

When providing play therapy services in a university based play therapy training clinic, one strategy for promoting social justice advocacy is to provide services at an affordable rate or through a sliding scale. Providing services using a sliding scale fee is common practice in university training centers (Aubrey, Hunsley, Josephson, & Vito, 2000). The sliding scale fee is typically set based on the client's income and number of people in the household. When clinics offer services at a reduced rate or pro bono, they enable access to play therapy for marginalized populations without creating a financial barrier. University based counseling clinics or play therapy training clinics often serve populations that belong to a lower socioeconomic social class bracket. When fees for services are adjusted to a level that is commensurate with the client or families' ability to pay, client attendance and outcome are not impacted (Clark & Kimberly, 2014). Some practitioners may argue against setting differential or sliding scale fees; however, the literature suggests that differential fees set according to income do not influence client attendance (Clark & Kimberly, 2014) or treatment outcomes (Aubrey et al., 2000) in any way. Therefore, offering a differential fee scale is a social justice approach to alleviate a financial burden to play therapy services for some clients.

Some strategies for supplementing fees in a university based play therapy clinic for clients with limited access to financial resources or in rural communities include eliciting gift funding from donors, applying for grant funding at the local, regional, state or federal level, or developing agreements with state agencies. Gift funding can be elicited by reaching out to the university foundation or advancement office as well as alumni from graduate programs. Previous or current faculty may be additional sources of gift funding to support play therapy services for low-income families in the training clinic. Clinic directors can also apply for grants from agencies such as the department of Health and Human Services, local and state Mental Health Boards, professional organizations, or private foundations to supplement fees for play therapy services in a university based training center. Finally, some state agencies such as Child Protective Services, departments of Child and Family Services, or state or local programs for children with disabilities may be able to support children by paying for play therapy services at a university based play therapy training clinic. Clinic directors can reach out to these partners and organizations to establish funding agreements, and this is a social justice advocacy approach given the potential to reduce financial barriers to play therapy services.

Clinic directors should also ensure play rooms at the clinic have diverse toys and toys that represent a variety of potential life experiences for children who may have experienced trauma (O'Connor, 2005). This is needed in social justice play therapy given disproportionate rates of adverse childhood experiences experienced by children of color and children living in poverty (Sacks & Murphy, 2018). For example, play rooms can include handcuffs, police cars, guns, and phones when working with children of incarcerated parents or victims of crime (Brown & Gibbons, 2018). Play rooms can be equipped with ethnically diverse dolls, foods, and dress up clothes to allow for expression for children of any culture (Davis & Pereira, 2014). Understanding individuals within their contexts and environments is a component of multicultural and social justice counseling (Ratts et al., 2016), so playrooms should be equipped with various toys connected to the child's related systems levels (O'Connor, 2016). Play therapy training clinic directors can help ready playroom materials for interns by considering diverse experiences of potential clients.

Before the intake session, clinic directors can develop culturally responsive organizational procedures that respect the diverse needs of clients. Culturally competent organizational procedures include offering cultural skills training for the administrative staff answering the phones in the training clinic, asking caregivers about therapist expectations and preferences, and offering intake forms in other languages (Whealin & Ruzek, 2008). Care must be taken in university play therapy training clinics to match children with play therapists with the experience and training to connect with diverse children and families. For example, if a child with a disability is referred to the training clinic for play therapy services, best practice would suggest that the child be matched with a practitioner who has experience or training in working with individuals with disabilities. Altogether, play therapists should be actively considering how diversity is connected to the experiences of the child and caregivers. It is important for children and caregivers to trust the play therapist's appreciation for the client's culture. Clinic directors can ensure multicultural training is a prerequisite for clinical experiences.

Clinical Skills and Supervision

Training clinics are likely the initial setting where graduate students provide play therapy services for actual clients. Therefore, interns will be providing play therapy with varying levels of competence and familiarity related to diverse demographic factors (e.g., ethnicity, nationality, religious orientation). For example, play therapists may have an initial encounter with children who are refugees in the university training clinic. In this scenario, play therapy interns should consider personal assumptions or perceptions about refugee status, build knowledge on the potential refugee experiences of oppression and advocacy needs faced by children and families, and review the literature on play therapy with refugee populations (e.g., Schottelkorb, Doumas, & Garcia, 2012) to apply this knowledge and skills with clients. All of this clinical work should be done with an awareness of social justice advocacy.

Evaluating clinical skill development is a crucial component of university play therapy training connected to clinical services. As students provide play therapy services in university clinics, instructors and supervisors must provide feedback on their clinical skills. One approach to documenting skill development is through a skills checklist form to provide formative and summative evaluation data. Training programs can include social justice advocacy skills on these program checklists to monitor the development of these skills.

Social justice advocacy competencies for play therapists include skills and actions needed for working with and on behalf of individuals, family systems, institutions, communities, and beyond (Ratts et al., 2015). Examples of these competencies are included in the Multicultural and Social Justice Counseling Competencies (Ratts et al., 2015). However, many of the recommended social justice focused conversations are beyond the scope of children receiving play therapy, so conceptualizing these competencies for play therapists requires using a family systems approach to clinical services. Ackerman (2017) provided a model for integrating social justice advocacy in child welfare that may prove helpful to play therapists when working with marginalized populations. Based on these recommendations, specific competencies for social justice advocacy should include the ability to initiate conversations with guardians about ways "culture, stereotypes, prejudice, discrimination, power, privilege, and oppression" may influence presenting problems and counseling relationships (Ratts et al., 2015, p. 11). Play therapists should be ready to explore with guardians the relationships children have with family, friends, and peers. Play therapists also need skills to empower children and caregivers to identify supportive adults at school, daycare, or other relevant settings who can address inequities in those settings (Ratts et al., 2015). Play therapists may need to provide information for supervisors to be able to evaluate competency for social justice advocacy skills as some of these actions may occur during phone consultations rather than video recorded sessions in the clinic.

All interns providing play therapy in the training clinic receive clinical supervision from an individual trained in supervision methods and skills. Clinic directors and affiliated program faculty often provide supervision for play therapists or for doctoral student supervisors who provide supervision for interns. Ideally, supervisors should have play therapy knowledge and experience to supervise play therapy interns in the university play therapy training clinic. Offering group supervision from a Registered Play Therapist-Supervisor (RPT-S) is recommended if individual supervisors are not trained in play therapy. Supervisors help play therapy interns understand privilege, marginalization, and the need for establishing supportive relationships with culturally diverse children, families, and communities (Ratts et al., 2016). Additionally, multiculturally competent play therapy supervision provides space for supervisors and supervisees to explore personal culture and views on play in a supportive environment (Drewes, 2008).

One model of social justice supervision recommends supervisors engage supervisees in Goodyear's (2014) pedagogical processes of modeling, feedback, direct instruction, and self-directed learning in each of three key areas: supervisory power relations, reflective practice, and advocacy skills (Asakura & Maurer, 2018). To foster the development of social justice advocacy, play therapy clinical supervisors should directly address issues of culture and power in the supervisory dyad, discuss supervisee's values and biases that influence perceptions and advocacy behaviors, and explore strengths and areas for growth as advocates (Glosoff & Durham, 2010). Additionally, supervisors can use questionnaires or structured measures, such as the Social Justice Advocacy Scale (Dean, 2009) and Social Justice Scale

(SJS; Torres-Harding, Siers, & Olson, 2012), to help play therapists explore social justice advocacy readiness and reactions to such instruments (Glosoff & Durham, 2010; Parikh et al., 2013). Play therapy supervisors help prepare play therapists to be social justice advocates.

ADVOCACY AND OUTREACH EFFORTS

There is a strong need for advocacy and outreach efforts in university based play therapy training clinics in order to both advocate for play therapy services and to advocate for marginalized populations. Advocacy involves using one's voice or standing to institute change (Wright & Jaffe, 2014). Advocacy is important in all aspects of mental health training, particularly when serving children who often lack the platform and power to change oppressive systems that are affecting them (Wright & Jaffe, 2014). Clinic directors have various ways in which they coordinate and provide social justice advocacy through promoting access to play therapy services, establishing community partnerships, and modeling best practices for child advocacy.

University programs increase access to play therapy services in school and clinical settings across their communities through the training of future play therapists. Social advocacy includes ensuring clients are aware of and have access to services within social institutions. University based play therapy training clinics provide access to services for clients when social institutions do not have a trained play therapist. Therefore, clinic directors should work to make other mental health providers aware of the play therapy services offered at the clinic. Clinic directors can promote awareness of services for marginalized populations by ensuring stakeholders have information about the training clinic and play therapy services. Providing flyers about play therapy services to local schools and non-profit agencies, such as those serving children and families experiencing poverty, neighborhood violence, relocation, or parental absence, may help disenfranchised families know about available low-cost play therapy services in the university training clinic.

Child Advocacy Efforts

Successful child advocacy includes efforts that seek to institute a positive change for children (Wright & Jaffe, 2014). There are different levels of advocacy depending on the population or system of professional focus. Advocacy for a particular child or small group of children is considered micro or case advocacy. Play therapists may engage in this advocacy by becoming an advocate for a child in a classroom or helping a guardian seek changes for their child. Community or group based advocacy is known as mezzo advocacy (Wright & Jaffe, 2014). Examples of mezzo level advocacy include leading a training on trauma for all educators in a school setting or advocating for a community through work at a university based play therapy training center. Advocates that work at the macro level seek to address a concern that affects a large group at the state, national, or international level. Before engaging in advocacy, it is important for clinic directors to identify end goals to appropriately identify advocacy targets (Wright & Jaffe, 2014).

Once a problem or concern has been identified for advocacy, clinic directors can determine resources necessary for an advocacy plan. The development of a coalition of allies is one way to help distribute the workload of advocacy within the organization and to recruit other professionals to help with the project. This could take the form of a board or committee, and is typically an alliance of individuals, organizations, or other like-minded individuals who are acting towards a common goal (Wright & Jaffe, 2014). Play therapy training clinic directors could be involved with a regional coalition of child and family mental health providers. Such groups could meet monthly or quarterly to discuss trends and support social change in the community. If seeking to start a coalition, clinic directors should identify potential partners (e.g., partnering school counselors, referral agency staff, program alumni, play therapists, and other faculty) and develop objectives for the coalition.

Elements of child advocacy include engaging allies, utilizing media, and blending micro and macro advocacy to institute change (Wright & Jaffe, 2014). Although there are various approaches to child advocacy described in the literature, organizational advocacy is the primary focus here given the scope of professional responsibilities for university based play therapy training clinic directors. Organization advocacy includes efforts by an individual within an organization (typically with a professional role) that aim to change practices for working with children or families.

Wright and Jaffe (2014) provided six steps for successful child advocacy developed from their professional experiences and practice in child advocacy. Following is a description of each step and potential application of each organizational or political advocacy step for university based play therapy training clinic directors.

Step 1: Knowing Your Issue

Knowledge is power when it comes to advocacy. Individuals cannot advocate for a population or change without fully understanding and knowing the important aspects of the situation. Advocates should be able to effectively and succinctly describe the issue to stakeholders, decision makers, gatekeepers, and others directly involved (Wright & Jaffe, 2014). For play therapy training clinic directors, this step involves determining which level of advocacy is most relevant (e.g. micro or macro) and the specific needs of the clients and potential clients in the center. For example, play therapy training clinic directors can use community data to identify a need in the community for access to mental health care for marginalized populations, including children. Based on the evident needs in the community, play therapy training clinic directors could determine a need to provide filial therapy groups to underserved caregivers in financial need in the community at no cost.

Step 2: Research for Background and Impact

Step 1 and Step 2 go hand-in-hand since research is necessary in order to have knowledge on the issue. The research step involves systematically gathering information to support the advocacy plan and to educate others about the issue. It is important to not only research the background of the issue but also the impact change could have on the community. Research can take the form of surveys, focus groups, previous research studies, interviews, census data, or demographic data (Wright & Jaffe, 2014). Following the example from Step 1, this step would involve researching funding sources at the community, state, or federal level that target services for children and that support your advocacy plan. The clinic director or group may need to research funding opportunities that support services for children and families.

Step 3: Preparing Effective Materials

Once the issue has been identified and research has been gathered, organizational advocates can prepare materials to distribute the information to decision makers, gatekeepers, team members, and allies. The development of a summary sheet is a succinct way to distribute the information to key stakeholders (Wright & Jaffe, 2014). Information can be shared in a variety of ways, including email distribution, town hall meetings, social media, or focus groups. The way that information is shared is not as important as ensuring that key stakeholders receive the information (Wright & Jaffe, 2014). Continuing the example provided in previous steps, the clinic director could prepare funding proposals or letters of intent, including proposed budgets, requesting financial support for clinic services or materials and submit these to potential funders.

Step 4: Making Meetings That Work

Organizational advocates can next plan strategic meetings focused on accomplishing the advocacy plan. It is important that the individuals involved in the meetings are key stakeholders (i.e., decision makers or gatekeepers with access to decision makers) who can help put the advocacy plan steps into motion. It is during this step that the work from the previous steps will pay off, as advocates who are knowledge about the plan, have researched both the issue and the impact of the solution, and have developed effective materials will be more successful at making the meetings work (Wright & Jaffe, 2014). For this step, the play therapy training clinic director would schedule meetings with potential donors of funding sources to present the materials. They may also meet with potential partners in the community to strategically develop partnerships, including referral sources or agencies that provide similar services.

Step 5: Conducting Strategic Follow-Up

In order to stay on the radar of decision makers and gatekeepers, organizational advocates must schedule strategic and appropriate follow-ups. Also, advocates need to understand the steps necessary for decision-making and action to reach the advocacy goals. Actions in this step include following up and providing updates to other key stakeholders, including fellow advocates and allies, on the progress of the project (Wright & Jaffe, 2014). Following the example, the clinic director could follow-up with the funding source on the decision of the funding or keep the funder appraised of the process of the application for funding or request for funding.

Step 6: Reinforcing Successful Advocacy Outcomes

Reaching step six implies that the advocacy plan has been either fully or partially successful. During this step the advocate works to ensure that lasting bonds are created with key stakeholders and that the advocacy project goals are reached. One way to maintain positive relationships with stakeholders is to thank them in a meaningful way. This could be as simple as a card or as elaborate as a press release. It is important to tactfully determine the appropriate way to thank stakeholders as some may require a public display of gratitude, via a press release or social media, while others may be embarrassed by such a public display and may wish to remain anonymous. It is imperative for future work together to determine the best way to recognize the key stakeholders for their work on the advocacy project (Wright & Jaffe, 2014). For example, play therapy training clinic directors may submit an announcement to the university marking team or campus news to publicize grant funding. Touting successes can generate awareness of play therapy clinical services and thank donors.

Altogether, these steps demonstrate the potential for university play therapy training clinic directors to engage in organizational advocacy within their roles and responsibilities. Training clinic directors may already be tasked with fundraising and developing community partnerships. Following these steps for child advocacy (Wright & Jaffe, 2014), university play therapy training clinic directors may be more cognizant of strategic social justice advocacy efforts that may expand play therapy services to marginalized children in the community.

Outreach Efforts

With awareness of the impact of oppressive systems on families and children, play therapy training programs and clinics may develop outreach efforts. Outreach efforts work to address the barriers experienced as a result of societal inequities while also highlighting the societal problems that impact children and families (Ratts et al., 2016). Clinic directors can further outreach efforts by integrating clinic services and programs into their local community. To help understand the needs of the community, clinic directors could invite members of the community to serve on the clinic's advisory board or could join community organizations. Another strategy for integrating the clinic into the community is to provide workshops or professional development opportunities to local educators, school counselors, or mental health providers. Clinic directors could also use the location of their clinic in the community to provide preventative outreach opportunities to families in the community. For example, directors could partner with local child care centers and preschools to provide outreach filial therapy groups for guardians to learn play therapy skills as a preventative and social justice strategy. Finally, training programs can work with schools and community mental health agencies to develop practicum or internship placements to provide play therapy services as center outreach and with center supervisors, especially in rural areas lacking supervisors with play therapy experience or the RPT-S credential.

Another example of how training clinics can facilitate outreach is through the development and use of mobile play therapy kits or portable play rooms. An example of this work occurred in Ferguson, Missouri as students and faculty provided a social justice outreach response by taking mobile sand trays and symbolic figurines into the community during a time of violence and community mourning (Bray, 2014). Students and faculty set up counseling tents to provide space for community members to talk and create scenes in sand trays, and community members were able to communicate their feelings and have space to be seen and heard. Community members were also provided information about free or low-cost counseling services in the university based training clinic or other local mental health agencies (Bray, 2014). This outreach work provided a way for students and faculty to be involved in social justice action in the community.

Finally, university based play therapy training clinics could coordinate play therapy outreach opportunities that offer mobile play therapy activities in the community. Outreach play therapy teams engage children and adults in brief play interventions, allow individuals opportunities for self-expression through play, and provide participants additional information about clinic services. Training clinics could assemble mobile play therapy kits with activities such as sand trays, story stones, or art making activities to engage individuals at community events or agencies. These mobile play therapy outreach efforts would require recruiting a team of students and faculty who have play therapy training. Ideally, the team members would be completing clinical coursework in the affiliated training program or be able to count the hours as direct client contact towards the Registered Play Therapist credential or licensure. It is important to ensure that all students and faculty interacting with individuals in the community on behalf of the clinic are carefully trained in play therapy and mobile play therapy techniques and under supervision while completing outreach interventions. To ensure appropriate outreach training, the training clinic director might host a targeted training for the team to learn the techniques that will be used. Potential settings where mobile play therapy outreach teams could have an outreach table or booth include back to school fairs at partnering schools, community mental health or health fairs, university sponsored events, and community events such as festivals with an area designated for children. Bringing play therapists from the clinic into the community increases visibility and access to services.

Case Example

Dr. Ana Griffin, Clinical Director of a university based play therapy center, was aware of the high rates of trauma exposure for children in a local school district that frequently hosted interns and employed graduates of the training program. Dr. Griffin met with school district administrators about available clinic services. Based on the mental health needs described by school district leaders, Dr. Griffin viewed expanding clinic play therapy services as a priority. Fitting with her professional role, she approached the steps to organizational child advocacy by gathering additional data from school district stakeholders (including administrators, counselors, teachers, and parents) about the needs of children. In addition to learning more about the prevalence of some trauma experiences, she learned that distance to the university clinic, transportation, and misinformation about mental health were reported barriers for services. With this knowledge, she researched grants that could expand play therapy services into schools during the school day to address distance and transportation concerns and prepared a funding proposal to purchase play therapy materials needed for expanding school-based services. Dr. Griffin also met with her advisory council and school district leaders to develop strategies for providing information about mental health to caregivers, and the team identified several outreach strategies, including running ads about the play therapy clinic in the local newspaper and hosting mental health focused parent workshops at schools, the library, and several churches across the region. The school leaders also planned to include professional development for teachers about mental health and provide teachers with strategies for talking about mental health concerns with caregivers during meetings or over the phone. Dr. Griffin organized a meeting with several community partners, including leaders from the county public health department, school district, child social services, and a few potential funding donors. At this strategic meeting, she presented demographic data on the community, mental health needs, strategies for addressing some of these needs, and a proposed budget. In the weeks following this successful meeting, she contacted donors and followed up with identified leaders on the various initiatives (e.g., workshops, professional development, advertising for clinic services). After six months, she secured a $10,000 donation to expand play therapy services in the schools and community. Dr. Griffin's leadership and partnerships with the school district stakeholders brought micro and mezzo level changes through increased play therapy services via interns at schools and affordable services at the university clinic. Also, this advocacy facilitated change for children and family systems as more caregivers received critical information about mental health through clinic outreach efforts.

IMPLICATIONS FOR CLINIC DIRECTORS

It is important to acknowledge these efforts to develop social justice advocacy take time and collaboration to implement. Although clinic directors may primarily interact with their program's graduate students in the clinic setting, the training for social justice advocacy work begins prior to clinical practice. Therefore, clinic directors need to build collaborative relationships with course instructors so that social advocacy is being promoted across the curriculum before play therapists see their first clients. To promote these efforts, clinic directors can share resources or ideas for class activities and service learning as outlined. Also, there may be varying attitudes and perceptions about the importance of professional social justice advocacy (Steele et al., 2014), so clinic directors may face resistance to proposed recommendations for a social justice advocacy curricular emphasis. Regardless, clinic directors can consider ways to partner with other faculty to further social justice advocacy before clinical interactions.

Clinic directors must also consider their resources and gather support for policy or practice changes in the clinic that further services to marginalized populations. Grounding these efforts in data is an important component of effective practice. Clinic directors could collect data (e.g., client demographic information, student perceptions of preparedness on social justice work, and clinic program evaluation data) to identify areas for social justice advocacy focus. Given the various responsibilities and demands on the clinic director's time, clinic directors may invite clinic workers or doctoral students to help plan play therapy continuing education events or organize outreach efforts at the onset of this work. Inviting doctoral students to help with these efforts also provides leadership and advocacy opportunities and can allow for easier implementation of large projects. Additionally, developing an advisory council that involves various stakeholders (e.g., community members, faculty, students, play therapist supervisors, representatives from partner agencies) provides guidance and accountability for social justice advocacy efforts as well as strengthens support for the training clinic. Involving these various stakeholders can help social justice advocacy development become a program initiative beyond the training clinic setting.

If serving marginalized children and families with a commitment to social justice advocacy, clinic directors need to be prepared for some of the barriers that may limit access or continuation of play therapy treatment. For instance, guardians may have difficulty arranging or bringing children for play therapy services due to access to transportation, communication methods, work schedules, language, or finances. With these barriers, clinic directors may notice premature termination of play therapy services. If clinic directors are committed to social justice advocacy, then they should consider how their clinic is accessible and approachable for diverse clients and families to potentially mitigate some of these barriers. There may need to be changes in policies and practices as clinic directors consider ways in which the play therapy training clinic can best serve marginalized populations.

Clinic directors are responsible for ensuring the best treatment for clients and optimal training experiences for play therapists. One training clinic procedure for monitoring client satisfaction with therapeutic services is using a self-report rating scale that measures client outcomes during therapy and the quality of the therapeutic alliance. Examples of these type of measures are the ORS (Outcome Rating Scale) and SRS (Session Rating Scale) (Duncan et al., 2003; Miller, Duncan, Brown, Sparks, & Claud, 2003). There are two versions of the rating scales designed for children (CORS/CSRS) and young children (YCORS/YCSRS). The CORS/CSRS has been normed for children ages 6 to 12 while the YCORS/YCSRS has been designed for children below 6 years of age (Bertolino, 2018). These evaluation procedures may need to be adapted when providing play therapy based on developmental level or other cultural factors of children. Given the developmental level of children, parents or guardians are likely better informants about child progress and behaviors outside of the playroom. If evaluation procedures are in use, clinic directors should review these report forms to monitor the effectiveness of play therapy for all clients.

Additionally, these types of evaluation procedures need to be considered from a social justice perspective. Ratts et al. (2016) outlined the importance of conceptualizing implications of power and oppression in the counseling relationship for various domains, including that of the privileged counselor and marginalized client. Regardless of theoretical approach to play therapy, there is an inherent power differential involved in play therapy given the play therapist's privilege of age, and many clients will have other marginalized identities. If using an evaluation procedure such as the CORS/CSRS or YCORS/YCSRS (Duncan et al., 2003; Miller et al., 2003) as a standard practice in the university training clinic, clinic directors should acknowledge that these evaluation forms may not provide accurate clinic data. Instead, they offer a tool for feedback that should be considered within a social justice paradigm. Children may not be ready or able to provide feedback about the work of the play therapist, and these types of procedures may not be congruent with the principles of some approaches to play therapy.

CONCLUSION

University based play therapy training clinics are critical settings for play therapist social justice advocacy development. Clinic directors can integrate social justice advocacy principles into the mission and work of the training clinic through play therapy training, clinical services, and outreach efforts. Just as suggested for play therapist social justice advocacy development, clinic directors can begin the process by reflecting on their personal social justice competence and advocacy action. Engaging in this reflective practice can help clinic directors determine priorities and create action plans for furthering the emphasis on social justice advocacy. Ultimately these efforts can help play therapists meet the needs of all children and families that can be served through university based play therapy training clinics.

REFERENCES

Ackerman, A. M. (2017). An integrated model for counselor social justice advocacy in child welfare. *The Family Journal (Alexandria, Va.)*, *25*(4), 389–397. doi:10.1177/1066480717736061

American Counseling Association. (2014). *ACA code of ethics*. Alexandria, VA: Author.

American Psychological Association. (2017). *Ethical principles of psychologists and code of conduct*. Washington, DC: Author.

Asakura, K., & Maurer, K. (2018). Attending to social justice in clinical social work: Supervision as a pedagogical space. *Clinical Social Work Journal*, *46*(4), 289–297. doi:10.100710615-018-0667-4

Association for Play Therapy. (2010). *Sample syllabus: Introductory graduate play therapy course*. Retrieved from https://cdn.ymaws.com/www.a4pt.org/resource/resmgr/Sample_Play_Therapy_Course_S.pdf

Association for Play Therapy. (2016). *Play therapy best practices: Clinical, professional & ethical issues*. Clovis, CA: Author.

Aubry, T. D., Hunsley, J., Josephson, G., & Vito, D. (2000). Quid pro quo: Fee for services delivered in a psychology training clinic. *Journal of Clinical Psychology*, *56*(1), 23–31. doi:10.1002/(SICI)1097-4679(200001)56:1<23::AID-JCLP3>3.0.CO;2-8 PMID:10661366

Baggerly, J. (2006). Service learning with children affected by poverty: Facilitating multicultural competence in counseling education students. *Journal of Multicultural Counseling and Development*, *34*(4), 244–255. doi:10.1002/j.2161-1912.2006.tb00043.x

Bertolino, B. (2018). *Effective counseling and psychotherapy: An evidence-based approach*. New York, NY: Springer. doi:10.1891/9780826141132

Bray, B. (2014, November 17). Storytelling and hope in Ferguson. *Counseling Today*. Retrieved from https://ct.counseling.org/2014/11/storytelling-and-hope-in-ferguson/

Brown, E. C., & Gibbons, M. M. (2018). Addressing needs of children of incarcerated parents with child-centered play therapy. *Journal of Child and Adolescent Counseling*, *4*(2), 134–145. doi:10.1080/23727810.2017.1381931

Carnes-Holt, K., & Bratton, S. C. (2014). The efficacy of child parent relationship therapy for adopted children with attachment disruptions. *Journal of Counseling and Development*, *92*(3), 328–337. doi:10.1002/j.1556-6676.2014.00160.x

Chang, C. Y., Crethar, H. C., Ratts, M. J., & Editors, G. (2010). Social justice: A national imperative for counselor education and supervision. *Counselor Education and Supervision*, *50*(2), 82–87. doi:10.1002/j.1556-6978.2010.tb00110.x

Clark, P., & Kimberly, C. (2014). Impact of fees among low-income clients in a training clinic. *Contemporary Family Therapy*, *36*(3), 363–368. doi:10.100710591-014-9303-9

Colby, S. L., & Ortman, J. M. (2015). *Projections of the size and composition of the U.S. population: 2014 to 2060, current population reports* (Report No. P25-1143). Washington, DC: U.S. Census Bureau.

Costas, M., & Landreth, G. (1999). Filial therapy with nonoffending parents of children who have been sexually abused. *International Journal of Play Therapy*, *8*(1), 43–66. doi:10.1037/h0089427

Davis, E., & Pereira, J. (2014). Child-centered play therapy: A creative approach to culturally competent counseling. *Journal of Creativity in Mental Health, 9*(2), 262–274. doi:10.1080/15401383.2014.892863

Dean, J. K. (2009). *Quantifying social justice advocacy competency: Development of the social justice advocacy scale* (Doctoral dissertation). Retrieved from http://digitalarchive.gsu.edu/cps_diss/40

Drewes, A. A. (2008). Culturally competent supervision of child and play therapists. In A. A. Drewes & J. A. Mullen (Eds.), *Supervision can be playful: Techniques for child and play therapist supervisors* (pp. 77–92). Lanham, MD: Jason Aronson.

Duncan, B. L., Miller, S. D., Sparks, J., Claud, D., Reynolds, L., Brown, J., & Johnson, L. (2003). The Session Rating Scale: Preliminary psychometric properties of a "working" alliance measure. *Journal of Brief Therapy, 3*, 3–12.

Glosoff, H. L., & Durham, J. C. (2010). Using supervision to prepare social justice counseling advocates. *Counselor Education and Supervision, 50*(2), 116–129. doi:10.1002/j.1556-6978.2010.tb00113.x

Goodyear, R. K. (2014). Supervision as pedagogy: Attending to its essential instructional and learning processes. *The Clinical Supervisor, 33*(1), 82–99. doi:10.1080/07325223.2014.918914

Harris, Z. L., & Landreth, G. L. (1997). Filial therapy with incarcerated mothers: A five week model. *International Journal of Play Therapy, 6*(2), 53–73. doi:10.1037/h0089408

Hill, N. R., Harrawood, L. K., Vereen, L. G., & Doughty, E. A. (2012). Advocacy training: Curriculum for professional and client advocacy. In C. C. Chang, C. A. Barrio Minton, A. L. Dixon, J. E. Meyers, & T. J. Sweeney (Eds.), *Professional counseling excellence through leadership and advocacy* (pp. 267–289). New York, NY: Routledge.

Landreth, G. L., & Bratton, S. C. (2006). *Child parent relationship therapy (CPRT): A 10-session filial therapy model*. New York, NY: Routledge.

Lee, C. C. (2012). Social justice as the fifth force in counseling. In C. C. Chang, C. A. Barrio Minton, A. L. Dixon, J. E. Meyers, & T. J. Sweeney (Eds.), *Professional counseling excellence through leadership and advocacy* (pp. 109–120). New York, NY: Routledge.

Miller, S. D., Duncan, B. L., Brown, J., Sparks, J., & Claud, D. (2003). The Outcome Rating Scale: A preliminary study of the reliability, validity, and feasibility of a brief visual analog measure. *Journal of Brief Therapy*, *2*, 91–100.

National Association of Social Workers. (2017). *Code of ethics*. Washington, DC: Author.

O'Connor, K. (2005). Addressing diversity issues in play therapy. *Professional Psychology, Research and Practice*, *36*(5), 566–573. doi:10.1037/0735-7028.36.5.566

O'Connor, K. (2016). Ecosystemic play therapy. In K. J. O'Connor, C. E. Schaefer, & L. D. Braverman (Eds.), *Handbook of play therapy* (2nd ed.; pp. 195–225). Hoboken, NJ: Wiley.

Parikh, S. B., Ceballos, P., & Post, P. (2013). Factors related to play therapists' social justice advocacy attitudes. *Journal of Multicultural Counseling and Development*, *41*(4), 240–253. doi:10.1002/j.2161-1912.2013.00039.x

Ratts, M. J., Singh, A. A., Nassar-McMillan, S., Butler, S. K., & McCullough, J. R. (2015). *Multicultural and social justice counseling competencies*. Retrieved from https://www.counseling.org/docs/default-source/competencies/multicultural-and-social-justice-counseling-competencies.pdf?sfvrsn=8573422c_20

Ratts, M. J., Singh, A. A., Nassar-McMillan, S., Butler, S. K., & McCullough, J. R. (2016). Multicultural and social justice counseling competencies: Guidelines for the counseling profession. *Journal of Multicultural Counseling and Development*, *44*(1), 28–48. doi:10.1002/jmcd.12035

Sacks, V., & Murphey, D. (2018, February). *The prevalence of adverse childhood experiences, nationally, by state, and by race/ethnicity* (Research Brief #2018-03). Retrieved from https://www.childtrends.org/wp-content/uploads/2018/02/ACESBrief_ChildTrends_February2018.pdf

Schottelkorb, A. A., Doumas, D. M., & Garcia, R. (2012). Treatment for childhood refugee trauma: A randomized, controlled trial. *International Journal of Play Therapy*, *21*(2), 57–73. doi:10.1037/a0027430

Smith, N., & Landreth, G. (2003). Intensive filial therapy with child witnesses of domestic violence: A comparison with individual and sibling group play therapy. *International Journal of Play Therapy*, *12*(1), 67–88. doi:10.1037/h0088872

Smith-Adcock, S., Davis, E., Pereira, J., Allen, C., Socarras, K., Bodurtha, K., & Smith-Bonahue, T. (2012). Preparing to play: A qualitative study of graduate students' reflections on learning play therapy in an elementary school. *International Journal of Play Therapy*, *21*(2), 100–115. doi:10.1037/a0026931

Steele, J. M., Bischof, G. H., & Craig, S. E. (2014). Political ideology and perceptions of social justice advocacy among members of the American Counseling Association. *International Journal for the Advancement of Counseling*, *36*(4), 450–467. doi:10.100710447-014-9217-0

Thanasiu, P. L., Rust, K. L., & Walter, S. M. (2018). Service learning and live supervision as early components in play therapy training. *International Journal of Play Therapy*, *27*(2), 103–113. doi:10.1037/pla0000069

Torres-Harding, S. R., Siers, B., & Olson, B. D. (2012). Development and psychometric evaluation of the social justice scale (SJS). *American Journal of Community Psychology*, *50*(1-2), 77–88. doi:10.100710464-011-9478-2 PMID:22080396

VanderGast, T. S., Post, P. B., & Kascsak-Miller, T. (2010). Graduate training in child-parent relationship therapy with a multicultural immersion experience: Giving away the skills. *International Journal of Play Therapy*, *19*(4), 198–208. doi:10.1037/a0021010

Whealin, J. M., & Ruzek, J. (2008). Program evaluation for organizational cultural competence in mental health practices. *Professional Psychology, Research and Practice*, *39*(3), 320–328. doi:10.1037/0735-7028.39.3.320

Wright, A. C., & Jaffe, K. J. (2014). *Six steps to successful child advocacy: Changing the world for children*. Thousand Oaks, CA: Sage. doi:10.4135/9781483387888

ADDITIONAL READING

Baggerly, J. (2006). Service learning with children affected by poverty: Facilitating multicultural competence in counseling education students. *Journal of Multicultural Counseling and Development*, *34*(4), 244–255. doi:10.1002/j.2161-1912.2006.tb00043.x

Ceballos, P. L., Parikh, S., & Post, P. B. (2012). Examining social justice attitudes among play therapists: Implications for multicultural supervision and training. *International Journal of Play Therapy*, *21*(4), 232–243. doi:10.1037/a0028540

Drewes, A. A. (2008). Culturally competent supervision of child and play therapists. In A. A. Drewes & J. A. Mullen (Eds.), *Supervision can be playful: Techniques for child and play therapist supervisors* (pp. 77–92). Landham, MD: Jason Aronson.

Glosoff, H. L., & Durham, J. C. (2010). Using supervision to prepare social justice counseling advocates. *Counselor Education and Supervision, 50*(2), 116–129. doi:10.1002/j.1556-6978.2010.tb00113.x

Parikh, S. B., Ceballos, P., & Post, P. (2013). Factors related to play therapists' social justice advocacy attitudes. *Journal of Multicultural Counseling and Development, 41*(4), 240–253. doi:10.1002/j.2161-1912.2013.00039.x

Ratts, M. J., Singh, A. A., Nassar-McMillan, S., Butler, S. K., & McCullough, J. R. (2016). Multicultural and social justice counseling competencies: Guidelines for the counseling profession. *Journal of Multicultural Counseling and Development, 44*(1), 28–48. doi:10.1002/jmcd.12035

VanderGast, T. S., Post, P. B., & Kascsak-Miller, T. (2010). Graduate training in child-parent relationship therapy with a multicultural immersion experience: Giving away the skills. *International Journal of Play Therapy, 19*(4), 198–208. doi:10.1037/a0021010

Wright, A. C., & Jaffe, K. J. (2014). *Six steps to successful child advocacy: Changing the world for children*. Thousand Oaks, CA: Sage. doi:10.4135/9781483387888

KEY TERMS AND DEFINITIONS

Advisory Council: A group of stakeholders who provide guidance and support for a program or initiative.

Advocacy: A practice of using one's voice to institute change at an individual, institutional, systemic, or political level.

Cultural Competence: The ability to recognize and understand personal culture and the complex ways this intersects with the client's culture and can influence the therapeutic relationship. Cultural competence includes recognizing and responding to different cultures and is a lifelong endeavor.

Marginalized Populations: Groups and communities which are discriminated against and excluded from mainstream social, economic, cultural, or political life based on a cultural identity or difference. Examples include, but are not limited to, race, religion, age, gender, or financial status.

Mobile Play Therapy: An approach offering play therapy outside of traditional office settings. The play therapist takes materials to client settings.

Multiculturalism: The development of a philosophy that encourages an understanding of diverse cultures along the lines of race, ethnicity, gender, social class, religion, age, or level of ability.

Outreach: The provision of services or activities to individuals with limited access or knowledge of services.

Service Learning: Activities that involve students in community experiences that benefit others, usually involving volunteer work followed by active reflection of the experience.

Social Justice: The concept of fair distribution of resources to all individuals.

Social Justice Advocacy: Intentional actions to meet the needs of disadvantaged groups and institute change based on an awareness of privilege, social inequality, and oppressive systems.

Chapter 8
Live Supervision in University-Based Play Therapy Training Clinics:
Roles, Process, and Considerations

Yi-Ju Cheng
Rider University, USA

Rochelle Ritzi
Independent Researcher, USA

Liz D. Ener
Jewish Family Service, USA

ABSTRACT

Experiential and contextualized learning experiences are essential for facilitating play therapy supervisees' skills development, understanding of play therapy, and self-insight necessary for growth. University-based training clinics have the capacities to provide such experiential learning opportunities; this setting, which often serves diverse community client populations, offers live supervision opportunities. To date, there is limited information available describing the process and procedure for providing live supervision in university-based play therapy training clinics. Therefore, the authors will discuss the functions of live supervision, the process and formats of live supervision, developmental stages of play therapy supervisees in live supervision, theoretical orientation and its impact on the play therapy live supervision process, additional considerations, and advantages and disadvantages of providing live supervision in this chapter all within the context of university-based training programs.

DOI: 10.4018/978-1-5225-8226-7.ch008

INTRODUCTION

In recent years, the demand for mental health services for children across academic and community settings has been increasing substantially (Bureau of Labor Statistics, 2018; Perou et al., 2013). Responding to such need, the profession of play therapy has experienced growth as evidenced by an increase in providers pursuing play therapist and play therapist-supervisor credentials in addition to play specific professional memberships, a developing play therapy research base, and the establishment of play therapy approved centers and training programs (Association for Play Therapy [APT], 2017a). According to the APT Annual Growth Report (APT, 2017a), about 100 graduate universities have provided play therapy specific internship opportunities for master's and doctoral level students since 2014, which reflects the importance of examining criteria and establishing consistency of play therapy training and supervision provided in university-based training clinics.

University-based training clinics often incorporate live supervision as a supervision modality (Mullen, 2016). While the simultaneous process and subsequent involved intricacies of both hands-on play therapy experience and live supervision requires specific considerations, the information describing the process and procedure for providing live supervision for play therapy within such setting is limited in the literature. In this chapter, the authors will firstly describe the roles of supervision in play therapy. By integrating the literature and research available in play therapy training and supervision and live supervision in counseling, the authors then will focus on the context of university-based play therapy training clinics and discuss the functions, process, format, and structure of play therapy live supervision; the developmental stages of play therapy supervisees in live supervision; theoretical orientation and its impact on the play therapy live supervision process; additional considerations; and advantages and disadvantages of providing live supervision.

ROLES OF SUPERVISION IN PLAY THERAPY

Supervision is an integral part of the mental health field and the preparation of mental health professionals (Barnett, Cornish, Goodyear, & Lichtenberg, 2007; Bernard & Goodyear, 2014). According to Bernard and Goodyear (2014), supervision is a process wherein a seasoned professional provides support, guidance, and intervention to a less experienced member of the same profession. Applying the key components of this definition to the context of play therapy supervision, the supervisor (a senior member of a particular profession who is trained in play therapy, has extensive play therapy related clinical experience, and appropriate supervisory training) ensures the competence of a supervisee who is therapeutically using play therapy techniques and paradigms through communicating, modeling, and teaching (APT, 2017b; Mullen, 2016). Within this evaluative and hierarchical relationship, the supervisor aims to promote the professional functioning of the supervisee, monitor client welfare, and evaluate supervisee performance (Bernard & Goodyear, 2014). Gibbs and Green (2008) noted that gatekeeping and protecting client care are particularly imperative and challenging when supervising mental health professionals who work with children given the vulnerability and unique needs of this population. Moreover, play therapy supervisors provide opportunities for supervisees to explore and integrate internal thoughts, feelings, values, and experiences into practice (Mullen, Luke, & Drewes, 2007; Ray, 2011). This emphasis on self-awareness is an important facet of the play therapy supervision process. In order for play therapy supervisors to fulfill the variety of responsibilities and roles from a place of expertise, they must receive additional targeted training and possess certain qualifications specific to the practice of play therapy. For example, APT (2017b) required play therapy supervisors to have additional clinical and play therapy experiences, supervision training, and ongoing play therapy education.

Supervision is a key requirement throughout play therapy training regardless of one's field of study (APT, 2017b). Play therapy supervision consists of specific considerations and approaches as well as developmental, theoretical, and educational perspectives required to facilitate necessary experiences and learning for play therapists (Landreth, 2012; Mullen, 2016; Ray, 2011; VanderGast et al., 2010). To date, play therapy literature has expanded to enhance understanding of the roles and concepts of supervision in play therapy. Literature has been published on topics such as supervision of basic and advanced play therapy skills (Ray, 2004), perceived training needs of supervisors (Fall, Drew, Chute, & Moore, 2007), the experiences and preferences of play therapists in clinical supervision (VanderGast et al., 2010), the impact of intensive supervision on child-centered play therapy training (Meany-Walen et al., 2013), helping supervisees understand genuineness (Blanco, Muro, & Stickley, 2014), predictors of satisfaction with play therapy supervision (VanderGast & Hinkle, 2015), and the incorporation of different approaches into the process of play therapy supervision (e.g., Glazer & Stein, 2015; Peabody, 2015; Purswell & Stulmaker, 2015). Additionally, Thanasiu, Rust, and Walter (2018) investigated service learning and live supervision in play therapy training and found that didactic instruction and live supervision with immediate feedback and direct modeling of play therapy skills correlate with an increase in self-perceived play therapy knowledge and competence.

Functions of Live Supervision in University-Based Play Therapy Training Clinics

Live supervision is a commonly employed supervision format in university-based training programs (Carlozzi, Romans, Boswell, Ferguson, & Whisenhunt, 1997; Mullen, 2016). According to Bernard and Goodyear (2014), the process of live supervision is unique from that of traditional supervision methods such as individual, triadic, or group supervision, because the role of supervisor extends to both coaching and co-therapist, which leads to a less distinct difference between therapy and supervision. In live supervision, the supervisor is able to directly observe and communicate with the supervisee through technological methods, which is often followed by discussion between the supervisor and supervisee that allows for reflection (Bernard & Goodyear, 2014; Clark, 2016; Thanasiu et al., 2018). Supervisors provide immediate feedback and have a greater degree of control over the course of therapy, which highlights the heightened teaching component that is encompassed in live supervision (Bernard & Goodyear, 2014; Mullen, 2016).

General counseling research (e.g., Koltz & Feit, 2012; Moody, Kostohryz, & Vereen, 2014) as well as play therapy literature (e.g., Bratton, et al., 1993; Guerney, 1978; Smith-Adcock et al., 2012; Thanasiu et al., 2018) supported the use of live supervision with supervisees providing counseling services. The process of experiential and contextualized learning experiences is essential for facilitating play therapy supervisees' skills development, understanding of play therapy, and self-insight necessary for growth (Bratton et al., 1993; Jones & Rubin, 2005; VanderGast et al., 2010). Live supervision is crucial for such in vivo practice experiences, especially when it involves children at risk for social and behavioral concerns (Smith-Adcock et al., 2012; Thanasiu et al., 2018). In addition, live supervision allows supervisors opportunities to safeguard client experiences in the present moment, which is particularly imperative while training beginning-level counseling and play therapy students (Koltz & Feit, 2012; Smith-Adcock et al., 2012; Thanasiu et al., 2018).

University-based training clinics provide opportunities for students to gain experiential learning, serve diverse client populations in the community, and receive live supervision that may broaden their clinical experience and cultivate their identity development (Hittner & Fawcett, 2011; Levinson, Black, Rafoth, & Slonim, 2010). After examining archival data from 364 children aged 3 to 10 years who were served in a university-based training clinic, Tsai and Ray (2011) proposed that training clinics bridge the gaps existing in children's needs for mental health services by making quality, low-cost services provided by graduate level counseling students under supervision, available to the community. The dual purpose of training and service is one of the characteristics of university-based training clinics that also contributes to the complexity of implementing live supervision within the setting. Therefore, it is essential for supervisors to understand the process, format, and structure of live supervision in order to utilize this modality appropriately and effectively.

PROCESS, FORMAT, AND STRUCTURE OF LIVE SUPERVISION IN UNIVERSITY-BASED PLAY THERAPY TRAINING CLINICS

Live supervision is an experiential learning modality that can provide trainees guidance and oversight in a live clinical setting. Thanasiu et al. (2018) suggested that live supervision may increase the effectiveness of services provided to the community. By engaging in live observation and supervision in play therapy, supervisors are better able to accurately assess and facilitate the supervisees capacities, interactions with child clients, integration of theory, and therapeutic dynamics. To effectively engage in live observation and supervision, supervisors must explore a number of aspects including the process, format, and structure specific to the practice of play therapy. As such, in efforts to aid in this process, the authors will discuss the process of live supervision, describe the formats and structure often used in live supervision of mental health professionals, and briefly apply these to play therapy supervision and training.

Process of Live Supervision

Although live supervision can lead to various levels of disruption to the therapeutic process, a review of the literature demonstrated that supervisory interruptions do not lead to significant disruptions to therapy sessions, the counselor-in-training, or the client (Champe & Kleist, 2003). Jakob, Weck, and Bohus (2013) suggested the process of live supervision may better safeguard clients; therefore, greater observational learning may occur using live supervision compared to post-session verbal feedback alone. Grainge, Bulmer, Flemming, and Allan (2013) suggested that live supervision lends to a decreased separation between teaching, learning, and supervision, which then leads to increased direct application of student learning. Beddoe, Ackroyd, Chinnery, and Appleton (2011) expressed the process one chooses to facilitate live supervision is as important as the format of live supervision. Therefore, supervisors should ensure the process of live supervision is deliberate and purposeful to facilitate a greater level of learning for the supervisee and bolster client care (Beddoe et al., 2011). In addition, Beddoe et al. suggested that the process of facilitating purposeful live supervision could be broken down into three stages: (1) before the session, (2) during the session, and (3) after the session.

The first stage should start with thoughtful preparation in creating the space for the observation and the session to occur. Whether using a viewing screen, two-way mirrors, video recording equipment in the therapy room to record the session, data storage, or a direct-line from the observation room to the therapy room, technical support will likely be required. After considering where and how to observe, the supervisor and supervisee should explore the criteria that form the basis of feedback for what will be observed. Removing ambiguity from this process can strengthen the supervisory relationship and decrease anxiety for the supervisee (Beddoe et al., 2011). For example, the supervisor and the supervisee should discuss what skills should be demonstrated by the supervisee, and if the session will be considered to be a formative or a summative assessment. The supervisor and supervisee should also discuss and practice the logistics of the chosen live supervision format. For example, practicing the use of the bug-in-the-ear, or to determine the room set up for in vivo supervision.

During the second stage, supervisors should be aware of their level of activity and the response from the supervisee and the client. Supervisors who are not active enough could lead supervisees to think there is something wrong with the equipment and/or their skills. Overly active supervisors can lead supervisees to believe the supervisor does not believe they are competent. Supervisees should also continue to manage their emotions proactively, as needed, during the session; supervisors should monitor supervisees levels of emotionality within session and determine if their emotionality is at a level that causes inappropriate or regressive interference in the therapeutic process.

The third stage happens after the session, when the supervisor and the supervisee should debrief and discuss feedback, allowing a deeper level of integration of the information and skills. Post-session debriefing is also a time to discuss issues and/or client conceptualization that was not able to be explored during live observation. Based on the feedback and debriefing, the supervisor and supervisee should begin planning for the next session.

Supervision Formats and Structure

Some formats of live supervision will lend to more effective play therapy supervision compared to other formats, depending on room or clinic set up, access to technology, and client needs. Therefore, when contemplating the format and structure of live supervision, play therapy program faculty must consider the formats through which live supervision can be provided. All of the formats outlined in this chapter consist of supervisors either observing the play therapist-in-training live from outside the room (i.e., behind a two-way mirror or in a separate room on a camera feed) or from inside the room.

Bug-in-the-Ear

When using the bug-in-the-ear format of live supervision, supervisees wear a wireless earbud through which they can hear their supervisor (Gallant & Thyer, 1989). The supervisor is then able to talk directly to the supervisee in real time throughout the session. The benefit of using the bug-in-the-ear format is there is no direct interference or interruption of the flow of the session; a disadvantage of this format is that supervisees can become distracted by their supervisor talking in their ear and may risk being disengaged from the child. However, in a play therapy session, it is common for the play therapist to observe the child's play behavior without the child talking (Landreth, 2012; Ray, 2011); therefore, the play therapist will be less likely to feel torn between who to listen to, as the child is not always communicating verbally. As a means of using this approach effectively, supervisors can be more intentional regarding the times they choose to speak to supervisees, such as opting for a time when the child is not actively verbal or focused directly on the play therapist. Hence, the supervisor can facilitate an immediate awareness of the child's play behavior and connect play behaviors to appropriate reflective responses and the supervisee's overall demeanor in the room (Ray, 2004).

In Vivo

In vivo supervision is when the supervisor is in the therapy room with the supervisee and client. The supervisor does not directly engage in therapy with the client; however, the supervisee is able to consult with the supervisor in real time, albeit in the presence of the client (Hunt & Sharpe, 2008). The benefit of in vivo supervision is that the supervisee can immediately pose a question to the supervisor, or the supervisor can offer immediate feedback without waiting until after the session, thereby directly influencing the outcome of the session. A disadvantage in using this format is that the client may view the supervisee as inferior to the supervisor, undermining the credibility and training of the supervisee and the quality of the therapeutic process. Specific to play therapy, a disadvantage that may occur is that the supervisor in the play therapy room who does not engage with a child client may lead to the child feeling rejected (Landreth, 2012). Young children will likely not understand the concept of in vivo supervision due to their developmental functioning (Ray, 2016).

Consultation Breaks and Phone-Ins

When utilizing a consultation break, the supervisor knocks on the door and the supervisee steps out of the room to receive instruction, or the supervisor phones in feedback or information directly to the supervisee (Borders & Brown, 2005). In either format, the client does not hear what is discussed between the supervisor and the supervisee. Another variation of consultation break is the use of a consultation team in which a team of professionals engage in the live observation process, often through the use of a camera or two-way mirror; they then can offer discussion-based feedback by having the supervisee go into the observation setting, or by phoning in information (Borders & Brown, 2005). An advantage of this format is that the client does not hear the supervisor. Therefore, the supervisor and/or team can offer instruction concretely and openly allowing for less ambiguity in the feedback process. A disadvantage is a greater risk of causing a disruption to the flow of therapy because the supervisee leaves the child in the playroom while meeting with the treatment team. In a play therapy session, the child client may use the disruption to break a limit or behave in a way that demonstrates frustration with the disruption, leading to difficulty differentiating between the original presenting concern and frustration with feeling disconnected from the play therapist (Ray, 2011). Child safety, attachment responses, feelings of abandonment, fear, and anxiety are important factors to consider when choosing to leave a child unattended in the playroom.

The Walk-In

The walk-in format is when the supervisor enters the therapy room at a deliberate time and interacts with both the supervisee and the client, and then leaves (Bernard, & Goodyear, 2014). Although entering the room may be common to offer support during a client crisis, the walk-in format utilizes the supervisor entering the room to redirect the session and/or to establish dynamics between the supervisor and the client, and/or between the therapist and the client. A benefit of the walk-in format is that the supervisor can immediately offer feedback and support to both the supervisee and the client. Similar to in vivo, a disadvantage in using the walk-in is that the client may view the supervisee as inferior to the supervisor, which could undermine the credibility of the supervisee. This type of intrusion may also disrupt the child's play. When working with an adult, a therapist can verbally redirect the client to return to the original topic; however, a play therapist cannot organically redirect a child to the same play behavior in the same way one can redirect an adult. However, a play therapist may be able to observe how a child adjusts from such disruptions and use reflection of immediacy to bring awareness to the child.

Computer or Tablet Assisted Live Supervision

The computer assisted live supervision format is often referred to as *bug-in-the-eye* because it has similar principles as the bug-in-the-ear format; however, the supervisee receives the information from his or her supervisor from a computer screen or tablet in view of only the supervisee (Machuca, Johnson, & Moro, 2016; Scherl & Haley, 2000). Advantages and disadvantages of the bug-in-the-eye format are similar to the bug-in-the-ear format. An advantage specific to the bug-in-the-eye, however, is that the supervisee can decide when to look at the feedback rather than the supervisor speaking in the supervisee's ear. The supervisee can therefore better minimize the possibility of distraction for both the supervisee and the client (Scherl & Haley, 2000). In a play session, however, placing an electronic device in the room may disrupt a child's play behavior. A child is typically free to move around the room and will likely notice when the supervisor types and the words appear on the screen, possibly drawing the child's attention. However, the play therapist can verbalize limits in regards to the child touching or playing with the computer or tablet, and the screen can also be placed in an area difficult for the child to view or reach. Also, the supervisor can use abbreviations and codes, such as RF for reflect feeling or RC for reflect content, just in case the child reads the screen (Machuca et al., 2016).

Selecting Supervision Formats

While the approaches differ based on tools, technology, and space needed to implement the approach, each method of live observation and supervision has both advantages and disadvantages that should be weighed when deciding which format to utilize. Most importantly, supervisors should consider the needs and goals of the play therapy programs and trainees being served against the available formats; some formats may be ill-suited for certain settings given that the technology and/or space may not be available or accessible. Another factor in deciding formats includes considering the population served. Because children may be more susceptible to being distracted by disruptions, supervisors may seek to employ less intrusive observation methods. Given that the population typically served by play therapy are minors, caregivers must be informed and give consent to the supervision procedures, which is an additional consideration.

Supervisors might decide to modify supervision formats or methods across the training process based on programmatic and trainee needs. For instance, as supervisees advance in their skill level, identified primary goals may change from assessing supervisee capacities to focusing more on facilitating therapeutic change or on assessing client and/or supervisee progress; therefore, live observation/supervision methods may change to more efficiently meet this new goal. Regardless of selected formats, supervisors need to consider the developmental stages of supervisees to structure the live supervision process.

DEVELOPMENTAL STAGES OF PLAY THERAPY SUPERVISEES IN LIVE SUPERVISION

To facilitate an effective supervision experience, supervisors should be knowledgeable about a supervisee's developmental level (Gibbs & Green, 2008). It is important to continuously assess a supervisee's level of experience, skills, worldview, and perception of counseling as he or she progresses (Gibbs & Green, 2008; Ray, 2011). Learning play therapy is a gradual, developmental process during which students often achieve emotional growth derived from internal and external experiences, self-evaluation, emergent confidence, an integration of skills and theoretical knowledge, and the development of a set of beliefs and attitudes essential for working with children (Aguilera, 2010; Kao & Landreth, 1997; Ray, 2011). Within the context of live supervision, Heppner et al. (1994) encouraged supervisors to mindfully balance the following dimensions: (1) providing explicit directions for supervisees versus suggesting minor adjustments to deepen an already moving emotional process for clients, (2) focusing on the content of the session versus encouraging emotional expression of clients, (3) confronting versus encouraging clients, (4) giving expert advice in a distant manner versus being emotionally connected to the supervisee and client, (5) reinforcing the needs and wants of supervisees versus challenging the supervisee to examine his or her own problems, and (6) engaging in the counseling process versus resigning from active intervention due to believing there was little that could be done. Regardless of the level of development, Champe and Kleist (2003) further proposed that developing a collaborative and supportive supervisory relationship is critical to providing an optimal live supervisory environment for all supervisees. As previously mentioned, supervisors are encouraged to hold an orientation prior to live supervision in which the supervisor is able to initiate an encouraging and open learning environment, to assess the supervisee's attitude toward live supervision, and to desensitize the supervisee to the uniqueness of live supervision (Bubenzer et al., 1987; Champe & Kleist, 2003). In university-based play therapy training clinics, it is also crucial that during the orientation, supervisors review the clinic policies, crisis management procedures, and paperwork requirements such as assessments and clinic forms.

The Integrated Developmental Model and Play Therapy Live Supervision

Several supervision models are available in the literature to serve as a roadmap to conceptualize play therapy supervisees' development and to provide matching interventions (Hartwig & Bennett, 2017). The integrated developmental model (IDM; Stoltenberg, 1981) is one of the most frequently cited supervision models in the play therapy literature (e.g., Blanco et al., 2014; Gibbs & Green, 2008; Hartwig & Bennett, 2017; Perryman, Moss, & Anderson, 2016). The IDM is a framework that emphasizes a safe supervisory relationship and describes supervisees' development as occurring through four levels (Stoltenberg, 1981). The authors aim to apply the IDM to the process of live supervision in play therapy as this has not been previously discussed.

Level 1

Level 1 is the stage in which the supervisee has limited training or experience and is dependent on the supervisor (Stoltenberg, 1981). During this early stage of training, supervisees are introduced to play therapy skills and theories as well as other pertinent subjects that aim to increase their intellectual understanding of the dynamics of play therapy, the play therapy process, and the role of play therapist. Although often rigorous in their pursuits to master the practice of play therapy, Level 1 play therapy supervisees often focus on their mistakes, which results in a lack of confidence and causes them to rely heavily on the advice and feedback from their supervisor in the live supervision process. This level of development is also characterized by a lack of awareness of self and others and a heightened level of anxiety originating from the anticipation of unknown experiences (Hartwig & Bennett, 2017; Smith-Adcock et al., 2012). The intervening or interruption proposed by the supervisor in this stage of live supervision might be perceived as a criticism that may elevate the supervisee's feelings of anxiety and apprehension (Moody et al., 2014; Mullen, 2016). Therefore, supervisors are responsible for recognizing and initiating conversations regarding the emotional reactions that supervisees experience to help them feel understood. Additionally, supervisees tend to operate under the belief that there is a perfect response to their child clients and may overly focus their attention on providing a perfect reflection, for example, without attending to the affect or energy level of the child client (Blanco et al., 2014; Ray, 2011).

The process of effective live supervision with Level 1 play therapists begins before the observation of the supervisee's clinical session (Beddoe et al., 2011). Supervisors and supervisees should discuss the child client's history and presenting issues and should review basic play therapy skills to prepare for the session (Ray, 2004). Considering the difficulties that novice play therapists experience, the authors encourage supervisors to provide direct and structured advice that is skill focused and to model basic play therapy skills, such as tracking behavior, reflecting content, reflecting feeling, returning responsibility, and esteem building, in live supervision (Ray 2004, 2011). For example, if a supervisee misses several opportunities to reflect feelings, the supervisor could cue the supervisee on when to reflect feelings. Novice play therapists may appear robotic while interacting with clients; therefore, supervisors could model appropriate body language such as leaning forward and presenting an open stance, and monitor supervisees' delivery of responses including rate and conciseness. Supervisors conveying empathic understanding can not only facilitate supervisees' confidence but also provide an opportunity for them to experience this fundamental attitudinal quality of play therapists (Ray, 2011). Frequency of interruption and intervening also requires an appropriate pace to avoid overwhelming supervisees. In addition, a certain degree of autonomy must be allowed for professional identity development to evolve at this level (Stoltenberg, 1981).

In the post-session meeting, in addition to positive and constructive feedback, a discussion on child development may further supervisees' recognition of the emotional and physical capabilities of the child (Blanco et al., 2014). Supervisors may also help play therapists to begin exploring internal reactions toward the therapy process, which includes the live supervision experience, by sharing observations of supervisees' nonverbal skills such as tone of voice and comfort level (Ray, 2004). Moreover, Moody et al. (2014) suggested that written feedback may enhance supervisees' learning and engagement in live supervision. Therefore, supervisors may consider using the Play Therapy Skills Checklist (PTSC; Ray, 2004) to supplement the live supervision process. PTSC has been used in play therapy training and supervision as an evaluative tool and in play therapy research as a treatment fidelity measure (Ray, 2004; Ray, Purswell, Haas, & Aldrete, 2017). PTSC consists of sections on nonverbal expressions, verbal skills, and open comments regarding overall impressions of the play therapy session and the strength and areas for growth for the play therapist (Ray, 2004; Ray et al., 2017). As a way to present concrete feedback, it would be helpful for the supervisor to complete all sections of the PTSC and discuss it with the Level 1 play therapy supervisee after each live supervision session.

It is worth noting that supervisees in this stage may include trainees who are new to the helping profession and those who are seasoned mental health professionals with mastered experience with a population other than children or are simply looking to develop a skill-set in the practice of play therapy (Gibbs & Green, 2008). The supervisees with the latter background may be especially challenged given the dichotomy between their sense of professional competence in one area and insecurity about their level of knowledge and skills in play therapy (Mullen, 2016). It is imperative for the supervisor to acknowledge the supervisee's struggle, address the possible tension in the supervisory relationship as a result of the challenge, and provide as much encouragement and understanding as possible.

When interacting with children, Level 1 play therapy supervisees are able to practice learned skills under the support of a trained supervisor, which may mitigate feelings of fear and foster exploration of their beliefs about children and the therapeutic relationship in play therapy (Smith-Adcock et al., 2012). The shift in emotional reactions from anxiety to excitement exemplifies the growth that occurs at this level.

Level 2

With growing self-awareness, supervisees struggle with dependence on supervisors while trying to develop a sense of autonomy as they move into Level 2 (Stoltenberg, 1981). Level 2 play therapy supervisees may desire to navigate their own individual identity as a play therapist and may become more self-assertive in choosing alternative techniques, behaviors, or styles available rather than imitating their supervisors. Stoltenberg (1981) stressed the importance of allowing supervisees in this level to have latitude, within limits, in a way that will benefit both the supervisees and the clients they serve.

Consequently, the authors suggest that the supervisor be prepared to address any conflict with the supervisee with an open and caring attitude while supporting their attempt to find a personal voice in the playroom. It is vital to recognize the supervisee's desire for independence as a part of development and to help him or her understand that although they are afforded the opportunity to investigate personal and professional values systems in play therapy practice, the safeguarding of child client's well-being and adherence to ethical standards serve as a boundary for permissibility (Ray, 2011). It is the responsibility of play therapy supervisors to help their supervisees navigate and balance their desire for self-exploration and the maintenance of client welfare and ethical practice. The live supervision provided during this level may be less directive. Supervisors may reduce the frequency of interruptions or intervening to allow more space for supervisees to assess their strengths and areas for growth. However, it is worth noting that dependency is still a struggle of supervisees during this stage and in the process of live supervision. Therefore, supervisors should continue to model new skills, provide advice or direction, and clarify questions when necessary. In the post-session meeting, in addition to demonstrating empathy and fostering self-awareness as before, supervisors may also celebrate how supervisees have discovered their own style of therapy because it allows the child client an opportunity to be served by a congruent play therapist (Blanco et al., 2014). The use of PTSC can still be particularly beneficial during this phase of live supervision (Ray, 2004). Supervisors and supervisees may fill out separate PTSC forms after each live supervision and compare and process them in the post-session meeting (Ray, 2004).

Level 3

Stoltenberg (1981) described Level 3 supervisees as showing an increased sense of professional identity and self-confidence with a greater level of empathy. Play therapy supervisees in this stage may become more aware of their conditional dependency on supervisors and appreciate different theoretical views and techniques (Blanco et al., 2014). As differences in expertise between supervisors and supervisees may diminish, the supervisory relationship transforms to a more peer-like relationship, with an emphasis on mutual sharing (Stoltenberg, 1981). The live supervision provided for Level 3 supervisees often involves more autonomy and less structure and instruction. Supervisors may intervene in the course of therapy only when attention is drawn to supervisees' advanced play therapy skills, such as enlarging the meaning of child's play and setting limits. Enlarging the meaning is an important advanced play therapy skill used to help children gain awareness or understanding of the patterns of their play by recognizing and reflecting the observed patterns (Ray, 2004). Role-playing the use of enlarging the meaning with the supervisor prior to the session may be beneficial (Ray, 2004).

In the post-session meeting, supervisors can occasionally review the basic play therapy skills but also support supervisees in understanding play behaviors, identifying play themes, and forming appropriate conceptualizations of clients to therapeutically converse about children and to communicate these observations and progress to parents (Ray, 2004). Supervisors are also encouraged to help supervisees transition to a deeper level exploration of the self and the therapeutic relationship with child clients. To support this process of exploration, supervisors can have supervisees complete the PTSC as a way to review and self-evaluate sessions of concern and can discuss it in the post-session meeting. Moreover, the occasional use of confrontation may deepen the development of genuineness of play therapy supervisees and expand the interactions between supervisors and supervisees to a more insightful level. This depth would also create more impactful interactions and connections between supervisees and their child clients (Blanco et al., 2014).

Level 4

Supervisees in Level 4 are defined as master counselors given their capability to practice independently with an adequate awareness of personal strengths and limitations (Stoltenberg, 1981). They are reflective, skilled, and knowledgeable practitioners who actively identify and address areas in their own performance that need improvement or guidance (Stoltenberg, 1981). The self-awareness and genuineness of Level 4 supervisees are well integrated into their way of being as play therapists (Blanco et al., 2014). Such play therapists have transformed into a valuable member of the play therapy field who might be able to serve as a supervisor for less advanced play therapists (Blanco et al., 2014). Given that supervisees on this level are able to function professionally and effectively in most settings, the supervisory relationship becomes collegial (Ray, 2011; Stoltenberg 1981). Since the play therapist has a significantly reduced need for structured, directive supervision, supervision sessions with live observation (i.e., observing without interacting with the supervisee; Bernard & Goodyear, 2014) may be more appropriate. The post-session meeting at this level may occur as consultation centering on how personal experiences influence the therapy process or a specific play therapy relationship (Ray, 2011). Supervisees spend attention and energy on exploring profound feelings of self in connection to play therapy and their role as a play therapist, as both their basic and advanced play therapy skills continue to develop (Ray, 2011). At Level 4, the frequent use of PTSC may no longer be required; rather, both supervisors and supervisees may decide when and how they would like to use it in the live supervision process to further monitor and advance the development of supervisees.

Anderson, Schlossberg, and Rigazio-DiGilio (2000) found drastic differences in supervisee perceptions of live supervision, as some refer to it as the best supervision experience and others identify it as the worst. Hence, acknowledging supervisees' developmental levels with an understanding of their degree of reactions to live supervision is fundamental to meaningfully engage them in the supervision process and productively supporting their growth in the personal and professional realms (Champe & Kleist, 2003).

THEORETICAL ORIENTATION AND ITS IMPACT ON PLAY THERAPY LIVE SUPERVISION PROCESS

The American Counseling Association (2014) code of ethics compels educators and supervisors to have "theoretical and pedagogical foundations" (p. 12) in their work with counselors-in-training, including the promotion of "the use of techniques/procedures/modalities that are grounded in theory and/or have an empirical or scientific foundation" (p. 14). The National Association of Social Workers (2008), the American Psychological Association (2010), and the American Association for Marriage and Family Therapy (2012) have similar ethical code requirements for their members. Therefore, regardless of field of study, supervisors in play therapy training programs must consider theoretical foundations when training play therapists.

Spruill and Benshoff (2000) suggested introductory level therapists should begin developing awareness about their personal beliefs and how such beliefs integrate with counseling theory. Therefore, consistent with the IDM (Stoltenberg, 1981), Level 1 play therapists may benefit from being introduced to two or three major play therapy theories; too much objective information may be overwhelming for supervisees to digest (Spruill & Benshoff, 2000). While Level 1 play therapists are learning the foundations of play therapy and basic play therapy skills (Ray, 2004), supervisors should encourage them to explore their own life experiences and how their experiences lead to the integration of a play therapy theory. Such exploration continues and serves as a foundation for play therapy supervisees progressing to

Level 2. Level 2 play therapists may start questioning whether a specific theory fits with their beliefs as they are navigating their own identity. Supervisors should be sensitive to the needs of supervisees at this level and provide opportunities where they can explore freely (Spruill & Benshoff, 2000). With increased experiences and continued self-reflection, Level 3 play therapy supervisees may begin to integrate their life and professional experiences, learning, and learned theories into practice. They may start to practice different play therapy approaches with appropriate intention. It is crucial for supervisors to involve supervisees in examining and discussing these experiences, including the use of theory to explore possible reflective responses, themes, and possible interventions to help them identify a guiding play therapy theory. This integration continues for Level 4 supervisees who practice and conceptualize play therapy sessions from a theory that is congruent to who they are as a professional and individual.

Applications of Play Therapy Theories to Live Supervision Process

Play therapy students should be encouraged to use the theoretical orientation they most closely identify with in the playroom, such as Child-Centered Play Therapy (CCPT; Landreth; Ray), Adlerian Play Therapy (AdPT; Kottman & Meany-Walen, 2016), or Cognitive Behavioral Therapy Play Therapy (CBT-PT, Knell, 1999, 2009). Although there are many theoretical orientations for play therapists to identify with, the authors will use CCPT, AdPT, and CBT-PT to discuss the role of the supervisor when training play therapists through live supervision.

While observing the session, supervisors providing advanced play therapy supervision to supervisees who identify with a CCPT approach should monitor for the supervisee's ability to reflect deeper meaning responses, such as identifying themes, limit-setting, and connecting with children to strengthen the therapeutic relationship (Ray, 2011). Supervisors providing advanced live supervision to supervisees who most closely align with an AdPT theoretical perspective should monitor the supervisee's ability to recognize and reflectively respond to the client's goals and the four therapy phases of therapy as outlined in the AdPT training manual (Wyatt & Seid, 2008). Supervisors observing supervisees who most closely identify with a CBT-PT approach should monitor the supervisee's ability to structure the session, including collaborating with the child and parents to determine homework/ tasks outside the therapy room (Knell, 1999, 2009). In each of these theoretical approaches, the supervisor should utilize the live supervision format to model the skills before, during, and after the session. This immediacy allows for greater integration of the skills compared to if the supervision session happens days later, as often the case with supervision models in a university training setting who do not use live supervision.

Lastly, just as supervisors should encourage and train their supervisees to be practicing from a sound theoretical orientation, play therapy supervisors should be grounded and intentional in their philosophical approach to play therapy supervision (Thomas, 2015). More specifically, Ray (2011) expressed that play therapy supervisors should possess the knowledge, skill, and experiences of an advanced clinician, as well as demonstrate the qualities of congruence, unconditional positive regard, empathetic understanding, supervision preparation, theory and practice education, supervision of supervision, and current and ongoing advanced play therapy experience. In sum, theory provides a framework for integrity between understanding, conceptualization, and, ultimately, action.

ADDITIONAL CONSIDERATIONS

Because of the inherent vulnerability of the clientele to be served compounded with the charge to facilitate trainees' educational experience and assess the application of trainee capacities, supervisors must attend to a number of considerations regarding live supervision of play therapy trainees. Such considerations include selecting appropriate volunteer clients for novice trainees, upholding client welfare while also facilitating trainees' development, balancing clinical procedural aspects (i.e., use of clinic space, quality childcare when trainees meet with parents, and equipping trainees with knowledge of clinic procedures in regards to appropriate use of space, maintaining playroom, and involvement of parents, amongst others.), quality of live supervision, and evaluation/assessment of student performance and capacities. Attending to all considerations can yield an impactful experience to clients, play therapy trainees, and supervisors.

Targeting appropriate clients and balancing client needs with capacities of trainees is an inherent responsibility of an informed supervisor; such responsibility is supported by theories of counselors-in-training overall maturational progression of practice and personal insight. That is, trainees earlier in their clinical development, such as those who are enrolled in an introductory play therapy course, must be well matched with child participants. Because of this notion, many well-established training programs often relies on volunteer child participants for these introductory courses. Instructors and supervisors of these courses work to screen these volunteer participants to ensure that they are generally well functioning (i.e., low risk, no history of mental health related struggles and/or trauma history, healthy attachment, etc.); this method affords trainees the opportunity to apply their skills in an experiential medium in which the focus is on demonstrating and cultivating basic play therapy capacities rather than on facilitating therapeutic outcomes of child clients. As trainees move along in their clinical sequences and strengthen their capacities, they are more prepared to work with clients who have increasing mental health related needs. Length of recommended treatment for the child and availability of the trainee is another aspect imperative for supervisors to consider when identifying appropriate child clients for trainees. For instance, children who have experienced the recent death of a loved one or are seeking treatment due to sexual abuse allegations would likely not be an appropriate fit for a trainee who would only be able to work with such a client for a short period of time. Pairing such a dyad together might exacerbate the child's struggles and/or be anti-therapeutic; a better solution might be to refer such clients to a clinic/agency/professional who could provide more long-term therapy due to continuity needs. Additionally, certain specified populations, such as sexually and/or physically abused children, parentally bereaved children, terminally ill children, and children in the foster care system, to name a few, require significantly more advanced training than an introductory play therapy course alone; advanced knowledge of such populations would also be required for working with caregivers and parents connected to child clients confronting such challenges. It would be imperative for supervisors to pair child clients presenting with such issues with more advanced supervisees who have the advanced training.

Maintaining client welfare is of utmost importance to supervisors as client welfare supersedes trainee educational and/or training needs (ACA, 2014). Occasionally, supervisors may be required to intervene directly or indirectly in a child's treatment in efforts to maintain client welfare. Indirect intervention occurs when supervisors affect treatment in a way that does not involve the clients (child or parents) directly, such as pulling the trainee aside and speaking with them explicitly about therapeutic direction; whereas direct intervention involves the supervisor having direct contact with the clients. Prior to intervening, supervisors should consider assessing if the intrusion is necessary, whether it would facilitate supervisee's sense of autonomy, and how the disruption would impact the pace of session (Borders & Brown, 2005, p. 49-50). Because intervening directly can be intrusive, highly disruptive, and even threatening to child clients specific to the use of in-vivo or walk-in methods of live supervision, the necessity of such intrusions should occur only after other avenues have been exhausted and/or the capacities of the trainee are in question. While in-vivo and walk-in methods of supervision are common practice in regards to live supervision, supervisors should consider rendering caution when employing such approaches and work to protect the child client's experience of the supervision process. Attending to when and how disruptions occur can help to minimize the negative impact of child clients in these instances of intrusion. Times to intervene might include when a child is indicating risk and a trainee freezes or begins to flounder beyond that which they might recover, begins mishandling the situation, and/or does not respond well to redirection. During the times of such intrusions, supervisors should introduce themselves to the child client, explain their role using developmentally appropriate language, and work to build rapport in developmentally appropriate means rather taking on an authoritative stance. It is imperative the supervisor communicates safety and handles the situation with the utmost respect for the child's therapeutic space; moreover, the supervisor is still in a teaching/modeling role when intervening as he or she must keep in mind that their trainee is observing their handling of the situation as well. Regardless of whether the supervisor intervenes directly and/or indirectly, the supervisor is encouraged to process the experience with the trainee and provide constructive feedback in a timely manner (Borders & Brown, 2005).

Evaluation is a fundamental responsibility of supervisors that requires them to have a solid understanding of overall student/supervisee readiness and the levels at which supervisees should be performing across their clinical development specific to the practice of play therapy (Borders & Brown, 2005; Ray, 2004). Although supervisors are responsible for facilitating supervisees' learning experiences and helping them to grow in their role as clinicians, supervisees also have responsibilities in demonstrating their capacities consistent with noted expectations and appropriate levels of development. Supervisors must clearly communicate the evaluation criteria and performance expectations as well as their assessment of student performance and engage in remediation as concerns arise. In the practice of play therapy, supervisees must not only develop an adequate skill-set in the active practice of play therapy, but also possess and demonstrate proficiency in child development, child assessment, and caregiver and teacher consultation, amongst others (Ray, 2011). As such, proficiency in skill development extends beyond the playroom as should supervisor evaluation of play therapy supervisees. Concerns should be addressed as early and often as possible to provide supervisees time to correct if the capacity to correct is present. Should the remediation plan require the supervisee to engage in personal counseling, the supervisor should take precaution to avoid engaging in dual relationships and/or violate the supervisee's privacy (ACES, 2011).

Gatekeeping, which is defined as "the evaluation of student suitability for professional practice" (Brear, Dorrian, & Luscri, 2008, p. 93), is a core responsibility of play therapy supervisors; ultimately, gatekeeping serves to protect the profession and community at large. Because of the inherent vulnerabilities of serving minors, gatekeeping responsibilities of play therapy supervisors are that much more augmented. Therefore, should a supervisor deem a play therapy supervisee to perform below level and/or demonstrate clinical impairment and/or the capacity to do harm, supervisors must take steps to remediate and/or dismiss when necessary (Glance, Fanning, Schoepke, Soto, & Williams, 2012). Supervisors should take note that although students may make progress across the semester toward meeting criteria, supervisees should not progress past training should criteria not be met or exceeded.

An aspect of gatekeeping specific to play therapy might involve discussing with supervisees other modalities or populations that might be better served with their skillset or discussing other occupations of better fit.

ADVANTAGES AND DISADVANTAGES OF PROVIDING LIVE SUPERVISION IN UNIVERSITY-BASED PLAY THERAPY TRAINING CLINICS

Conducting live supervision in university-based play therapy training clinics presents both advantages and disadvantages. One significant advantage is the opportunity for supervisees to experience and practice in a real-life setting that contributes to advancement in utilizing skills, application of theoretical knowledge, and trust in the therapeutic process (Kao & Landreth, 1997; Smith-Adcock et al., 2012; Thanasiu et al., 2018). Play therapy supervisees may also develop a sense of pride in overcoming the challenges involved with in vivo experiences (Muro et al., 2015). In addition, Thanasiu et al. (2018) proposed that structured live supervision makes service learning a feasible teaching modality for early play therapy training. The coaching component embedded in the function of live supervision amplifies the likelihood of positive outcomes for not only therapy for the child clients but also the learning experiences of the supervisees (Bartle-Haring, Silverthorn, Meyer, & Toviessi, 2009; Bernard & Goodyear, 2014; Landis & Young, 1994). Specifically, live supervision with direct modeling and immediate concrete feedback helps supervisees recognize and address transference and countertransference, reduce anxiety, and develop confidence (Thanasiu et al., 2018). With input from supervisors, supervisees are able to witness and experience how a therapy process systematically and therapeutically unfolds (Bernard & Goodyear, 2014). Moreover, under the structure of university-based training clinics and live supervision, clients are protected directly and promptly by supervisors' intervening, which is of particular importance in child counseling (Bernard & Goodyear, 2014; Koltz & Feit, 2012; Smith-Adcock et al., 2012). As a result of this function, the quality of service is improved accordingly (Bernard & Goodyear 2014).

The disadvantages of providing live supervision in university-based play therapy training clinics include training in the live supervision modality and the use of technology (Champe & Kleist, 2003), demands on the time of supervisors (Lee & Everett, 2004; Yu, 2012), the cost of facilities, the complexity of scheduling appropriate clients, and the potential negative reactions of clients and supervisees (Bernard & Goodyear, 2014). Researchers also have proposed that a potential disadvantage is that live supervision may impede supervisees' initiative or creativity in relation to self-sufficiency throughout the course of therapy (Lee & Everett, 2004; Lee, Nichols,

Nichols, & Odom, 2004; Thomas, 2010). In other words, supervisees may develop excessive dependency on their supervisor rather than appropriate self-confidence if supervisors do not encourage and allow for greater autonomy (Bernard & Goodyear, 2014; Lee & Everett, 2004). These challenges highlight the necessity for supervisors to pursue continued education and professional development in the subject of live supervision and other fundamentals of supervision to be able to conduct intentional and impactful live supervision for supervisees across different developmental levels (Champe & Kleist, 2003).

CONCLUSION

Universities have been a common setting for providing play therapy training to both novice and experienced clinicians (Ray, 2010; Ray, 2011; Smith-Adcock et al., 2012) as they provide both experiential learning and live supervision opportunities and serve diverse and underrepresented client populations in the community (Levinson, Black, Rafoth, & Slonim, 2010). Within this chapter, emphasis has been placed on providing guidelines, describing the process of live observation and supervision of play therapy trainees, and exploring advantages and disadvantages.

The use of live supervision within a university-based play therapy training clinic contributes to the development and competence of play therapy supervisees by going beyond play therapy skills and knowledge to ensure the safety and welfare of clients in an immediate manner. As live supervision is unique in its format and delivery, it is accompanied by specific advantages and challenges. To maximize the potential benefits and manage the expected difficulties, supervisors must consider the impact of theoretical orientation and developmental levels on supervisees' goals and experiences in the live supervision process. It is also vital for supervisors to help both supervisees and clients understand the modality of live supervision to reduce any negative emotional reactions, such as the feeling of insecurity and apprehensiveness toward live supervision. Essentially, developing a safe and encouraging supervisory relationship serves as a foundation for implementing a positive and effective live supervision experience for play therapist trainees in university-based training clinics.

REFERENCES

Aguilera, M. E. (2010). An exploratory study of the developmental experience of novice play therapists. *Dissertation Abstracts International; Section A, 70,* 3352.

American Association for Marriage and Family Therapy. (2012). *AAMFT code of ethics*. Alexandria, VA: Author.

American Counseling Association. (2014). *ACA code of ethics*. Alexandria, VA: Author.

American Psychological Association. (2010). *Ethical principles of psychologists and code of conduct*. Washington, DC: Author.

Anderson, S. A., Schlossberg, M., & Rigazio-DiGilio, S. (2000). Family therapy trainees' evaluations of their best and worst supervision experiences. *Journal of Marital and Family Therapy*, *26*(1), 79–91. doi:10.1111/j.1752-0606.2000.tb00278.x PMID:10685354

Association for Counselor Education and Supervision (ACES) Taskforce on Best Practices in Clinical Supervision. (2011, April). *Best practices in clinical supervision*. Retrieved June 30, 2013, from http://www.acesonline.net/wp-content/uploads/2011/10/ACES-Best-Practices-in-clinical-supervision-document-FINAL.pdf

Association for Play Therapy. (2017a). *APT annual growth report by CEO*. Retrieved from https://cdn.ymaws.com/www.a4pt.org/resource/resmgr/about_apt/Website_version.pdf

Association for Play Therapy. (2017b). *Credentialing guide: Registered play therapist (RPT) & supervisor (RPT-S)*. Retrieved from: https://cdn.ymaws.com/www.a4pt.org/resource/ resmgr/Credentials/RPTS_Guide_Dec_2017.pdf

Barnett, J. E., Cornish, J. A. E., Goodyear, R. K., & Lichtenberg, J. W. (2007). Commentaries on the ethical and effective practice of clinical supervision. *Psychology: Research and Practice*, *38*, 268–275.

Bartle-Haring, S., Silverthorn, B. C., Meyer, K., & Toviessi, P. (2009). Does live supervision make a difference? A multilevel analysis. *Journal of Marital and Family Therapy*, *35*(4), 406–414. doi:10.1111/j.1752-0606.2009.00124.x PMID:19785698

Beddoe, L., Ackroyd, J., Chinnery, S., & Appleton, C. (2011). Live supervision of students in field placement: More than just watching. *Social Work Education*, *30*(5), 512–528. doi:10.1080/02615479.2010.516358

Bernard, J. M., & Goodyear, R. K. (2009). *Fundamentals of clinical supervision* (4th ed.). Upper Saddle River, NJ: Pearson Education.

Bernard, J. M., & Goodyear, R. K. (2014). *Fundamentals of clinical supervision* (5th ed.). Boston, MA: Pearson Education.

Blanco, P. J., Muro, J. H., & Stickley, V. K. (2014). Understanding the concept of genuineness in play therapy: Implications for the supervision and teaching of beginning play therapists. *International Journal of Play Therapy*, *23*(1), 44–54. doi:10.1037/a0035478

Borders, L. D., & Brown, L. L. (2005). *The new handbook of counseling supervision*. New York, NY: Routledge.

Bratton, S., Landreth, G., & Homeyer, L. (1993). An intensive three day play therapy supervision/training model. *International Journal of Play Therapy*, *2*(2), 61–79. doi:10.1037/h0089366

Bratton, S., Ray, D., & Landreth, G. (2010). Play therapy. In A. Gross & M. Hersen (Eds.), Handbook of clinical psychology: Vol. 2. Children and adolescents. New York, NY: John Wiley & Sons.

Bratton, S., Ray, D., Rhine, T., & Jones, L. (2005). The efficacy of play therapy with children: A meta-analytic review of the outcome research. *Professional Psychology, Research and Practice*, *36*(4), 376–390. doi:10.1037/0735-7028.36.4.376

Brear, P., Dorrian, J., & Luscri, G. (2008). Preparing our future counseling professionals: Gatekeeping and implications for research. *Counselling & Psychotherapy Research*, *8*(2), 93–101. doi:10.1080/14733140802007855

Bubenzer, D. L., Mahrle, C., & West, J. D. (1987). *Live counselor supervision: Trainee acculturation and supervisor interventions*. Paper presented at the American Association for Counseling and Development Annual Convention, New Orleans, LA.

Bureau of Labor Statistics. (2018). *Occupational outlook handbook*. Retrieved August 1, 2018, from https://www.bls.gov/ooh/

Carlozzi, A. F., Romans, J. S. C., Boswell, D. L., Ferguson, D. B., & Whisenhunt, B. J. (1997). Training and supervision practices in counseling and marriage and family therapy programs. *The Clinical Supervisor*, *15*(1), 51–60. doi:10.1300/J001v15n01_04

Champe, J., & Kleist, D. M. (2003). Live supervision: A review of the research. *The Family Journal (Alexandria, Va.)*, *11*(3), 1–8. doi:10.1177/1066480703252755

Clark, G. (2016). Using technology to enhance supervision at the University of Southern California. In S. Goss, K. Anthony, L. S. Stretch, & D. M. Nagel (Eds.), *Technology in mental health: Applications in practice, supervision and training* (pp. 366–377). Springfield, IL: Charles C. Thomas.

Deaver, S. P., & Shiflett, C. (2011). Art-based supervision techniques. *The Clinical Supervisor*, *30*(2), 257–276. doi:10.1080/07325223.2011.619456

Donald, E. J., Culbreth, J. R., & Carter, A. W. (2015). Play therapy supervision: A review of the literature. *International Journal of Play Therapy*, *24*(2), 59–77. doi:10.1037/a0039104

Fall, M., Drew, D., Chute, A., & Moore, A. (2007). The voices of registered play therapists as supervisors. *International Journal of Play Therapy*, *16*(2), 133–146. doi:10.1037/1555-6824.16.2.133

Gallant, J., & Thyer, B. (1989). The "Bug-in-the-ear" in clinical Supervision. *The Clinical Supervisor*, *7*(2-3), 43–58. doi:10.1300/J001v07n02_04

Gibbs, K. A., & Green, E. J. (2008). Sanding in supervision. In A. A. Drewes & J. A. Mullen (Eds.), *Supervision can be playful: Techniques for child and play therapist supervisor* (pp. 27–38). Plymouth, UK: Jason Aronson.

Glance, D., Fanning, G., Schoepke, A., Soto, W., & Williams, M. A. (2012). *Gatekeeping in counselor education*. Retrieved from http://www.counseling.org/resources/library/vistas/ vistas12/Article_11.pdf

Glazer, H. R., & Stein, D. (2015). Mindfulness and the play-therapist supervisor: A study in transformative learning. *International Journal of Play Therapy*, *24*(1), 41–53. doi:10.1037/a0038663

Grainge, A. S., Bulmer, C., Fleming, M., & Allan, R. (2013). Using live supervision to deliver family intervention training. *Mental Health Practice*, *16*(9), 12–18. doi:10.7748/mhp2013.06.16.9.12.e828

Guerney, L. (1978). Training and evaluation of students as consultants in an adult-child relationship enhancement program. *Professional Psychology*, *9*, 193–198.

Hartwig, E. K., & Bennett, M. M. (2017). Four approaches to using sandtray in play therapy supervision. *International Journal of Play Therapy*, *26*(4), 230–238. doi:10.1037/pla0000050

Heppner, P. P., Kivlighan, D. M., Burnett, J. W., Berry, T. R., Goedinghaus, M., Doxsee, D. J., …Wallace, D. L. (1994). Dimensions that characterize supervisor interventions delivered in the context of live supervision of practicum counselors. *Journal of Counseling Psychology, 41*(2), 227-235.

Hittner, J., & Fawcett, M. (2011, October 27). Developing a counselor education training clinic: The first year. In *Ideas and research you can use: VISTAS 2012*. Retrieved from: https://www.counseling.org/resources/library/vistas/vistas12/Article_22.pdf

Hunt, C., & Sharpe, L. (2008). Within-session supervision communication in the training of clinical psychologists. *Australian Psychologist, 43*(2), 121–126. doi:10.1080/00050060801933402

Jakob, M., Weck, F., & Bohus, M. (2013). Live supervision: From the one-way mirror to video-based online supervision. *Verhaltenstherapie, 23*, 170–180. doi:10.1159/000354234

Jones, L., & Rubin, L. (2005). PT 101: Teaching introduction to play therapy at the graduate level. *International Journal of Play Therapy, 6*, 1–20. doi:10.1037/h0088899

Kao, S., & Landreth, G. L. (1997). Evaluating the impact of child-centered play therapy training. *International Journal of Play Therapy, 6*(2), 1–20. doi:10.1037/h0089405

Knell, S. M. (1999). Cognitive behavioral play therapy. In S. W. Russ & T. Ollendick (Eds.), *Handbook of psychotherapies with children and families* (pp. 385–404). New York, NY: Plenum. doi:10.1007/978-1-4615-4755-6_20

Knell, S. M. (2009). Cognitive behavioral play therapy. In K. J. O'Connor & L. D. Braverman (Eds.), *Play therapy theory and practice: Comparing theories and techniques* (pp. 203–236). Hoboken, NJ: Wiley.

Koltz, R. L., & Feit, S. S. (2012). A phenomenological study: The experience of live supervision during a pre-practicum counseling techniques course. *Qualitative Report, 17*(80), 1–24.

Kottman, T., & Meany-Walen, K. (2016). *Partners in play: An Adlerian approach to play therapy* (3rd ed.). Alexandria, VA: American Counseling Association.

Landis, L. L., & Young, M. E. (1994). The reflecting team in counselor education. *Counselor Education and Supervision, 33*(3), 210–218. doi:10.1002/j.1556-6978.1994.tb00287.x

Landreth, G. (2012). *Play therapy: The art of the relationship*. New York, NY: Taylor and Francis Group. doi:10.4324/9780203835159

Lee, R. E., & Everett, C. A. (2004). *The integrative family therapy supervisor: A primer*. New York, NY: Brunner-Routledge.

Lee, R. E., Nichols, D. P., Nichols, W. C., & Odom, T. (2004). Trends in family therapy supervision: The past 25 years and into the future. *Journal of Marital and Family Therapy*, *30*(1), 61–69. doi:10.1111/j.1752-0606.2004.tb01222.x PMID:14763209

Levinson, E. M., Black, L., Rafoth, M. A., & Slonim, J. E. (2010). Community collaboration and university-based clinics in school counseling. In E. M. Levinson (Ed.), *Handbook of education, training, and supervision of school psychologists in school and community* (Vol. 2, pp. 291–305). New York, NY: Routledge.

Lin, Y. W., & Bratton, S. (2015). A meta-analytic review of child-centered play therapy approaches. *Journal of Counseling and Development*, *93*(1), 45–58. doi:10.1002/j.1556-6676.2015.00180.x

Machuca, R., Johnson, T., & Moro, R. R. (2015). Tablet-assisted live supervision: Eye-bug supervision. In *Ideas and research you can use: VISTAS 2016, Article 55*. Retrieved from https://www.counseling.org/docs/default-source/vistas/article_5547f227f16116603abcacff0000bee5e7.pdf?sfvrsn=4

Meany-Walen, K. K., Lindo, N. A., Turley, E., Chung, C., Akay, S., Cheng, Y. J., & Chen, S. Y. (2013). Evaluating the impact of intensive supervision of child-centered play therapy training. *British Journal of Play Therapy*, *9*, 16–25.

Moody, S., Kostohryz, K., & Vereen, L. (2014). Authentically engaged learning through live supervision: A phenomenological study. *Counselor Education and Supervision*, *53*(1), 19–33. doi:10.1002/j.1556-6978.2014.00046.x

Mullen, J. A. (2016). Play therapy supervision. In K. J. O'Connor, C. H. Schaefer, & L. D. Braverman (Eds.), *Handbook of play therapy* (2nd ed.; pp. 549–560). Hoboken, NJ: John Wiley & Sons.

Mullen, J. A., Luke, M., & Drewes, A. A. (2007). Supervision can be playful, too: Play therapy techniques that enhance supervision. *International Journal of Play Therapy*, *16*(1), 69–85. doi:10.1037/1555-6824.16.1.69

Muro, J. H., Holliman, R. P., Blanco, P. J., & Stickley, V. K. (2015). Exploring play therapy training: An investigation on the impact of practice on attitude, knowledge, and skills with master's level students. *International Journal of Play Therapy*, *24*(4), 234–247. doi:10.1037/a0039811

Murrell, E., Steel, Z., Gaston, J., & Proudfoot, H. (2002). Training the clinical psychologist: Profile of a university-based clinic. *Australian Psychologist*, *37*(2), 123–128. doi:10.1080/00050060210001706766

National Association of Social Workers. (2008). *Code of ethics of the national association of social workers*. Washington, DC: Author.

Peabody, M. A. (2015). Building with purpose: Using LEGO SERIOUS PLAY in play therapy supervision. *International Journal of Play Therapy*, *24*(1), 30–40. doi:10.1037/a0038607

Perou, R., Bitsko, R. H., Blumberg, S. J., Pastor, P., Ghandour, R. M., Gfroerer, J. C., … Huang, L. N. (2013, May). Mental health surveillance among children-United States, 2005-2011. *MMWR Supplements*, *17*(62), 1-35. Retrieved from: https://www.cdc.gov/mmwr/preview/mmwrhtml/su6202a1.htm?s_cid=su6202a1_w

Perryman, K., & Doran, J. (2010). Guidelines for incorporating play therapy in the schools. In A. A. Drewes & C. E. Schaefer (Eds.), *School-based play therapy* (2nd ed.; pp. 61–86). Hoboken, NJ: John Wiley & Sons. doi:10.1002/9781118269701.ch3

Perryman, K. L., Moss, R. C., & Anderson, L. (2016). Sandtray supervision: An integrated model for play therapy supervision. *International Journal of Play Therapy*, *25*(4), 186–196. doi:10.1037/pla0040288

Purswell, K. E., & Stulmaker, H. L. (2015). Expressive arts in supervision: Choosing developmentally appropriate interventions. *International Journal of Play Therapy*, *24*(2), 103–117. doi:10.1037/a0039134

Ray, D. C. (2004). Supervision of basic and advanced skills in play therapy. *Journal of Professional Counseling, Practice, Theory, & Research*, *32*(2), 28–41. doi:10.1080/15566382.2004.12033805

Ray, D. C. (2010). Challenges and barriers to implementing play therapy in schools. In A. A. Drewes & C. E. Schaefer (Eds.), *School-based play therapy* (2nd ed.; pp. 87–106). Hoboken, NJ: John Wiley & Sons. doi:10.1002/9781118269701.ch4

Ray, D. C. (2011). *Advanced play therapy: Essential conditions, knowledge, and skills for child practice*. New York, NY: Routledge. doi:10.4324/9780203837269

Ray, D. C. (Ed.). (2016). *A therapist's guide to child development: The extraordinary normal years*. New York, NY: Routledge.

Ray, D. C., Purswell, K., Hass, S., & Aldrete, C. (2017). Child-centered play therapy-Research integrity checklist: Development, reliability, and use. *International Journal of Play Therapy*, *26*(4), 207–271. doi:10.1037/pla0000046

Scherl, C., & Haley, J. (2000). Computer monitor supervision: A clinical note. *The American Journal of Family Therapy*, *28*(3), 275–282. doi:10.1080/01926180050081702

Smith-Adcock, S., Davis, E., Pereira, J., Allen, C., Socarras, K., Bodurtha, K., & Smith-Bonahue, T. (2012). Preparing to play: A qualitative study of graduate students' reflections on learning play therapy in an elementary school. *International Journal of Play Therapy*, *21*(2), 100–115. doi:10.1037/a0026931

Spruill, D. A., & Benshoff, J. M. (2000). Helping beginning counselors develop a personal theory of counseling. *Counselor Education and Supervision*, *40*(1), 70–80. doi:10.1002/j.1556-6978.2000.tb01800.x

Stoltenberg, C. D. (1981). Approaching supervision from a developmental perspective: The counselor complexity model. *Journal of Counseling Psychology*, *28*(1), 59–65. doi:10.1037/0022-0167.28.1.59

Stulmaker, H. L., Lertora, I., & Garza, Y. (2015). Facilitating empathic perspective taking in beginning child-centered play therapists: The role of supervision. *International Journal of Play Therapy*, *24*(4), 177–189. doi:10.1037/a0039330

Thanasiu, P. L., Rust, K. L., & Walter, S. M. (2018). Service learning and live supervision as early components in play therapy training. *International Journal of Play Therapy*, *27*(2), 103–113. doi:10.1037/pla0000069

Thomas, D. A. (2015). Intentionality in supervision: Supervising play therapy interns and practitioners. In *Ideas and research you can use: VISTAS Online, Article 38*. Retrieved from: https://www.counseling.org/docs/default-source/vistas/article_387a5c21f16116603 abcacff0000bee5e7.pdf?sfvrsn=6

Thomas, J. T. (2010). *The ethics of supervision and consultation: Practical guidance for mental health professionals*. Washington, DC: American Psychological Association. doi:10.1037/12078-000

Tsai, M., & Ray, D. C. (2011). Play therapy outcome prediction: An exploratory study at a university-based clinic. *International Journal of Play Therapy*, *20*(2), 94–108. doi:10.1037/a0023441

VanderGast, T. S., Culbreth, J. R., & Flowers, C. (2010). An exploration of experiences and preferences in clinical supervision with play therapists. *International Journal of Play Therapy*, *19*(3), 174–185. doi:10.1037/a0018882

VanderGast, T. S., & Hinkle, M. S. (2015). So happy together? Predictors of satisfaction with supervision for play therapist supervisees. *International Journal of Play Therapy*, *24*(2), 92–102. doi:10.1037/a0039105

Wyatt, R. C., & Seid, E. L. (2008). Instruction's manual for Adlerian play therapy with Terry Kottman, PhD. Mill Valley, CA: Psychotherapy.net.

Yu, A. (2012). *iSupe: An innovation in live supervision*. Presented at the *Eighth International Interdisciplinary Conference on Clinical Supervision*, Garden City, NY.

Section 3

Contemporary Applications

This section offers contemporary applications to setting up supervision as well as a specified focus populations in setting up play therapy clinics in the university setting as well as outside the university. Considerations, set up, and facilitation methods are reviewed and offer the reader essential aspects when developing a play therapy clinic.

Chapter 9
Live Play Therapy Supervision

Raul Machuca
Barry University, USA

ABSTRACT

In this chapter, the author introduces live play therapy supervision as a complementary method to the traditional ways in which play therapy supervision is done, particularly in the context of play therapy training clinics. As conceived here, live play therapy supervision represents a valuable addition to the clinical supervision practices employed in the training of future play therapy practitioners. Specifically, this chapter proposes a working definition of live play therapy supervision, presents the advantages and disadvantages of using this model, explores some methods as well as techniques of live play therapy supervision, and describes the process of live play therapy supervision. Finally, the profile and role of the live play therapy supervisor is defined, the supervisory relationship is described, as well as the implications and future research possibilities in this area.

INTRODUCTION

The training of competent clinicians, and play therapists in particular, involves the convergence of specific learning conditions. Such conditions include the use of best practices in clinical education and supervision specifically designed for the training of play therapists, as well as the fulfillment of ethical mandates that safeguard a comprehensive system of learning and care. In addition, the use of methods that most clearly facilitate the training and supervision of play therapists becomes paramount given the uniqueness of this clinical specialty, and the level of vulnerability of the populations play therapists typically serve. As such, a case is made here about the relevance of using a supervision method which has the potential to facilitate and

DOI: 10.4018/978-1-5225-8226-7.ch009

significantly enhance the play therapy supervision process, while attending to the uniqueness of the play therapy experience, the live play therapy supervision method.

In its current state, there appears to be limited research related to the supervision of play therapists, with most of the literature around the topic being the result of very valuable, yet mainly anecdotic experiences, or conceptual elaborations (Donald, Culbreth & Carter, 2015). In addition, there is still a need for a more clearly defined theory, as well as methods or models of play therapy supervision; particularly one that integrates the traditional models of supervision with the uniqueness, creativity and expressiveness of play therapy (Hudspeth, 2015).

In this chapter, the author introduces live play therapy supervision as a complementary method to the traditional ways in which play therapy supervision is done such as self-report, live observation, video reviews, asynchronous supervision, etc. As conceived here, live play therapy supervision actually implies the use of direct assessment and intervention by the supervisor during a live observation of a play therapy session; therefore, live play therapy supervision represents a valuable addition to the clinical education and supervision practices employed in the training of future play therapy practitioners. This chapter also represents a contribution to the very limited body of knowledge that exist about live play therapy supervision.

Specifically, this chapter proposes a working definition of live play therapy supervision, presents the advantages and disadvantages of using this model, explores some methods as well as techniques of live play therapy supervision, and describes the process of live play therapy supervision. Finally, the profile and role of the live play therapy supervisor is explored, the supervision relationship is discussed, and the implications and future research possibilities in this area are presented.

LIVE SUPERVISION

Live supervision involves the direct observation of a counselor-in-training's session, and the synchronous intervention and guidance of a seasoned clinical supervisor (Bernard and Goodyear, 2014; Machuca, Johnson & Moro, 2016). By its very definition, live supervision is an experiential supervision method that provides both supervisor and supervisee the opportunity to interact in real time. Live supervision is different from other methods of supervision in that it allows the supervisor to provide direct guidance and intervention to the supervisee during the course of a counseling session. This is a very common method of supervision in counselor education and supervision settings (Koltz & Feit, 2012; Moody & Vereen, 2014), as well as other clinical programs with on-campus training clinics.

Live supervision has evolved following a somewhat parallel process to the development and subsequent advantages provided by modern computer and communication technologies. In addition, different modalities, structures and logistic variations have been used in the process of providing live supervision. Historically, the observation of live counseling sessions has been done through one-way mirrors, closed circuit camera systems, web-based live observation systems, as well as in-room observations and co-therapy modalities. Consequently, the direct provision of clinical guidance and supervision interventions has been done through walk-in, phone-in or call-in methods, by scheduling breaks or summoning the clinician in training to the observation room at critical points or during scheduled session breaks, bug-in-the ear methods (Boylston & Tuma, 1972), bug-in-the eye methods (Klitzke & Lombardo, 1991; Machuca, Johnson & Moro, 2016; Neukrug, 1991), and through direct supervisor in-the room guidance and modeling (Levinger, 1994). The choice of a method of observation and communication during live supervision has depended on the level of obstruction and interruption allowed and desired, the developmental level of the supervisee, the counseling modality, counseling specialty, theoretical orientation, technology available, familiarity of supervisor with technology, skills and methods used, and the theory of supervision, among other variables. These live supervision methods will be discussed in greater detail in terms of play therapy below.

PLAY THERAPY SUPERVISION

Play therapy supervision is an essential requirement in the training of play therapy practitioners. It is also qualitatively unique and needs to be considered differently from the general model of clinical supervision (Donald, Culbreth & Carter, 2015). Part of what makes play therapy supervision a unique experience has to do with the creativity and expressiveness of the play therapy experience, its theoretical underpinnings, the logistics involved, the language used, the populations typically served and many other factors (Donald, Culbreth and Carter, 2015; Hundspeth, 2015). To attend to the uniqueness of the play therapy process, play therapy supervision requires the development of a supervision model that not only addresses the unique factors stated before but that, as Teufel (2007) stated, goes beyond case conceptualization, and involves a more intentional and focused effort on intervention skills, treatment planning, ethics, assessment, and theoretical orientation.

Borrowing from the general definition of supervision (Bernard and Goodyear, 2014), and based on the characteristics of the play therapy supervision experience, and the role of the supervisor and the supervisee (Donald, Culbreth & Carter, 2015), play therapy supervision can be defined as the systematic process in which a seasoned play therapy practitioner supervisor facilitates the development of basic and advanced play therapy techniques, as well as the overall personal and professional development of a beginner play therapy practitioner. Given the particular nature of play therapy, the play therapy supervision process involves a comprehensive and holistic approach that requires for the supervisor to have a clear professional identity and expertise as a play therapist, and for the supervisee to be able to learn specific play therapy techniques, demonstrate creative and expressive skills in the process of working with children, as well as the capability to trust and rely on the play therapy process.

Models of Play Therapy Supervision

Several models for the provision of play therapy supervision have been documented in the literature. Some of them are the Intensive Three-day Play Therapy Supervision Model (Bratton, Landreth & Homeyer, 1993), the 15-week Child-Centered Self-Reflective Play Therapy Supervision Model (Giordano, 2000), and the Three Step Model (Allen, Folger & Pehrsson, 2007). The Intensive Three-Day Play Therapy Supervision/Training Model involves an individual and group live supervision component, as well as post session feedback and synchronous and asynchronous observation. The live component of this developmental model is done through a one-way mirror and the communication between supervisors and supervisees occurs at scheduled breaks in which the supervisee walks out of the play therapy room and the client waits in the waiting room (Bratton, Landreth & Homeyer, 1993). In the 15-week Child-Centered Self-Reflective Play therapy Supervision Model, doctoral students with vast play therapy experience provide supervision to play therapists in training using a manualized approach (Giordano, 2000). In the Three Step Model, a developmental approach is used to facilitate the learning and practice of play therapy skills, which are presented to the supervisee in a series of steps and corresponding with the child's progression of play (Allen, Folger & Pehrsson, 2007). Live supervision using this model typically involves being present during the play therapy session, and or providing feedback and direct guidance during the play therapy session (Smith-Adcock, Shin & Pereira, 2015).

LIVE PLAY THERAPY SUPERVISION

Applying, once again, the overall definition of supervision (Bernard and Goodyear, 2014) to the live play therapy supervision process, we can say that live play therapy supervision refers to the experiential process in which an experienced play therapy supervisor provides synchronous guidance, feedback and intervention to a play therapist-in-training during the course of a play therapy session. A defining characteristic of this method of play therapy supervision is that the play therapy supervisor has the possibility of immediately addressing and intervening on any aspect of the play therapy session as it occurs. For the supervisee, it represents an opportunity to receive immediate feedback, to apply it right away, and to experience instant support. This last element is very important in live supervision because feeling supported by the supervisor during the play therapy session is, perhaps, the most significant factor in effective live play therapy supervision.

Extrapolating the general goals of play therapy supervision, the main goals of live play therapy supervision are to improve play therapy skills and techniques, adapt play therapy process to specific clients, develop conceptualization skills, develop self-awareness, receive professional support, and minimize possibilities of supervisee burnout (VarderGast & Hinkle, 2015). Other goals of live play therapy supervision are to provide immediate feedback, facilitate faster guided implementation of feedback, as well as to facilitate an encourage a supportive environment for beginning supervisees. Guerney (1978) highlighted early on the importance of using live play therapy supervision consistently in the effective training of play therapists.

Methods of Live Play Therapy Supervision

Live supervision methods are particularly useful and appropriate during the early stages of the play therapy supervisee's professional development (Koltz & Feit, 2012; Smith-Adcock, et al., 2012). There are several methods of live play therapy supervision which are used depending on the supervisee, supervisor and client needs. The use of a live play therapy supervision method also depends on the level of intrusiveness that is appropriate for the play therapy session being conducted, as well as the logistics and technological resources available for the supervision process. The methods described here correspond to those most commonly described in general supervision (Bernard & Goodyear, 2014), and play therapy supervision literature (Bratton, Landreth & Homeyer, 1993; Levinger, 1994), as well as other methods of live supervision that can be easily adopted for the play therapy supervision process. The general logistics for the use of the methods described below may involve one or two separate rooms, depending on where the supervisor and the supervisee are located. If located in separate rooms, the observation and listening to the live play therapy session can be done through a one-way mirror or a closed-circuit audiovisual system.

Co-Play Therapy Supervision

Described as two therapists working together, one acting as supervisor and the other one as supervisee. In this method, there is a division of the therapeutic role, with one therapist supervisee working with the child, and the other one commenting on their interaction and setting limits (Levinger, 1994). Co-play therapy supervision can be used also in the context of a tandem play therapy process where the supervisor can take the lead initially, and gradually allows for the play therapy trainee to assume a more active and central role as therapist. Using this model, the supervisor who is located in the play therapy room with the supervisee and the child, can model live for the supervisee the use of specific play therapy techniques. Once the play therapy trainee takes the lead in the session, the supervisor may track the therapist/child interaction and intervene at crucial points as needed.

Participant Supervision

Originally described as a model for co-therapy (Yerushalmi, 2001) and similar to the co-play therapy method, in participant supervision the play therapy supervisor can play the role of therapeutic player for structured or unstructured play therapy. For instance, throughout the play therapy session, the supervisor may ask the child about any way in which the child can be assisted in the play, and the supervisor will assume the roles assigned by the child as appropriate. With the supervisor assisting in the child's play, the supervisee can focus on practicing any necessary skills, techniques or interventions. This method of live play therapy supervision is ideal if the supervisee is working with a child who may need a higher level of attention or response by the supervisee and or the supervisor. Since the supervisor is already in the room, any critical incidents can be attended immediately.

Bug-in-the-Ear

This method of live play therapy supervision involves the use of a voice communication device, typically a headphone or headset as the primary mechanism for the provision of feedback. The supervisor, situated in an adjacent observation room, uses a microphone to communicate with the play therapist. At any point during the play therapy session, the supervisor provides verbal input to the supervisee as needed in the form of directions, suggestions, comments, examples, specific statements to be used, etc. It is very important for the supervisor to make sure the provision of feedback does not interfere with the play therapy supervisee's capability to attend to the child. As described in its original version (Boylston & Tuma, 1972) this method of live supervision was highly advantageous because it represented a less intrusive aid for the supervisee and for the therapeutic alliance. However, it also introduced the challenge for the supervisee of attending to both the supervisor and the client at the same time, as well as the risk of over-instruction from the supervisor (Scherl

& Haley, 2000). This method of live supervision can be done using a one-way observation window or a closed-circuit audiovisual system.

Bug-in the-Eye

The bug-in-the-eye method uses visual forms of communicating feedback to the supervisee. The traditional method involves the use of computer-based communication devices where the supervisor types the feedback into a computer board located in the observation room and the feedback is displayed for the supervisee on a screen located in the therapy room (Klitzke & Lombardo, 1991).

Eye-Bug Supervision

Also known as tablet-based play therapy supervision and a form of bug-in-the-eye supervision method, this is a most convenient form of communication between the supervisor and the supervisee involving the use of tablets. When using this method, the supervisor located in an observation room sends visual messages to the supervisee using various tablet-based technological applications (Machuca, Johnson & Moro, 2016). A one-way observation window or a closed-circuit audiovisual system can be used for all bug-in-the-eye methods described.

Walk-In Supervision

When using this method, the supervisor leaves the observation room and walks in the play therapy room in order to provide any needed re-direction and or feedback to the supervisee. Most typically used during more pressing critical incidents in supervision, this method may also involve the supervisor switching from play therapy observant to co-play therapist if the play therapy process calls for it. A common form of live supervision used in training clinics, this is also considered a therapy intervention where the supervisor enters the therapy room spontaneously or at a pre-arranged time at intervenes with both the supervisee and the client (Bernard & Goodyear, 2014).

Walk-Out Supervision Method

This method of live supervision refers to spontaneous and or scheduled breaks taken by the supervisee in the course of a therapy session. The goal of the walk-out is for the supervisor and the supervisee to discuss any critical incidents happening in the counseling session. It is most commonly described as an interruption of the counseling session, in which the supervisee leaves the client in the counseling room or the waiting room and goes to the observation room where the supervisor is located. The walk-out method is used by the Intensive Three Day Play Therapy Supervision/ Training Model (Bratton, Landreth & Homeyer, 1993). In this model, there is a scheduled 30-minute feedback sessions with the supervisee during the course of a play therapy session, with the child client in the waiting room.

Phone-In Supervision Method

This method of live play therapy supervision requires the use of a phone system for communication between the observation room and the play therapy room. When required, the supervisor uses a phone to call to communicate any immediate feedback that may be useful to the supervisee working with the child. As originally described, this method of live supervision may be used during critical incident moments of the counseling session for the supervisor to call-in to provide immediate input to the supervisee (Bernard & Goodyear, 2014).

Although some methods of live play therapy supervision can be more distracting to the child and or intrusive for the play therapy process, it is up to the supervisor to decide the most appropriate and comprehensive way to deliver the best supervision experience to the live play therapy supervisee. Paraphrasing Machuca, Johnson and Moro (2016), and applying their ideas to the live play therapy supervision process, it is possible to affirm that each method of live play therapy supervision has advantages and disadvantages. Text-based, or visual supervision methods seem more efficient in comparison with auditory methods as they may be less distracting and intrusive for child clients. Auditory methods such as bug-in-the-ear allow the supervisor to provide a faster and better detailed input in the shortest time. It also allows for the input to be modeled right in the moment for the supervisee. As mentioned before, it also requires the play therapist to attend to the child client and the supervisor at the same time, and if not done appropriately, it could be highly distracting and could interfere with the play therapist's ability to maintain awareness and focus. According to Miller, Miller & Evans (2002), visual-based interventions have the advantage of being delivered in a non-intrusive manner, as well as providing the opportunity for the supervisee to apply feedback given during a session with minor disruption in the counseling process. Machuca, Johnson & Moro (2016) also warn about the high costs and sometimes complex logistics associated to visual-based interventions using teleprompters or computer monitors. These authors however make a case for the advantages introduced by the latest technology of wireless internet and tablet computers, which facilitate a combination of minimally-intrusive and simple to set up live supervision experiences.

Techniques and Interventions in Live Play Therapy Supervision

Play therapy supervision techniques, and particularly, live play therapy supervision techniques are used with the purpose of facilitating awareness (Bratton, Ceballos, & Sheely, 2008), improving the development of basic and advance play therapy skills, and promoting overall growth of the supervisee (Mullen, Luke, & Drewes, 2007). According to Borders and Leddick (1987), the choice of interventions depends on the supervisee's goals, developmental level, experience, and learning style. It also depends on the supervisor's theoretical orientation, assessment of supervisee skills (goals), and purpose of the supervisory experience. Although they were originally employed for assessment of the play therapy supervisee's skills, some instruments were also identified as play therapy supervision interventions by Donald, Culbreth, & Carter (2015) in their play therapy supervision review of literature. Their list includes the Play therapy Observer (PLATO) by Tanner & Mathis (1995), the Play Therapy Skills Checklist (PTSC) by Ray (2004), and the eight principles for non-directive play therapy by Axline (1969).

In the process of providing live play therapy supervision, however, the supervisor may use multiple techniques and interventions in addition to those specifically described for play therapy supervision. The identification of specific live play therapy supervision techniques and interventions may facilitate a more wholistic and comprehensive supervision experience for the supervisee. Some live play therapy techniques can be implemented during the delivery of the feedback through audiovisual means such as voice, texts and images to facilitate confidence building and encouragement to the supervisee. The use of universal symbols of approval such as the thumbs up and the happy face are example of these. In addition, live play therapy techniques such as tracking supervisee's behavior during the play therapy session can be used as well to help increase awareness, for modeling of skills, and to provide instant identification of skills being displayed by supervisees in their play therapy session.

The supervisor may also employ different interventions such as introducing a parallel process between the supervisee and the client, and the supervisor and the supervisee (Mullen, Luke, & Drewes, 2007). When employing a parallel process, and taking into account the attention capabilities of the supervisee, the supervisor may provide feedback to the supervisee that represents examples of the basic and advanced skills the supervisee could use with the child. More specifically, live feedback from the supervisor may include actual ways of responding, tracking, reflecting, returning responsibility, and identifying themes, which the supervisee can use right away with the client. Ray (2004) calls for some caution when facilitating some advanced play therapy skills with the supervisee during live supervision. An example is that of a supervisor facilitating the identification of themes during live supervision. According to this author, when play therapists attempt to analyze play themes during play therapy, they might lose sight of connecting with the child in the moment (Ray, 2004). Other techniques that can be unique to the live play therapy supervision experience involve the provision of specific key comments and responses to the supervisee to be immediately employed with the child. The input provided by the supervisee can also convey specific examples of skills, model therapeutic affect to be used with the child, as well as to model the provision of both basic and advanced skills (Mullen, Luke, & Drewes, 2007).

ADVANTAGES AND DISADVANTAGES OF THE LIVE PLAY THERAPY SUPERVISION EXPERIENCE

The use of live play therapy supervision has both advantages and disadvantages when used in the training of play therapists. The advantages of using this method of play therapy supervision vastly outnumber the challenges, particularly when live play therapy supervision is used by highly qualified supervisors with knowledge of and access to appropriate technological resources. Most of the advantages and disadvantages of the live play therapy supervision process described below were taken or adapted from the general literature on clinical supervision (Bernard & Goodyear, 2014), some of the literature on play therapy supervision (Bratton, Landreth & Homeyer, 1991; Donald, Culbreth & Carter, 2015; Hudspeth, 2015; Stulmaker, Lertora & Garza, 2015; Ray, 2004), the very small body of literature on live play therapy supervision (Thanasiu, Rust & Walter, 2018), and others as specifically cited.

Advantages of Live Play Therapy Supervision

The use of live play therapy supervision has multiple advantages. In general, live play therapy supervision adds a sense of immediacy to both the assessment and intervention processes of supervision. It also provides specific advantages to the personal and professional development of the supervisee, the quality of care for the clients, and the nature of the supervision relationship. The following are more specific ways in which the use of live play therapy supervision represents a clear strength in the training and supervision of play therapists:

Early and Immediate Assessment

The use of live play therapy supervision facilitates the immediate assessment of the play therapy supervisee's development and skills, as well as the timely assessment of the play therapy process as it occurs. This assessment can be done using play therapy supervision instruments like the ones mentioned by Donald, Culbreth, & Carter, (2015), or by direct observation of the supervisee's behavior and skills. Using the Play Therapy Skills Checklist (Ray, 2004), a supervisor can verify instantaneously the use of specific skills by the supervisee, as well as to provide a more focused feedback on any skills in need of improvement. The use of the PTSC is recommended to be employed during asynchronous as well as live play therapy supervision (Ray, 2004). The live play therapy supervision experience facilitates earlier recognition of strengths and areas for growth as well as earlier introduction of necessary supervision interventions.

Immediate Feedback

In live play therapy supervision, the feedback or input can be given to the supervisee immediately and as needed throughout the play therapy session. With the use of live play therapy supervision, the supervisor does not have to wait until the post session review of a play therapy session to provide feedback, to provide guidance, or to implement a supervision intervention with the play therapist in training. A live play therapy supervision method allows the supervisor to receive immediate information on the play therapist-in training's performance and to act accordingly (Machuca, Johnson & Moro, 2016).

Immediate Implementation

Live play therapy supervision allows for the play therapy supervisee to implement the feedback provided by the supervisor as it occurs. For instance, a supervisor may ask the supervisee to use a specific skill or technique, or point out specific key elements of the process as they occur. Since the supervisor is able to provide timely feedback to the supervisee, it significantly closes the time gap between assessment and implementation of corrective feedback (Machuca, Johnson & Moro, 2016).

Extension of Supervisor's Expertise

Since the play therapy supervisor is able to interact with the supervisee during the play therapy session, there is a more direct extension although somewhat limited, of the play therapy supervisor's expertise into the work of the play therapist in training. Understandably, the presence of the play therapy supervisor increases the likelihood that certain aspects of the play therapy process, which could be missed by beginning play therapist will be both identified and addressed. Acting as an extension of the supervisor's expertise also facilitates an earlier introduction of advanced and more challenging play therapy skills such as enlarging meaning, since the live play therapy supervisor can determine the appropriateness of its use, and closely guide the delivery of it.

Improvement of Supervisees' Perceptions, Attitudes and Identity

Play therapist in training who receive live supervision report increased levels of perceived support and confidence (Smith-Adcock, Shin & Pereira,2015). In addition, counselors-in-training receiving live supervision have reported increased development of their identity as counselors (Koltz & Feit, 2012; Moody & Vereen, 2014). The use of live play therapy supervision has also been beneficial in increasing perceived knowledge and skills, as well as improvement in attitudes about play therapy among supervisees (Thanasiu, Rust & Walker, 2018).

Increased Availability of Interventions

Depending on the live play therapy supervision method used, there is an increased numbert of supervision interventions the supervisor can use during the play therapy supervision process. For example, when using tablets as the primary communication device between supervisor and supervisee, the supervisor can resource to multiple ways of providing guidance such as text, sound, images, and even emojis to convey information and feedback to the supervisee (Machuca, Johnson & Moro, 2016).

Client Welfare

Ensuring client welfare is also a very important advantage of live play therapy supervision. Bernard & Goodyear (2014) stated the purposes of supervision as fostering the supervisee's professional development and ensuring client welfare. This statement is particularly true during live play therapy supervision given the immediacy with which the supervisor can attend to any remediation needs on the part of the play therapy supervisee. In addition, Jordan (1999), Koltz & Feit (2012), and Smith-Adcock et al., (2012) as cited by Thanasiu, Rust & Walker (2018) agreed on the idea that when beginning play therapy supervisees provide play therapy, live supervision is used as a way of protecting the clients.

Working Alliance

Live supervision that focuses on modeling, support, and immediate, concrete feedback has been also recognized as a very useful instrument in facilitating the supervisor and supervisee working alliance (Thanasiu, Rust & Walker, 2018).

Disadvantages of Live Play Therapy Supervision

There are some disadvantages associated to the use of this method of supervision. In general, the weaknesses of this method may vary depending on the level of supervisors' technology proficiency, their openness to new methods of supervision, as well as the availability of resources at the training facilities. Some of the specific disadvantages in the use of live play therapy supervision are:

Technology Requirements and Knowledge

Some methods of live play therapy supervision may require the use of specific technology to which both the supervisor and supervisee need to have access and be familiar. Some level of technological proficiency and training is a necessary requirement for both the play therapy supervisor and the supervisee.

Cost

The use of technology and the incorporation of more sophisticated methods of observation and feedback delivery may represent a significant investment. For example, the use of the eye-bug supervision method requires the use of at least two tablets, as well as the acquisition of additional technological applications to be used during the live supervision process (Machuca, Johnson & Moro, 2016).

Limited Mobility

Play therapy often requires for the supervisee to be able to move frequently around the play room, as well as to be able to change activities depending on the child's process. Some methods of live play therapy supervision delivery, even those that facilitate more mobility such as tablets, may involve the additional task of having to change their placement frequently during the play therapy session.

Risk of Interruption or Distraction

The choice of a method for live play therapy supervision delivery may depend on the level of interruption and or distraction a particular method could place on the flow of a play therapy session. Even one of the least intrusive methods such as eye-bug supervision would require for the supervisee to attend to the tablet occasionally, which could be distracting for both the supervisee and the client.

Over-Reliance on Supervisor

An additional challenge to overcome when using live play therapy supervision is the possibility of the supervisee to become over-reliant on the supervisor. Another side of this challenge is the risk of the supervisor to over-extend the frequency and amount of guidance, feedback and or interventions used during the play therapy session.

The Process of Live Play Therapy Supervision

Preparation

The provision of live play therapy supervision requires some training and logistical preparation. Prior to the live play therapy supervision experience, play therapy supervisees need to receive enough training in play therapy for them to perform autonomous play therapy sessions with their clients. The ideal model for play therapy training as described by Bratton, Landreth & Homeyer (1993), involves a process of training, application and supervision. We argue that in the case of live play therapy supervision the application and the supervision can happen simultaneously. A combination of both asynchronous and live play therapy supervision would be ideal in the training of beginning play therapist. This model is ideal because live play therapy supervision facilitates the direct observation of the play therapy process, the provision of immediate feedback and the timely implementation of interventions. The use of asynchronous play therapy supervision facilitates the processing of the play therapy experience, the discussion of the supervisor and the supervisee' assessment, as well as the case conceptualization and future planning. The combination of asynchronous and live play therapy supervision can take the form of live observation of a play therapy session followed by a feedback session. It can also happen as a combination of live observation and observation of recorded sessions by the supervisor with both live feedback being offered as well as after-session feedback.

In terms of logistics, it is recommended live play therapy supervision be provided using an observation room adjacent or as close as possible to the play therapy room. The required technology depends on the live play therapy supervision method used, and it may vary from using direct observation through a one-way mirror, to closed circuit television monitoring, as well as audiovisual communication with the supervisee using computers and display screens, as well as headphones and tablets.

Technological Requirements

Technological requirements for the provision of live play therapy supervision also depends on the type of supervision experience that is most accessible to play therapy training and supervision facilities. Technology employed can be very simple such as one-way audio communication devises or as complex as live observation and feedback using a secure web-based monitoring system. We advocate for the use of a tablet-based system like the one used in the eye-bug supervision method describe by Machuca, Johnson & Moro (2016). Live play therapy supervision can be provided using one tablet situated in the observation room and one tablet situated in the play therapy room. The tablet in the play therapy room can be moved and position in different places, or it can be held by the play therapy supervisee. Ideally, it should facilitate the supervisee's mobility in the room and an easier view of the visual feedback sent by the supervisor. The use of eye-bug supervision in play therapy also requires connection to internet signal, as well as access to safe technological applications for text messaging and communication such as the Tigerconnect app formerly known as Tigertext.

Supervision Recommendations

The process of implementing live play therapy supervision should start with an orientation to the method for both the supervisees and their clients. As expected, and depending on the method used, the presence of a particular communication devise in the play therapy session for instance, may provoke initial curiosity on the child. An honest and transparent socialization of the method is usually enough to respond to the child's curiosity and to start or continue with a regular play therapy process.

The following is an adaptation to the live play therapy supervision process of some of the recommendations for the eye-bug live supervision method originally presented by Machuca, Johnson & Moro (2016). In the process on implementing live play therapy supervision, supervisors will be better served if they make sure to:

- Become familiar with all the possibilities that the method of live play therapy supervision employed may offer to the supervision experience. This may include things from demonstrating, modeling, and changing roles in co-play therapy supervision, to the use of alternative forms of feedback like emojis, images, and links to specific information made possible by the tablet-based methods.
- Prefer the use of short and concrete feedback. Developing a list of code words is recommended prior to the start of the live play therapy supervision experience. This is also important as a way of modeling for the supervisee how to communicate their intent to their child clients in as few words as possible. For this purpose, we adhere to the idea of providing feedback of a maximum of ten words as a good rule of thumb (Ray, 2004).

- Be aware of the play therapist's developmental level as this may determine the type of feedback you are to send from providing verbatim expressions to use with clients, to more general directives. Ray (2004) recommends the presentation of concrete categories of verbal responses from which supervisees may become aware of the variety and effect of responses. In addition, it is important to know that play therapy supervisees at initial levels of professional development may benefit better from more teaching and direction in supervision, as well as from verbatim presentation of responses (Stulmaker, Lertora, and Garza, 2015).
- Make sure to convey feedback that you are perfectly comfortable socializing with clients. In the course of the play therapy session, children may have spells of curiosity about what is being communicated and the supervisee should be able to share the content on the screen with their clients in the most open and transparent way possible.

The Live Play Therapy Supervisor

Like all play therapy supervisors, live play therapy supervisors should have extensive training and experience in play therapy. They also need to be structured, organized, and should provide supervision within the limits of the theoretical model of play therapy in which they have been trained (Ray, 2004).

Supervisees value the play therapy training and experience of their supervisor (Aguilera, 2009; VanderGast, Culbreth, & Flowers, 2010). In fact, the most important factors related to supervisee satisfaction with supervision are supervisor professional identity as a play therapist and supervisee years of play therapy experience (VanderGast & Hinkle, 2015). More experienced supervisors, such as those with a clear professional identity as play therapist as well as those who hold play therapy supervision credentials such as registered play therapy supervisors (RPT-S) are preferred by supervisees and would be able to offer more effective and targeted feedback to them (Donald, Culbreth, & Carter, 2015). The professional identity of live play therapy supervisors is crucial as this characteristic would serve as the primary tool to facilitate the development of a play therapist's professional identity (Donald, Culbreth, & Carter, 2015).

Live play therapy supervisors are to focus both on the personal and professional development of the supervisees, as well as in the development of their skills (Landreth, 2012). Since there is extensive focus of play therapy supervision on conceptualization skills, a balance between the focus on awareness, development, skills and conceptualization is highly recommended. Supervisors must be also highly organized, concrete, and flexible to attend to the needs of each supervisee (Bratton, Landreth & Homeyer, 1996).

Other desirable characteristics of live play therapy supervisors, in addition to the ones more recently described in the literature for play therapy supervisors (Donald, Culbreth & Walker, 2015) are sense of immediacy, attention to detail, resourcefulness and creativity. Finally, given the technological demands of today's world, a live play therapy supervisor needs to be highly proficient in the use of technology, as well as in the employment of a more diverse set of technological tools. Familiarity with technological applications as well as other technological aids is highly recommended.

The Supervisory Relationship in Live Play Therapy Supervision

In addition to factors that play a role in the supervisory relationship as described in the general supervision literature such as gender and sexual identity, race, ethnicity, supervisor's style, age, personality characteristics, developmental level, supervision approach, etc., (Bernard & Goodyear, 2014), and the more specific factors associated to the play therapy supervisory relationship such as the importance of the supervisor credentials and training, as well as the positive perception of the supervisory relationship (Donald, Culbreth & Carter, 2015), there are some factors that may be unique to the supervisory relationship, in the context of live play therapy. These additional supervisory relationship factors in live play therapy supervision are related to the unique conditions involved in live play therapy supervision. Things like being observed live, being given immediate feedback for performance in play therapy sessions, as well as having to implement feedback right away, on top of being assessed live during the whole process, demands the existence of a very special relationship between live play therapy supervisors and their supervisees.

In response to initial research efforts or in anticipation of what further research may clarify on the matter, some authors have highlighted the need for a strong supervisory working alliance (Thanasiu, Rust and Walter, 2018), as a *sine qua non* condition for the implementation of this supervision method. This is a relationship characterized by clear recognition of the supervisor's competence, mutual respect, and a very high level of support offer and perceived (Ray, 2011; VanderGast, Culbreth & Flowers, 2010). For the success of the live play therapy supervision experience, and for a stronger supervisory relationship, there is a need for a supervisor to be highly trained and with specific supervision credentials in play therapy. Supervisee's perception of a clear professional identity of their supervisors as play therapists is preferred and seems to influence a more positive experience for supervisees (VanderGast, Culbreth & Flowers, 2010) In addition, the supervisor must be willing to step in, literally and figuratively, and to be equally exposed in the demonstration and modeling of play therapy skills for their supervisees (Kratz & Lund, 1994). The supervisees on the other hand need to be comfortable with their own vulnerability and open to feedback and to its immediate implementation. Finally, the live play therapy supervisory relationship should be a playful experience (Donald, Culbreth & Carter, 2015), an experience that parallels the play therapy experience.

IMPLICATIONS FOR PLAY THERAPY TRAINING, SUPERVISION, AND PRACTICE

Given the limited documentation and research related to play therapy supervision, and the almost non-existent research and information on live play therapy supervision, it is imperative for training programs and play therapy training facilities to include specific training modules on play therapy supervision. The training on play therapy supervision should also include specific experiential learning around the use of live play therapy supervision methods, techniques and interventions. The recommendation of more targeted focus on live play therapy supervision training is particularly important for both on campus and off campus counseling training clinics. Anywhere there is a play therapy room and an observation room available, the possibility of a more wholistic and comprehensive live play therapy supervision training experience awaits.

An important aspect of the training of play therapy supervisors is the incorporation of specific training in the implementation of technology in supervision. Play therapy supervisors will benefit greatly from learning and implementing specific technological applications, using various forms of observation and communication equipment, as well as learning the necessary requirements and skills for new modalities of play therapy supervision such as online supervision. It is also desirable for live play therapy supervisors to be aware of the latest and safest technological applications that can be used and in accordance to the existing resources in their training settings.

Live play therapy supervision represents a vast and somehow unexplored field. Its use will add significantly to the field of play therapy practice, particularly when employed in combination with effective training and with asynchronous methods of play therapy supervision. The use of live play therapy supervision would have a significant impact in the practice of play therapy, particularly by novice play therapists. No other method offers the possibility of directly extending the knowledge and experience of the play therapy supervisor onto the supervisee as fast as live play therapy supervision. It also facilitates more effective and immediate attention to any critical incidents that surface during the play therapy session, including issues of competence, gatekeeping, ethical behavior, safety, and many others.

ETHICAL CONSIDERATIONS

Some of the most important ethical issues involved in live play therapy supervision are related to the ethical mandate to be fully trained and to receive play therapy supervision as part of the requirements for play therapy practitioners (APT, 2013). The literature on play therapy supervision however speaks of the fact that there may be many play therapists who may not be getting supervision (Donald, Culbreth, & Carter, 2015).

The ethical training and supervision mandate also apply for play therapy supervisors. The literature in this area also speaks of the lack of play therapy supervisors, as well as the existence of play therapy supervisors with limited supervision training, including training in specific models of supervision (Fall et al., 2007).

As such, it is very important for play therapy supervisees, play therapy practitioners and play therapy supervisors to adhere to the general code of ethics of their professions particularly in terms of competence, as well as to the ethical and best practice guidelines provided by the professional organizations for play therapy.

FURTHER RESEARCH

Given the small body of knowledge on live play therapy supervision that is available further research on the general experience of implementing this method of supervision is needed. It is also needed further research in more specific applications of the live play therapy supervision experience such as the effects of employing specific techniques and interventions, the effects of live play therapy supervision on diverse supervisee variables, the use of live play therapy supervision with more advanced play therapy practitioners, as well as the effects of technology in the live play therapy supervision process.

Some other areas of research as it relates to live play therapy supervision are:

- Group play therapy live supervision
- Supervision of live play therapy supervision
- Live play therapy supervision and its effects on clients (e.g., a comparative client outcomes research between play therapy supervision and live play therapy supervision)
- Play therapy supervisee's perceptions of live play therapy supervision. The research on the use of live play therapy supervision may also improve the perception and preference that play therapy supervisees may have about this

modality of supervision. According to VanderGast, Culbreth, & Flowers (2010), live play therapy supervision was not ranked among the top supervision formats of interest by participants without Registered Play Therapist (RPT) or Registered Play Therapist Supervisor (RPT-S) credentials.

CONCLUSION

Live play therapy supervision represents a very valuable alternative and a great complement to play therapy supervision mostly based on observation and video recording. Some examples of its implementation have been described, and they illustrate its usefulness in facilitating the development of awareness and play therapy skills. Live play therapy supervision enables the implementation of both simple and more complex supervision interventions. The use of a parallel process between supervisor, supervisee and clients is an example of the later.

Live play therapy supervision facilitates an extension of the knowledge, skills and experience of the supervisor to the supervisee in a more immediate and effective manner. Play therapy clients whose beginning play therapists received live play therapy supervision will benefit immediately from this more immediate extension of the supervisor into the play therapy session. Counselors do not need to wait until some of their skills are fully integrated in their tool box in order to present them to their clients.

There is a highly recognized need for more research in the area of play therapy supervision. This need is even more significant as it relates to live play therapy supervision methods, interventions and techniques. The research about the relationship between multiple supervisee and client variables in the context of play therapy supervision and live play therapy supervision is also in its infancy.

REFERENCES

Aguilera, M. E. (2009). *An exploratory study of the developmental process of novice play therapists* (Doctoral dissertation). Retrieved from ProQuest dissertations & theses. (UMI Number 3376769)

Allen, V. B., Folger, W. A., & Pehrsson, D. E. (2007). Reflective process in play therapy: A practical model for supervising counseling students. *Education*, *127*, 472–479.

Association for Play Therapy. (2013). *RPT/S credentialing guide: Registered play therapist (RPT) & Supervisor (RPT-S).* Retrieved from http://c.ymcdn.com/sites/www.a4pt.org/resource/resmgr/ RPT_and_RPT-S_Credentials/RPTS_Guide.pdf

Axline, V. M. (1969). *Play therapy*. New York, NY: Ballantine Books.

Bernard, J. M., & Goodyear, R. K. (2014). *Fundamentals of Clinical Supervision* (5th ed.). Boston: Pearson.

Borders, L. D., & Leddick, G. (1987). *Handbook of counseling supervision*. Alexandria, VA: American Counseling Association.

Boylston, W., & Tuma, J. (1972). Training of mental health professionals through the use of the 'bug in the ear'. *The American Journal of Psychiatry, 129*(1), 92–95. doi:10.1176/ajp.129.1.92 PMID:5034190

Bratton, S., Ceballos, P., & Sheely, A. (2008). Expressive arts in a humanistic approach to play therapy supervision: Facilitating therapist self-awareness. In A. A. Drewes & J. A. Mullen (Eds.), *Supervision can be playful: Techniques for child and play therapist supervisors* (pp. 211–232). Lanham, MD: Rowman & Littlefield.

Bratton, S., Landreth, G., & Homeyer, L. (1993). An intensive three day play therapy supervision/ training model. *International Journal of Play Therapy, 2*(2), 61–79. doi:10.1037/h0089366

Donal, E., Cunbreth, J., & Carter, A. (2015). Play therapy supervision: A review of the literature. *International Journal of Play Therapy, 24*(2), 59–77. doi:10.1037/a0039104

Fall, M., Drew, D., Chute, A., & More, A. (2007). The voices of registered play therapists as supervisors. *International Journal of Play Therapy, 16*(2), 133–146. doi:10.1037/1555-6824.16.2.133

Giordano, M. A. (2000). *Effectiveness of a child-centered self-reflective play therapy supervision model* (Doctoral dissertation). Retrieved from ProQuest dissertations & theses. (UMI Number 3064391)

Guerney, L. (1978). Training and evaluation of students as consultants in an adult-child relationship enhancement program. *Professional Psychology, 9*, 193–198.

Hudspeth, E. F. (2015). An Introduction to Clinical Supervision in Play Therapy: Research, Practice, and Application. *International Journal of Play Therapy, 24*(2), 55–58. doi:10.1037/pla0000011

Klitzke, M. J., & Lombardo, T. W. (1991). A "bug-in-the-eye" is better than a "bug-in-the-ear": A teleprompter technique for on-line therapy skills training. *Behavior Modification*, *15*(1), 113–117. doi:10.1177/01454455910151007 PMID:2003846

Koltz, R. L., & Feit, S. S. (2012). A phenomenological study : The experience of live supervision during a pre-practicum counseling techniques course. *Qualitative Report*, *17*(80), 1–24.

Kranz, P. L., & Lund, N. L. (1994). Recommendations for supervising play therapists. *International Journal of Play Therapy*, *3*(2), 45–52. doi:10.1037/h0089168

Landreth, G. (2012). *Play therapy: The art of the relationship*. New York, NY: Taylor and Francis Group, LLC. doi:10.4324/9780203835159

Levinger, A. (1994). Co-play therapy. *International Journal of Play Therapy*, *3*(2), 53–62. doi:10.1037/h0089127

Machuca, R., Johnson, T., & Moro, R. (2016). Tablet-based live supervision: Eye-Bug Supervision. VISTAS 2016 Summer Ed.

Miller, K. L., Miller, S. M., & Evans, W. J. (2002). Computer-assisted live supervision in college counseling centers. *Journal of College Counseling*, *5*(2), 187–192. doi:10.1002/j.2161-1882.2002.tb00221.x

Moody, S., Kostohryz, K., & Vereen, L. (2014). Authentically engaged learning through live supervision: A phenomenological study. *Counselor Education and Supervision*, *53*(1), 19–33. doi:10.1002/j.1556-6978.2014.00046.x

Mullen, J. A., Luke, M., & Drewes, A. A. (2007). Supervision can be playful, too: Play therapy techniques that enhance supervision. *International Journal of Play Therapy*, *16*(1), 69–85. doi:10.1037/1555-6824.16.1.69

Neukrug, E. S. (1991). Computer-assisted live supervision in counselor skills training. *Counselor Education and Supervision*, *31*(2), 132–138. doi:10.1002/j.1556-6978.1991.tb00151.x

Ray, D. (2004). Supervision of basic and advanced skills in play therapy. *Journal of Professional Counseling, Practice, Theory, & Research*, *32*(2), 28–41. doi:10.1080/15566382.2004.12033805

Ray, D. (2011). Supervision of play therapy. In D. Ray (Ed.), *Advanced play therapy: Essential conditions, knowledge, and skills for child practice*. New York, NY: Routledge. doi:10.4324/9780203837269

Scherl, C., & Harley, J. (2000). Computer monitor supervision: A clinical note. *The American Journal of Family Therapy*, *28*(3), 275–282. doi:10.1080/01926180050081702

Smith-Adcock, S., Davis, E., Pereira, J., Allen, C., Socarras, K., Bodurtha, K., & Smith-Bonahue, T. (2012). Preparing to play: A qualitative study of graduate students' reflections on learning play therapy in an elementary school. *International Journal of Play Therapy*, *21*(2), 100–115. doi:10.1037/a0026931

Smith-Adcock, S., Shin, S. M., & Pereira, J. (2015). Critical incidents in learning child-centered play therapy: Implications for teaching and supervision. *International Journal of Play Therapy*, *2*(2), 78–91. doi:10.1037/a0039122

Stulmaker, H., Lertora, I., & Garza, Y. (2015). Facilitating emphatic perspective taking in beginning child-centered play therapist: The role of supervision. *International Journal of Play Therapy*, *24*(4), 177–189. doi:10.1037/a0039330

Tanner, Z., & Mathis, R. D. (1995). A child-centered typology for training novice play therapists. *International Journal of Play Therapy*, *4*(2), 1–13. doi:10.1037/h0089316

Teufel, L. A. (2007). *Clinical supervision of child and adolescent counselors in residential foster care: A collective case study.* Graduate Thesis and Dissertations. Retrieved from Scholar Commons. http://scholarcommons.usf.edu/etd/2383

Thanasiu, P. L., Rust, K. L., & Walker, S. M. (2018). Service learning and live supervision as early components in play therapy training. *International Journal of Play Therapy*, *27*(2), 103–113. doi:10.1037/pla0000069

VanderGast, T. S., Culbreth, J. R., & Flowers, C. (2010). An exploration of experiences and preferences in clinical supervision with play therapists. *International Journal of Play Therapy*, *19*(3), 174–185. doi:10.1037/a0018882

VanderGast, T. S., & Hinkle, M. S. (2015). So happy together? Predictors of satisfaction with supervision for play therapist supervisees. *International Journal of Play Therapy*, *24*(2), 92–102. doi:10.1037/a0039105

Yerushalmi, K. (2001). Participant supervision in co-therapy. *The Israel Journal of Psychiatry and Related Sciences*, *38*(2), 102–114. PMID:11475912

Chapter 10
Play-Based Bereavement Centers for Children and Families

Renee Turner
University of Mary Hardin-Baylor, USA

ABSTRACT

This chapter outlines the structure and therapeutic foundation for a play-based bereavement center geared toward children and families experiencing grief. Organizational structure and duties are discussed along with information regarding developing a playful facility including art/expressive writing, music, drama, symbolic play, and emotional regulation and release therapeutic opportunities. The author focuses on the supervision and training of community volunteers and counselors-in-training to increase positive outcomes and drive sustainability.

INTRODUCTION

In recent years, services for bereaved children have increased; however, most communities still lack appropriate resources for this specific population. Bereavement-based play therapy clinics can be a viable and sustainable option for most communities to fill this need. Bereavement-based play therapy clinics differ from non-bereavement counseling clinics in the depth of grief services provided by specialty staff in an environment which supports connection, wonder, and the supportive, playful exploration of grief and the soul's journey.

DOI: 10.4018/978-1-5225-8226-7.ch010

While the precise number of children impacted by bereavement is unknown, "an estimated 1 out of 15 children in the U.S. will experience the death of a parent or sibling before they reach the age of 18" (Judi's House/JAG Institute, 2018). It is also difficult to identify reliable statistics regarding the number of children who experience the loss of any significant loved one before adulthood; even the term "significant" is nebulous and subject to debate as family structures vary considerably. The pain and impacts associated with childhood grief, on the other hand, are evident. Short-term impacts on bereaved children may include increased behavioral and academic issues (Holland, 2001; Worden, 1996), reduced self-esteem, symptoms of depression and anxiety, psychosomatic complaints, and physical illness (Worden, 1996), while long-term impacts may include attachment issues (Field & Filanosky, 2010), substance use and related disorders (Holland, 2001), along with anxiety, depression, and other psychiatric and behavioral disorders (Worden, 1996) which may continue into adulthood. According to Dowdney (2000), the majority of children return to baseline functioning within one year, with only an approximated 20% of children requiring mental health intervention. Fortunately, even brief bereavement support after the loss of a parent is shown to reduce the likelihood of severe long-term issues (Bergman, Axberg, & Hanson, 2017). Bereavement support may occur in many formats to include individual, family, and group therapy.

Grief support groups are the most widely cited form of bereavement support (Bergman et al., 2017) and have been shown to reduce isolation and provide a vital support network (Leick & Davidsen-Nielsen, 1991; Hopmeyer & Werk, 1994; Siddaway, Wood, Schulz, & Trickey, 2015), reduce educational issues and behavioral concerns in youth (Tonkins & Lambert, 1996), improve sense of self, and increase resiliency. The group setting provides a space for children to learn about grief and connect with other bereaved children, thereby normalizing their experiences (Siddaway et al., 2015). From a social learning perspective, observational experiences encourage growth through vicarious learning and processing. For many children, this experience returns the child to a sense of normalcy in peer groups, creating a sense of belonging, a vital aspect of child development. Moreover, peer support groups may serve as additional support for caregivers who are unable to provide children with the support needed due to the weight of their own grief (Dopp & Cain, 2012). Therefore, grief support groups may also provide a sacred and supportive space for children to share emotions and thoughts which may make family members and other non-grievers uncomfortable (Worden, 1996).

This chapter explores various options for the structure and therapeutic foundation of bereavement-based play therapy clinics geared toward children experiencing grief with an emphasis on group play therapy.

Play Therapy and Bereavement

Children experience and process bereavement differently from their adult counterparts (Cohen, Mannarino, & Knudsen, 2004; Webb, 2003); therefore, clinicians must carefully consider a child's developmental level before applying interventions. Based on their developmental level, children may be unable to cognitively understand the process and permanency of death (Crenshaw, 1995) or verbally express their emotions (Landreth, 2012). Moreover, current literature suggests children with trauma histories, such as traumatic bereavement, may have inhibited language capacity and ability to verbally process traumatic events (Porges, 2011; Van der Kolk, 2015). For these reasons, children are more likely to process grief through symbolic representation and metaphor (Creshaw, 1995; Webb, 2003), which naturally occurs during the process of play therapy.

Play therapy is developmentally matched to meet the complex emotional needs of grieving children (Creshaw, 1995; Webb, 2003). Because play is considered the universal language of children (Landreth, 2012), it is a natural medium for problem-solving and self-soothing. Play therapy provides children the opportunity to process and play out their feelings and experiences, including grief, using their natural language (Axline, 1969; Kottman & Meany-Walen, 2015; Landreth, 2012). Through metaphors and stories, children project and explore life, death, abandonment, and grief without directly talking about the experience (Green & Connolly, 2009). Webb (2003) suggests play therapy is effective for individuals, groups, and families, and it is the optimal therapy for bereaved children.

Play therapists align with a range of theoretical orientations; however, there is currently no evidence to indicate that any specific theoretical orientations are superior when working with grieving children. Despite a lack of empirical evidence in support of specified theoretical orientations, it appears that non-directive play therapy approaches are favored when working with grieving children (Green & Connolly, 2009; Webb, 2003), particularly during the early phases of the therapeutic process. The literature consistently highlights the importance of establishing a safe, trusting relationship (Green & Connolly, 2009; Landreth, 2012; Webb, 2003) and providing children the opportunity to explore and express feelings associated with grief (Green & Connolly, 2009; Reddy, Files-Hall, & Schaefer, 2005; Webb, 2002). Given the need for theoretical flexibility, throughout this chapter, conceptual frameworks and general insights are provided instead of specific interventions to encourage clinical staff to employ individualized, theoretically-driven play therapy.

Building a Playful Facility

Literature offers scant resources for creating play-based bereavement clinics, and insufficient research exists to support a single standardized model. Clinics will need to adjust services based on available space, funding, the volume of children seeking services, and community needs. For example, in a military-based community, a stronger emphasis on military service loss and suicide best aligns with the community's grief experience (Sories, Maier, Beer, & Thomas, 2015). Structure aside, foundational to a bereavement-based play therapy clinic is creating a space in which children are invited into a world of healing. This goal is achieved by intentionally building a playful facility which includes therapeutic toys and varied opportunities for expressive engagement.

Toy Selection

Appropriately selected materials are essential for clients to navigate their therapeutic work. In general, toy selection should include a range of toys which facilitate symbolic and therapeutic play (Landreth, 2012). Guidelines for toy inclusion vary by theoretical orientation, but it is generally agreed that toys should be durable, simple to use, attractive to children in different developmental stages (Kottman & Meany-Walen, 2015; Landreth, 2012; Ray et al., 2013), and culturally sensitive (Drewes, 2005). However, the literature offers inconsistent information regarding the inclusion and exclusion of specific toys and categories based on theoretical orientation and population. In a study examining the most frequently used toys in Child-Centered Play Therapy, Ray et al. (2013), found the top 11 toys (sandbox, arts/crafts, paint and easel, water, kitchen, puppets, bop bag, hats, and big aggressive animals) were used by 25% or more of children in the sample (p. 52). Despite these results, Ray et al. cautioned play therapists against making uniform decisions regarding toy choice, instead encouraged play therapists to include toys based on the needs of individual children. Therefore, intentional selecting, not collecting, of toys (Landreth, 2012) asks the question, "what does this facilitate?" More specifically, when working with grieving children, "how does this toy facilitate *grief*?" While toys are a fundamental part of the therapeutic play process, it is essential to also consider in what method, or modality, toys will be used and available therapeutic space.

Therapeutic Modalities

While no therapeutic modality is shown to be more effective than others with grieving children, many therapeutic modalities and interventions are generally accepted. These include (but are not limited to) expressive arts and written expression (Malchiodi,

2011), dramatic play (Weber & Haen, 2005), and traditional symbolic play (Webb, 2002). In addition to these therapeutic modalities, the inclusion of space for physical and emotional self-regulation is suggested as trauma and attachment-related concerns which often accompany grief (Badenoch, 2008). In large clinics, it is reasonable to assume that separate rooms would house each of these therapeutic opportunities. However, in the case of smaller clinics, these therapeutic opportunities may be condensed or scheduled based on weekly topics or emphases. Furthermore, while each modality is supported by empirical research that demonstrates its effectiveness with bereavement populations, it is not critical to offer each modality when funds and space are limited. When these practical constraints limit therapeutic opportunities, this author recommends minimally providing symbolic and dramatic play areas.

Please note that each of the therapeutic opportunities listed above has an associated specialty designation (e.g., Registered Drama Therapist, Registered Art Therapist) which requires significant modality-specific training and supervision. To ensure that modalities are ethically and correctly applied, the clinic director should obtain ongoing training, supervision, and consultation in areas that fall outside of their scope of competency. Details and rationales for each of these rooms/specialties follow.

Art and Creative Writing

Art is a powerful tool for bereavement because the pain of grief is often unspeakable (Malchiodi, 2011; Rozman, 2015). Therapeutic art is an example of a creative intervention that facilitates opportunities for the child to express deep pain without the use of concrete language (Edgar-Bailey & Kress, 2010; Webb, 2002; Webb, 2003). According to Van der Kolk (2015), grief and trauma experiences are encoded in the body as sensory memories and experiences. The practice of creating art enables individuals to connect with this embodied sensory experience as they explore, process, understand and recover from grief (Steele & Malchiodi, 2012). Because children naturally engage in this medium with little prompting or intervention, it is an obvious choice for bereavement-based play therapy clinics.

Visual arts encompass a broad range of expression including collage, painting, drawing, scrapbooking, sculpting, art/craft making, and multi-media creations. Written expression including poetry and story writing, integrate easily into this room and may be utilized as a multi-modal form of therapeutic intervention. Specific art interventions to process grief include scrapbooking (King, Prout, Stuhl, & Nelson, 2016), creating memory books and other memorial creations, doll-making (Feen-Calligan, McIntyre, & Sands-Goldstein, 2009), visual representations of the deceased, and so on. Simple prompts with as few directions as possible, provide children permission to choose, therefore increasing the child's sense of control (Edgar-Bailey & Kress, 2010; Rozman, 2015). For example, the play therapist might say, "we can make a memory book about your mom, or we can make something else out of these supplies. You get to choose." This approach echoed in the literature, provides a safe place for the grief narrative to arise (Stutey, Helm, LoSasso, & Krieder, 2015) when the child is ready to process.

Art supplies in a room designed for this modality may include:

- Finger paints and other washable-style paints for children or acrylics for adolescents;
- Various materials to serve as a base or canvas (e.g., construction paper, scrapbooking paper, stretched canvas);
- A range of developmentally-appropriate writing and drawing utensils
- Miscellaneous craft supplies (e.g., ribbon, pom-poms, glue, glitter, scissors, art paper, dowels, sequins, beads, yarn, feathers);
- An easel;
- Various types of clay and Play-Doh;
- And magazines and poster board for collages (Kottman & Meany-Walen, 2018).

Consider the age and developmental level of children utilizing this therapeutic modality and select art materials which are attractive to the specified age group. Finally, art rooms need smocks, plastic table covers, durable and easy-to-clean surfaces, and a large assortment of brushes. Additional information regarding art room set-up and therapeutic practices are found in Malchiodi (2011).

Dramatic Playroom

Drama therapy creates an "embodied, experiential process that draws on the patient's capacity for play" (Haen, p.236, 2015) which promotes insight, resolve conflict, and changes cognitive structures (Haen, 2015). Using dramatic play, children create and act out stories about their world in an attempt to make sense of life events using fantasy, metaphor, storytelling, enactment, and dress-up (Cattanach, 2007). Weber & Haen (2005) suggest very young children respond positively to dramatic play as it requires no verbalization; with a mere costume change, children are transported to another time, place, or, version of self through a "double reality. For example, a pair of nursing scrubs and stethoscope allows the child to become a nurse or physician and "cure" the patient's cancer. However, dramatic play is not always so apparent due to the need for emotional distance. In the example provided, the nurse may represent a nurturing or caregiver theme; the same theme is present when the child pretends to be a veterinarian tending to a sick animal. The second example, on the other hand, allows the child to enact nurturing/rescue without directly considering a hospital scene or people, thereby creating emotional distance (Haen, 2015). It is not uncommon, therefore, for bereaved children to use dramatic play to act out illness, death, funerals, and other specific bereavement-related events.

Dramatic playrooms vary based on the size of the bereavement clinic and the number of group participants. Due to a lack of empirical support for bereavement-based dramatic play, the following is based on the author's clinical observation in bereavement-based play clinics. An elaborate center may include a stage with production-quality lights, sound, smoke machine, and so forth; however, most small or start-up centers will operate on a significantly smaller scale and budget. In these settings, a mirror with dress-up items serves as a sufficient base. For purposes of simplicity, dramatic play items are divided into two broad categories: interactive items (e.g., hands-on, dress-up items) and support items. Interactive items serve as the foundation for dramatic play; support items enhance the dramatic process. Bereavement play requires specific interactive items including medical kits/supplies (e.g., stethoscope, band-aids, gauze, surgical masks), judge's gavel, tombstones, scrubs in varying sizes, capes of varying colors and sizes (e.g., superhero, judge's robe), miscellaneous fabric in varying materials (e.g., gauze, silk), magic wands and crowns, rescue worker hats and jackets (e.g., EMS, Police), and military-related items. While this list may be expanded to match the culture and clients of the center, these items will facilitate most bereavement-based play. Support items include a director's clapboard, mirror(s), writing supplies, director's chair, seating for audience members, and various props (e.g., clock, puppets, masks). Additional information regarding drama therapy and dramatic play is found in Weber and Haen (2005).

Symbolic Playroom

This room is best viewed as a "traditional" play therapy room. As previously stated, play is the language of children and toys are their words (Landreth, 2012) therefore, including a room which facilitates symbolic play therapy is necessary for young children to process their grief. The recommended toys to facilitate symbolic play vary by theoretical orientation. Both Landreth (2012) and Kottman and Meany-Walen (2018) provide comprehensive lists of toys needed to facilitate symbolic play.

Therapists should ensure that the room includes a balanced selection of toys across each toy category for the optimal choice of expression (Landreth, 2012) while providing ample choices increases the likelihood that the child will have what they need to process their grief (Edgar-Bailey & Kress, 2010). Nurturing toys allow the child to nurture self and others using a) babies and baby items (e.g., cradles, blankets, clothes, baby bottles); b) stuffed animals; c) domestic animal figures (e.g., cow, dog, cat); d) child-sized cozy blankets and pillows. Real-life play items mirror everyday life and include a) dollhouses with dolls and furniture; b) domestic items (e.g., dishes, food, child-sized brooms, dustpans, play kitchens); c) phones and other play electronic devices; d) doctor's kits; and e) transportation toys (e.g., ambulance, fire truck, police car, military vehicles). Scary toys are crucial for bereaved children including a) monsters; b) figures that defy death (e.g., zombies, mummies, vampires); c) sharks and alligators; d) snakes and insects; e) ghosts and demons; and f) mystical items (e.g., ogre, Cerberus, Chimera, dragon). Finally, aggressive toys provide a vital opportunity for energetic release (Oaklander, 2006) and mastery. Aggressive items include a) punching bag or bop bag; b) foam swords and soft bats; c) toys soldiers; and d) weapons (e.g., rubber knives, retractable knives, play gun, dart gun, rope).

The symbolic playroom may also include a sandbox, which is among the most frequently used play therapy toys (Ray et al., 2013). This author has observed bereaved children frequently use the sandbox as a valuable backdrop for burial play. In this form of play, children can bury and resurrect figures (e.g., dolls, zombies) and create tombs and crypts (e.g., graves, Egyptian pyramids) as they gain an understanding of death permanency and process funeral processions.

Self-Regulation: Physical Release

In some children, processing grief increases difficult emotions like abandonment, anxiety, and anger. As children process grief, it is not uncommon for dysregulation to occur (Badenoch, 2008) as the child embodies the grief experience. As a result, it is not uncommon to observe an increase in children's kinesthetic energy and desire to release this energy through movement or physical aggression as they experience hyperarousal (Warner, Cook, Westcott, & Koomar, 2014). Therefore, clinics are encouraged to minimally provide an outlet through which children can release a sympathetic charge. In line with findings by Ray et al. (2013), the bop bag is a popular aggression/emotional release toy utilized by grieving children, especially boys. However, other options achieve the same goal and are more conducive to group interactions. Group activities which involve the movement of the whole body are excellent methods of for regulation for children in a hyperactive state (Warner et al., 2014). Consider installing a basketball hoop (if sufficient outdoor space is available) or including items such as jumping balls, a beach ball, a small trampoline, or other therapeutic movement-based interventions.

When space allows larger clinics may further consider designing a designated physical release regulation room. For example, a room with padded the walls, foam wedges and bolsters, weighted blankets, foam swords, and physioballs of varied size (Warner et al., 2014). As a safety measure, maintain low ratios of children to facilitators (e.g., 1:3) and post at least one facilitator any time the room is in use. Some children will neither need nor desire participation in a physical release room and may benefit from a calming room, as described below.

Self-Regulation: Relaxation Room

The purpose of a relaxation room is to return the child to the here-and-now, promote integration, and create a felt sense of safety (Badenoch, 2008). This room is useful for a variety of therapeutic interventions. First, children may need a respite from the chaos of everyday life and experience the room as a space for reconnection, grounding, and centering before beginning any depth processing (Green & Myrick, 2014). This room may also serve as a grounding tool for children who have become activated during their bereavement play (Badenoch, 2008; Warner et al., 2014). Features of this room may include comfortable seating, items scented with aromatherapy, sensory toys, cozy blankets, plush pillows, a small play tent, and low lighting. If smaller facilities are unable to designate an entire room for relaxation, facilitators can adjust the curriculum and add relaxation time to the closing group activity. Closing group activities may include deep breathing, grounding activities (e.g., sensing feet on the ground, progressive relaxation), or group connection activities (e.g., singing a song, huddles).

As previously mentioned, the set-up of a bereavement-based play therapy clinic is dictated by the facility's size, funding, and the volume of children receiving services; therefore, the preceding information should serve as a general guide that is open to adaptation. Based on the size of the facility, the rooms described above may exist separately or combined into one or two multi-purpose therapeutic rooms. A topical description of possible organizational structures follows.

Organizational Structure

Many organizational and program options exist for providing bereavement-based play therapy support based on setting and community needs. When a university setting houses the counseling clinic and part of a counselor training program, a clinic director or appointed faculty supervisor is likely responsible, whereas, in a community-based setting, the responsibility falls to either an executive or clinical director. To determine the most sustainable structure, clinical directors must consider 1) funding, 2) clinical staffing, and 3) community needs.

Funding

As one would imagine, building a play-based center has significant upfront costs. While funding is critical to the success of any clinic, it is rarely discussed in the literature. Competing and dissimilar accreditation and licensure paths further complicate determining a clear funding path. Helm, O'Halloran, and Kahlo (2010) encourage pursuing endowments and grant and creating community partnerships.

In consideration of community partnerships, clinical staff may provide bereavement training to area agencies, conduct in-service training for school administrators, or offer assessment and screening services to local mental health authorities. This author also recommends creating community partnerships with area churches, hospitals, and hospices. It is further recommended to "outsource" services as a method of cost sharing while still meeting community needs (for an elaborated discussion, see Helm et al., 2010).

Clinical Staffing

Equal in importance to funding is an adequately trained clinical staff. The clinical director or whoever is deemed responsible for the treatment aspect of the center, oversees program design, supervision of students, and community outreach. As the most critical member of the clinic, the clinical director must possess a clinical license and have ample experience working with play therapy and bereavement. Moreover, for ethical purposes, this author strongly recommends that the clinical director also hold the Registered Play Therapist-Supervisor designation. Additionally, many bereavement center models operate as non-profits with minimal paid staff and volunteer support. The use of counselors-in-training (discussed later) may reduce financial burdens, fill clinical needs, and provide invaluable clinical training.

Community Needs

Groups should serve the needs of their communities. Therefore, consider administering a community needs assessment to determine the types of services that best meet the unique needs of the grief community. For example, in some communities, individual play-based bereavement services may exist, but not group therapy opportunities. In other communities, group therapy may exist for one group but not for others. Create therapeutic programs which match the strongest needs, and add additional programs as needed. Also, consider the culture in which the clinic is based to determine if individual or family services best meet the community's needs.

Therapeutic Program Groups

Many play therapy experts support the use of play therapy with bereaved children (Green & Connolly, 2009; Reddy et al., 2005; Webb, 2002); however, most literature is anecdotal. Unfortunately, there is scant research regarding models for play-based bereavement clinics, and no data is available regarding the impact of long-term bereavement group effectiveness. Nonetheless, between expert opinion and available research, play-based bereavement therapy groups are supported. One study examined children's response to three intensive group therapy "workshops" using play therapy on consecutive weekends, lasting three to five hours each (Siddaway et al., 2015). This study demonstrated a reduction in psychiatric symptoms (i.e., depression and anxiety); however, that children who had experienced the death of a parent benefitted significantly less from the workshops than those who had experienced the death of an extended family member. Siddaway et al. (2015) suggest that this difference to the degree of secondary losses (i.e., change of schools and financial status) and the intensity of losing an attachment figure. In another study, researchers conducted a meta-analysis analyzing grief camps that used play therapy for periods ranging from two to five days (Clute & Kobayashi, 2013). While the study found an overall increase in coping skills and feelings of connectedness, there was no significant differences in PTSD scales or long-term behavior. It is reasonable to assume that a longer-term evaluation period is needed to yield these changes. Finally, another study analyzed short-term play therapy grief groups (eight-week duration), which were found to significantly reduce grief symptomology in children aged seven through eleven (Tonkins & Lambert, 1996).

Group Play Therapy

Group play therapy is the primary format of therapy services at most bereavement centers and echoed in the literature (Bergman et al., 2017). In a grief group setting, play therapy is thought to provide a mix of engagement and avoidance, enabling children to better assimilate the processing of grief (Clute & Kobayashi, 2013). According to Ray (2011), the benefits of group play therapy include increased comfort and participation of the child, vicarious and induced catharsis, vicarious and direct learning, therapist observation of social interaction, social reality testing and limit setting, and positive social interactions (for a comprehensive review of group play therapy, see Sweeney, Baggerly, & Ray, 2014). The frequency of each group depends upon participant/facilitator ratios, type of death loss, and community needs. Ideally, bereavement clinics should have multiple programs based on types of loss and participants' age.

Screening and Selection

Group dynamics are driven by the participating members therefore, it is critical to screen potential group members (Corey, Corey, & Corey, 2018). Setting, theoretical orientation, group function and member demographic/population all impact the inclusion or exclusion of potential group members (Corey, et al., 2018; Sweeney, Baggerly, & Ray, 2014). In general, screening for children should include (a) the child's social ability to participate in a group, (b) the child's ability to maintain their safety and the safety of others, (c) recent hospitalizations and self-harming behaviors, and (d) amount of one-on-one attention required. Bereavement specific considerations include the type of death loss and the degree of trauma associated with the loss (Worden, 2009). Because traumatic losses are positively correlated with increased levels of anxiety and elevated symptoms of PTSD, children who have experienced a highly traumatizing loss, such as a loved one's death by homicide or suicide, are more likely to need 1:1 support. However, rather than automatically screening children out of the group process, consider lowering the facilitator to child ratio to support or adding additional facilitators to provide individual support as needed. If a child is screened out of the group process, the child should be referred for individual counseling within the clinic if possible until they are ready for the group process. Ray (2011) and Sweeney, et al., (2014) offer additional guidelines for screening play therapy groups.

Group Type

Because children bereaved by different death loss types have been found to grieve in different ways, the literature supports a division of grief types into separate groups (Worden, 1996; Worden, 2009). In a start-up bereavement clinic or small bereavement clinic in which participant numbers are low, consider dividing participants into two primary groups: sudden death/accident or terminal/chronic illness. The sudden/accidental death group includes car accidents, drowning, heart attacks, suicide, and homicide, while the terminal/chronic illness group includes death due to cancer, advanced age, and so on. This division is not ideal, however, as suicide and homicide grievers are shown to experience different grief trajectories that people grieving other types of sudden death; among these differences, people who have lost a loved one to suicide or homicide are at increased risk for complicated grief (Currier, Neimeyer, & Bergman, 2008). In larger bereavement centers with more funding and clinical support, a more specific division may include:

- Sudden/accidental death,
- Death from a terminal or chronic illness,
- Death of an extended family member,
- Sibling loss,
- Death by suicide,
- Death by homicide (Wordon, 2009) and
- Military-related loss (Sories et al., 2015).

Age

Children benefit most from the group therapy process when they are placed with children of similar age (Sweeney, et al., 2014). This remains true for grieving children as their developmental understanding of death is dictated in part by their cognitive development (Crenshaw, 1995). According to Ray (2011), it is generally recognized to match children within one year of age. While this suggestion is the optimal choice, given the specialized nature of grief groups, clinics may need to expand the age range slightly. Therefore, it is useful to consider the overall match between the personalities and therapeutic needs of included children more so than chronological age (Ray, 2011).

Group Structure

While ample literature exists regarding adults in group therapy, there is very little research regarding group *play* therapy or clear suggestions for best managing the group process with children. Therapeutic groups with adults generally run for 60 to 90 minutes in length (Corey, et al., 2018), however, based on this author's clinical observations, groups longer than 45 minutes will likely fall outside the threshold of the developmentally appropriate attention span for children. Due to a lack of available literature of bereavement-based play groups, the following is a sample format based on the author's clinical observations, which should be adjusted based on the developmental age of the children, facilitator ratio, and theoretical orientation of the group:

- **30 minutes**: Pre-group with facilitators/clinical staff.
- **15-30 minutes:** Ice breaker and group process (depending on age).
- **15-30 minutes:** Non-directive play (depending on age).
- **15 minutes:** Group closing.
- **45 minutes:** Post-group process.

The described hypothetical structure allows for adequate supervision of counselors-in-training, therapeutic intervention, and group management. *Pre-group* includes facilitators and the clinical director with a discussion regarding known case changes, the theme of the group, and so forth. During the *group process*, children meet together for check-in, centering, and connection with a light discussion or overview of the group topic. *Non-directive play* immediately follows the group process. In non-directive play therapy groups, it is optimal to have a 1:2 or 1:3 ratio (Ray, 2011) of children to group facilitators. During this phase, children may float between rooms/modalities at their discretion. *Group closing* is meant to bring the group together, ground children in reality, and close the group session. Closing rituals are soothing for children; therefore, consider how the group may close in the same way each week. Finally, the *post-group process* is intended for group facilitators and the clinic director (who may or may not take part in the group facilitation process) to come together and process the group session. Not only is this helpful for the clinic director to understand group members' progress; it is also a vital part of the supervisory process (discussed later).

Bereavement-Based Play Therapy Training and Supervision

Thus far, this chapter has provided a rationale for bereavement-based play therapy clinics, recommended toys and materials for setting up bereavement-based play therapy groups, and discussed options for therapeutic programs, however, the best-organized clinic is only as effective as its therapeutic staff. Facilitating play therapy groups is considered an advanced skill (Ray, 2011); therefore, facilitators should demonstrate solid play therapy knowledge before facilitating group therapy. Additionally, this author recommends facilitators have a basic understanding of the developmental aspects of grief, loss, and trauma. Finally, facilitators should also explore their personal grief histories, as well as strategies for self-care and burnout prevention.

Grief Training

Because the Council for Accreditation of Counseling and Related Programs (CACREP) does not explicitly require grief training as part of their standards (CACREP, 2016), it is reasonable to assume that not all counselor preparation programs require this material as part of standard coursework. Therefore, this author recommends that clinics address the following topics during training: 1) the history of grief counseling and grief counseling models, 2) circumstances of death, 3) developmental reactions to grief, and 4) personal grief histories. A working knowledge of these areas expands conceptualization capacity. In turn, this capacity may improve empathetic understanding and therapeutic presence, both of which are critical components of play therapy (Ray, 2004).

Grief Models

Although not play therapy specific, facilitators should possess a working knowledge of grief counseling fundamentals to include the evolution of grief through historical and cultural contexts, as well as grief recovery models. Elizabeth Kubler-Ross paved the way for grief therapists with her ground-breaking book, *On Death and Dying* (1969). While this book was seminal to the field of bereavement, linear multi-stage models such as the one described by Kubler-Ross have subsequently received criticism, as grief is generally not linear in its progression. In addition, early authors minimized the grief experience in children. In the last thirty years, clinicians have moved away from stage models of grief and toward task models (Worden, 1996; Worden, 2009), meaning-making models (Neimeyer, Burke, Mackay, & van Dyke Stringer, 2010; Wong, 2008), attachment models, and embodiment models (Turner, 2017). Worden (1996) provides an excellent foundation for understanding the developmental aspects of children's grief and conceptualizing the contextual components of systemic grief.

Circumstances of the Death

Grief reactions vary based on the circumstances surrounding the death; therefore, these circumstances should influence the topics addressed within the group process, as well as interventions applied. Bereavement resulting from a terminal or chronic illness creates contradictory feelings of relief and sadness, which may create minor levels of guilt. Generally, terminal and chronic illness death increase the opportunity for saying good-bye, whereas sudden deaths (e.g., accident, drowning, heart attack) often have a degree of suddenness and violence (Worden, 1996; Worden, 2009). Violent death losses (e.g., suicide, homicide) are shown to increase a child's risk for substance abuse, mental health problems, and physical health problems (Burke, Hellman, Scott, Weems, & Carrion, 2011; Mersky, Topitzes, & Reynolds, 2013). Children bereaved by suicide and homicide are also more likely to experience symptoms of complicated grief (Currier, Neimeyer, & Bergman, 2008; Kristensen, Weisaeth, & Heir, 2012). Prigerson et al. (1995) describe complicated grief as bereavement that is accompanied by elevated and persistent distress about death separation, impaired functioning, disbelief, and difficulty moving forward with life without the person who died. The bereavement experiences of children whose parents die by violent means (e.g., suicide or homicide) are distinctive in many ways, including increased feelings of rejection/abandonment, shame, and guilt (Worden, 2009); difficulty with attachment; difficulty with continuing bonds (Currier, Irish, Neimeyer, & Foster, 2015; Field & Filanosky, 2010; Hunt & Hertlein, 2015); and difficulty establishing trust in adult relationships.

Developmental Reactions to Grief

To effectively facilitate bereavement play, facilitators need an understanding of expected developmental behaviors associated with grief. While there is no standard trajectory for grief recovery, Piaget's theory of cognitive development (Piaget & Inhelder, 1969) is a useful guide for understanding children's ability to understand and process grief. Children two to seven years of age have a relatively small working concept of death. Cognitively, children at this stage are egocentric with minimal ability to think outside themselves. In a world governed by fantasy, children at this stage may create faulty beliefs regarding their ability to cause death. For example, a five-year-old may conceptualize the death of a loved one as a direct result of the child's negative behavior (Piaget & Inhelder, 1969). Children at this stage need simple, clear, consistent, and honest descriptions of death (Crenshaw, 1995). Children eight to eleven years of age generally have a working concept of death; however, their understanding may be based on television and video games, which inaccurately depict the permanence of death. Due to the concrete nature of cognitive processing among children in this age group, facilitators should expect children to ask specific, fact-driven, and often detailed questions about the process of death and dying. Such questions may create emotional surges for the facilitator; thus, it is critical that facilitators understand and have processed their personal grief histories.

Personal Grief Histories

Therapists who are self-aware are thought to have increased empathetic understanding, unconditional positive regard, and congruence (Ray, 2011). While training facilitators does not require deep emotional processing of grief experiences, which is more in line with personal therapy, facilitators should demonstrate emotional awareness regarding their loss history, as well as an ability to explore their grief without emotional or physical dysregulation. In essence, the more self-aware facilitators are, the more likely they are to effectively support the therapeutic relationship. This author recommends engaging trainees in an experiential grief activity, such as creating a grief timeline, in order to explore their personal grief histories and beliefs about death, dying, and the afterlife. Children notoriously ask questions like, "What happens after you die?" and "is Heaven real?" Self-understanding of personal beliefs increases the likelihood student facilitators will remain present and genuine in the therapeutic relationship during these difficult moments (Blanco, Muro, & Stickley, 2014).

Bereavement-Based Play Therapy Training

As previously mentioned, it is recommended that facilitators have basic play therapy training before facilitating bereavement-based play therapy groups. While foundational play therapy skills are critical for practice, this section focuses on advanced play therapy skills as they relate to bereavement-based play therapy: conceptualization, enlarging meaning, identifying play themes, and connecting with children (Ray, 2004).

Conceptualization of the Whole Child

The death of a loved one, particularly a parent, has far-reaching impacts. In addition to bereavement, the child is likely to experience a cascade of losses including potential changes in residence, changes in economic status, separation of parents, change of school, loss of friends, and so forth (Worden, 1996). Focusing solely on the death loss does not meet the needs of the whole child. Supervisors are encouraged to ask supervisees questions which facilitate conceptualization of the whole child. The following questions facilitate the whole child conceptualization.

- "What else has changed in the child's life?"
- "What somatic complaints or behavioral issues have occurred since the death?"
- "Is the child depressed?"
- "What did the child lose when they lost (the person who died)?".

Thorough case conceptualization drives effective treatment strategies and plans; in the context of play therapy, it also facilitates identifying play themes and enlarging meaning.

Enlarging Meaning

Enlarging meaning occurs across theoretical orientations and is intended to facilitate understanding and insight of the child (Landreth 2012; Kottman & Meany-Walen, 2018). Enlarging meaning occurs through identifying and verbalizing patterns in play or verbalizing play themes which are foundational to the presenting issue. Play therapists may enlarge meaning, or increase awareness of emotions, core beliefs, values, meaning, relationships, or other theoretically-based concepts, through well-timed facilitative responses. While enlarging meaning increases a child's insight, poor timing may disrupt the therapeutic relationship (Ray, 2004) or give the child an impression that the therapist is not attuned or "listening" (Badenoch, 2008). Determining what content to bring to the child's awareness can be a challenge, as competing theoretical orientations offer different stances on directive versus non-directive application of play (Yasenik & Gardner, 2012). Since literature does not support a specific theoretical application, the Play Therapy Dimensions Model (PTDM) by Yasenik and Gardner (2012) may serve as a useful guide for facilitators and supervisors. In the PTDM model, there are two dimensions, consciousness and directiveness, that drive degree and type of responding, therapist participation, and open discussion and exploration.

Identifying Play Themes

Play themes help conceptually identify the child's communication during a play therapy session. According to Ray (2011), very little literature is available regarding identifying play themes; however, they remain central to client conceptualization and tracking play therapy progress. Ray encourages play therapists to demonstrate solid play therapy skills and self-awareness before interpreting play themes to avoid potential disruptions in the therapeutic relationship. Therefore, play theme identification should occur under the context of supervision. This author recommends focusing on this aspect of training during *post-group*.

While numerous play themes exist, the most commonly identified are a) protection, b) relationship, c) mastery, d) nurturing, e) grief/loss/abandonment, f) helpless/inadequate, g) power and control, h) aggressive, and i) safety and security (Ray, 2004). As expected, grief and loss are prominent themes in bereavement play; however, in this author's clinical observations, bereavement play is subject to producing all play themes at various points in the healing process (for an extensive review, see Ray, 2011). Grief is associated with many primary and secondary losses (Worden, 2009) and reducing the child's pain to the experience to death loss, discredits the child's whole experience and may limit their opportunity for growth.

Connecting With Children

Connecting with children means being fully present (Kestly, 2016) and bearing witness to the stories they tell (Weber & Haen, 2005). The use of non-directive play therapy and expressive therapy interventions with bereaved children is underscored in the literature for several reasons. Primarily, demonstrating therapeutic presence or a "be with" attitude (Landreth, 2012) means the connection is valued over performance or therapeutic progress. Despite theoretical orientation, a warm and genuine therapeutic relationship is regarded as central for progress to occur (Blanco et al., 2014; Landreth, 2012; Kottman & Meany-Walen, 2018; Yasenik & Gardner, 2012). In a group setting, "being with" instead of "doing" may mean giving children opportunities to experience joy in a social context again without needing to worry about others. Specifically, for grieving children, the group process may be one of few venues in which the child is viewed independently from their grief. This author does not encourage facilitators to force children to name the deceased loved one. Group experts emphasize 'passing' and silence are a natural part of the initial group stages and necessary to build trust within the therapeutic relationship and the group (Corey et al., 2017); grieving children deserve the same regard. When the therapist is attuned to the needs of the child, rapport and relational connection still occur (Badenoch, 2008).

Supervision of Student Facilitators

Empirical research supporting the effectiveness of play therapy is steadily growing; however, there remains a dearth of literature regarding the process and practice of play therapy supervision. In a review of the literature, Donald, Culbreth, and Carter (2015) found that parallel to the child-therapist relationship, most current approaches to play therapy supervision focus on the relationship as the cornerstone for growth. In addition, exploring the person of the therapist is of equal importance to learning play therapy specific skills to enforce the importance of self and genuineness in the therapeutic relationship, especially in the early phases. Furthermore, VanderGast and Hinkle (2015), found a key aspect of supervisory satisfaction is working with a supervisor who has a clear identity as a play therapist and fosters a play therapy identity in others. Therefore, it is crucial for play therapy supervisors to create a safe space for empathy and unconditional positive regard (Donald, et al., 2015; Ray, 2011)

To achieve this goal, a combination of individual, group, and live supervision provide varied opportunities for facilitators to learn through direct mentorship and peer support. Individual supervision is necessary to focus on individual student progress, however, live, and post-group supervision serves multiple purposes. First, observation of the overall group process keeps the clinic director alert to the clinical activity of individual children. Second, post-group supervision that occurs immediately after the group session which allows the student facilitator to reflect on the child's progress, their performance and conceptualize the child at a deeper level. The immediacy of live/post-group supervision drives the effectiveness of the feedback and learning (Thanasiu, Rust, & Walter, 2018). To increase skills and growth, a play therapy skills checklist (for sample checklists, see, Ray, Purswell, Haas, & Aldrete, 2017) and peer-rating feedback (Swank, 2018) are helpful additions to the play therapy supervision process.

Supervision Content Areas

Content areas such as client progress, theoretical application, therapeutic interventions, and ethics are standard components of supervision (for an extensive review, see Bernard & Goodyear, 2018 or Drewes & Mullen 2008). However, supervision in bereavement-based play therapy clinics requires additional focus. The following areas are the most consistent areas of supervision content in the author's clinical observations.

Countertransference

According to Elliot (2016), countertransference with child clients is a larger ethical issue than of confidentiality. Countertransference may be related to maternal or paternal instincts, feelings toward the caregiver, or the supervisees lack of self-awareness. While there is a lack of research regarding countertransference with childhood grief, this author has observed supervisees experience discomfort with death-related content, have emotional reactions to a death story, or attempt to shield their child clients from pain. One way in which it may occur is via redirection or minimization of play themes related to specific death-related content. For example, if a child experiences an emotional reaction during a medical reenactment play (for instance, as the child attempts to perform CPR on a doll), a facilitator may point that child to another play area rather than tracking and reflecting. Indications that a supervisee may be experiencing countertransference during a session include being unable to recall session events (disassociation), feeling emotionally overwhelmed during the retelling of the session events (personalization), over-focusing on one client, avoiding a particular child/situation, or becoming angry at a caregiver. Supervisory questions such as "What about this case is hard?" or pointed observations such as "I notice you do not like to talk about this case" or "It seems your grief is clouding your view" can facilitate self-awareness for the supervisee.

Self-Care

Holding space and maintaining a therapeutic presence for children with grief and trauma has all-encompassing impacts. Burnout impacts emotional, physical, cognitive, relational, and spiritual wellness which in turn impair therapists' empathy and judgment. While all therapists are at risk for developing burnout and impairment, the risk increases when a significant portion of client present with trauma and crisis (Iqbal, 2015; MacKay, 2017). For these reasons, recent literature suggests, self-care is vital to trauma training programs (Iqbal, 2015; MacKay, 2017). Working with children may be especially taxing due to the degree of presence, attunement, and attachment required for effective play therapy (Meany-Walen et al., 2018). At the time of this writing, only one research study has explored the self-care of play therapists. Participants in this study overwhelmingly reported that wellness and self-care were not sufficiently addressed in their graduate programs (Meany-Walen et al., 2018). Supervisors can thus assume that student supervisees have a limited understanding of wellness, methods for assessing wellness and burnout, and ways to maintain self-care over the long term. Based on this data, supervisors have an ethical obligation to explore self-care and wellness strategies with their supervisees on an ongoing basis.

Termination

Endings and goodbyes are painful, particularly for children with death or abandonment histories (Worden, 1996). If parents are absent or unavailable due to their grief, children may crave attuned connection. In these cases, it is not uncommon for children to develop deep attachments with facilitators. Given the high degree of attachment that can characterize the therapeutic relationship, ongoing discussions of termination are warranted to prevent the child from perceiving the termination of that relationship as another painful loss (Gil & Crenshaw, 2015). Planned terminations which therapeutically processed may provide a corrective experience for children in need of healthy good-byes (Garcia, 2012). Two parties may terminate the therapeutic relationship: child/family and facilitators. Caregiver psychoeducation regarding attachment and good-byes may reduce the number of premature terminations but avoiding all premature termination is unavoidable. However, regarding facilitators, it is vital that clinical staff set clear expectations of facilitators and plan therapeutic programs that align with the natural ebb and flow of facilitator seasons, such as an academic semester.

CONCLUSION

Grief is an unfortunate experience for many children, which can have significant long-term impacts (Worden, 2009). Fortunately, bereavement-based groups have many demonstrated positive impacts (Bergman et al., 2017; Tonkins & Lambert, 1996). During their time of confusion and sorrow, children positively respond to the support and normalization bereavement groups provide (Siddaway et al., 2015), and because play therapy is empirically supported for children, it is a natural match for the complex emotional needs of grieving children (Creshaw, 1995; Webb, 2003). By developing a play-based bereavement clinic, grieving children receive a place to therapeutically engage in developmentally appropriate methods of healing in connection with other grieving children. However, building a successful bereavement-based play clinic requires more than stocking therapeutic toys. The development of a successful bereavement-based play therapy clinic requires clear vision, funding support, an understanding of the community's needs, and a willingness to engage with community partners. Most importantly, a successful clinic must provide thorough grief and play therapy training and supervision. Building a bereavement-based play therapy clinic can have long-lasting impacts that shape children and families for generations. While this vision may seem daunting, it is entirely possible to realize it with a clearly defined organizational model, well-trained clinical staff, and above all, a shared commitment to the therapeutic effects of play.

REFERENCES

Association for Play Therapy. (1997). A definition of play therapy. *The Association for Play Therapy Newsletter*, *16*(1), 7.

Axline, V. (1964). *Dibs in search of self*. New York, NY: Ballantine.

Axline, V. (1969). *Play Therapy*. New York, NY: Ballantine.

Badenoch, B. (2008). *Being a brain-wise therapist*. New York, NY: Norton.

Bergman, A., Axberg, U., & Hanson, E. (2017). When a parent dies: A systematic review of the effects of support programs for parentally bereaved children and their caregivers. *BMC Palliative Care*, *16*(39). doi:10.118612904-017-0223-y PMID:28797262

Bernard, J. M., & Goodyear, R. K. (2018). *Fundamentals in Clinical Supervision* (6th ed.). New York, NY: Pearson Publishing.

Blanco, P. J., Muro, J. H., & Stickley, V. K. (2014). Understanding the concept of genuineness in play therapy: Implications for the supervision and teaching of beginning play therapists. *International Journal of Play Therapy*, *23*(1), 44–54. doi:10.1037/a0035478

Burke, N. J., Hellman, J. L., Scott, B. G., Weems, C. F., & Carrion, V. G. (2011). The impact of adverse childhood experiences on an urban pediatric population. *Child Abuse & Neglect*, *35*(6), 408–413. doi:10.1016/j.chiabu.2011.02.006 PMID:21652073

Cattanach, A. (2007). *Narrative approaches in play with children*. London: Jessica Kingsley.

Clute, M. A., & Kobayashi, R. (2013). Are children's grief camps effective? *Journal of Social Work in End-of-Life & Palliative Care*, *9*(1), 43–57. doi:10.1080/15524256.2013.758927 PMID:23438644

Cohen, J. A., Mannariron, A. P., & Knudsen, K. (2004). Treating childhood traumatic grief: A pilot study. *Journal of the American Academy of Child and Adolescent Psychiatry*, *43*(10), 1225–1233. doi:10.1097/01.chi.0000135620.15522.38 PMID:15381889

Corey, M. S., Corey, G., & Corey, C. (2017). *Groups: Process and Practice* (10th ed.). NY: Brooks/Cole Publishers.

Council for Accreditation for Counseling and Related Programs. (2016). *2016 CACREP Standards*. Retrieved from http://www.cacrep.org/wp-content/uploads/2018/05/2016-Standards-with-Glossary-5.3.2018.pdf

Crenshaw, D. A. (1995). *Bereavement: Counseling the grieving throughout the life cycle*. New York, NY: Continuum Press.

Currier, J. M., Irish, J. E. F., Neimeyer, R. A., & Foster, J. D. (2015). Attachment, continuing bonds, and complicated grief following a violent loss: Testing a moderated model. *Death Studies*, *39*(1), 201–210. doi:10.1080/07481187.2014.975869 PMID:25551174

Currier, J. M., Neimeyer, R. A., & Berman, J. S. (2008). The effectiveness of psychotherapeutic interventions for the bereaved: A comprehensive quantitative review. *Psychological Bulletin*, *134*(5), 648–661. doi:10.1037/0033-2909.134.5.648 PMID:18729566

Donald, E. J., Culbreth, J. R., & Carter, A. W. (2015). Play therapy supervision: A review of the literature. *International Journal of Play Therapy*, *24*(2), 59–77. doi:10.1037/a0039104

Dopp, A. R., & Cain, A. C. (2012). The role of peer relationships in parental bereavement during childhood and adolescence. *Death Studies*, *36*(2), 41–60. doi:10.1080/07481187.2011.573175 PMID:24567994

Dowdney, L. (2000). Annotation: Childhood bereavement following parental death. *Journal of Child Psychology and Psychiatry, and Allied Disciplines*, *4*(7), 819–830. doi:10.1111/1469-7610.00670 PMID:11079425

Drewes, A. A. (2005). Appendix: Multicultural play therapy resources. In E. Gil & A. A. Drewes (Eds.), *Cultural issues in play therapy* (pp. 72–95). New York, NY: Guilford Press.

Drewes, A. A., & Mullen, J. A. (2008). *Supervision can be playful: Techniques for child and play therapist supervisors*. Lanham, MD: Jason Aronson, Inc.

Edgar-Bailey, M., & Kress, V. E. (2010). Resolving child and adolescent traumatic grief: Creative techniques and interventions. *Journal of Creativity in Mental Health*, *5*(2), 158–176. doi:10.1080/15401383.2010.485090

Elliott, V. S. (2016). Ethical challenges and considerations in the treatment of children. *Modern Psychoanalysis*, *41*(2), 93–112. Retrieved from http://dewey.umhb.edu:2048/login?url=http://search.ebscohost.com/login.aspx?direct=true&db=pbh&AN=131626916&site=eds-live

Feen-Calligan, H., McIntyre, B., & Sands-Goldstein, M. (2009). Art therapy applications of dolls in grief recovery, identity, and community service. *Art Therapy: Journal of the American Art Therapy Association, 26*(4), 167–173. doi:10.1080/07421656.2009.10129613

Field, N. P., & Filanosky, C. (2010). Continued bonds, risk factors for complicated grief, and adjustment to bereavement. *Death Studies, 34*(1), 1–29. doi:10.1080/07481180903372269 PMID:24479173

Garcia, F. (2012). Healing good-byes and healthy hellos: Learning and growing from painful endings and transitions. *Transactional Analysis Journal, 42*(1), 53–61. doi:10.1177/036215371204200107

Gil, E., & Crenshaw, D. (2015). *Termination challenges in child psychotherapy*. New York, NY: Guilford Press.

Green, E. J., & Connolly, M. E. (2009). Jungian family sandplay with bereaved children: Implications for play therapists. *International Journal of Play Therapy, 18*(2), 84–98. doi:10.1037/a0014435

Green, E. J., & Myrick, A. C. (2014). Treating complex trauma in adolescents: A phase-based, integrative approach for play therapists. *International Journal of Play Therapy, 23*(3), 131–145. doi:10.1037/a0036679

Haen, C. (2015). Vanquishing monsters: Group drama therapy for treating trauma. In C. Malchiodi (Ed.), *Creative interventions traumatized children* (pp. 235–257). New York, NY: Guilford Press.

Haine, R. A., Wolchik, S. A., Sandler, I., Millsap, R. E., & Ayers, T. S. (2006). Positive parenting as a protective resource for parentally bereaved children. *Death Studies, 30*(1), 1–28. doi:10.1080/07481180500348639 PMID:16296557

Helm, H. M., O'Halloran, M. S., & Kahlo, D. (2010). Funding training clinics. In A. K. Mobley & J. E. Myers (Eds.), *Developing and maintaining counselor education laboratories* (2nd ed.). Alexandria, VA: Association of Counselor Education and Supervision.

Holland, J. (2001). *Understanding children's experiences of parental bereavement*. London, England: Jessica Kingsley Publishers.

Hopmeyer, E., & Werk, A. (1994). A comparative study of family bereavement groups. *Death Studies, 18*(3), 243–256. doi:10.1080/07481189408252657 PMID:10135136

Hunt, Q. A., & Hertlein, K. M. (2015). Conceptualizing suicide bereavement through an attachment lens. *The American Journal of Family Therapy, 41*(1), 16–27. doi:10.1080/01926187.2014.975651

Iqbal, A. (2015). The ethical considerations of counselling psychologists working with trauma: Is there a risk of vicarious traumatisation? *Counselling Psychology Review, 30*(1), 44–51. Retrieved from https://www.researchgate.net/publication/284154295_The_ethical_considerations_of_counselling_psychologists_working_with_trauma_Is_there_a_risk_of_vicarious_traumatisation

Judi's House/JAG Institute for Grieving Children and Families. (2018). *Understanding childhood grief in the U.S.* Retrieved from https://www.judishouse.org/cbem/

Kestly, T. A. (2016). Presence and play: Why mindfulness matters. *International Journal of Play Therapy, 25*(1), 14–23. doi:10.1037/pla0000019

King, J., Prout, B., Stuhl, A., & Nelson, R. (2016). Scrapbooking as an intervention to enhance coping in individuals experiencing grief and loss. *Therapeutic Recreation Journal, 50*(2), 181–185. doi:10.18666/TRJ-2016-V50-I2-7308

Kottman, T., & Meany-Walen, K. (2015). *Partners in Play: An Adlerian approach to play therapy* (3rd ed.). Alexandria, VA: American Counseling Association. doi:10.1002/9781119272205

Kottman, T., & Meany-Walen, K. (2018). *Doing play therapy: From building the relationship to facilitating change.* New York, NY: Guilford Press.

Kristensen, P., Weisaeth, L., & Heir, T. (2012). Bereavement and mental health after sudden and violent losses: A review. *Psychiatry, 75*(1), 76–97. doi:10.1521/psyc.2012.75.1.76 PMID:22397543

Kubler-Ross, E. (1969). *On death and dying.* New York, NY: MacMillan Press.

Landreth, G. (2012). *The art of the relationship* (3rd ed.). New York, NY: Routledge. doi:10.4324/9780203835159

Leick, N., & Davidsen-Nielsen, M. (1991). *Healing pain: Attachment, loss, and grief therapy.* New York, NY: Routledge.

Machiodi, C. A. (2015). Neurobiology, creative interventions, and childhood trauma. In C. Malchiodi (Ed.), *Creative interventions traumatized children* (pp. 3–23). New York, NY: Guilford Press.

MacKay, L. M. (2017). Differentiation of self: Enhancing therapist resilience when working with relational trauma. *Australian and New Zealand Journal of Family Therapy*, *38*(4), 637–656. doi:10.1002/anzf.1276

Malchiodi, C. A. (2011). *Handbook of Art Therapy* (2nd ed.). New York, NY: Guilford Press.

Meany-Walen, K., Cobie-Nuss, A., Eittreim, E., Teeling, S., Wilson, S., & Xander, C. (2018). Play therapists' perceptions of wellness and self-care practices. *International Journal of Play Therapy*, *27*(3), 176–186. doi:10.1037/pla0000067

Mersky, J. P., Topitzes, J., & Reynolds, A. J. (2013). Impacts of adverse childhood experiences on health, mental health, and substance use in early adulthood: A cohort study of an urban, minority sample in the U.S. *Child Abuse & Neglect*, *37*(11), 917–925. doi:10.1016/j.chiabu.2013.07.011 PMID:23978575

Neimeyer, R. A., Burke, L. A., Mackay, M. M., & van Dyke Stringer, J. G. (2010). Grief therapy and the reconstruction of meaning: From principles to practice. *Journal of Contemporary Psychotherapy*, *40*(2), 73–83. doi:10.100710879-009-9135-3

Oaklander, V. (2006). *Hidden treasures: A map to the child's inner self.* New York, NY: Routledge.

Piaget, J., & Inhelder, B. (1969). *The psychology of the child* (2nd ed.). New York, NY: Basic Books.

Porges, S. W. (2011). *The Polyvagal Theory: Neurophysiological foundations of emotions, attachment, communication, and self-regulation*. New York, N.Y: W. W. Norton.

Prigerson, H. G., Maciejewski, P., Reynolds, C. III, Bierhals, A., Newsom, J., Fasiczka, A., ... Miller, M. (1995). Inventory of complicated grief. *Psychiatry Research*, *59*(1-2), 65–79. doi:10.1016/0165-1781(95)02757-2 PMID:8771222

Ray, D. C. (2004). Supervision of basic and advanced skills in play therapy. *Journal of Professional Counseling, Practice, Theory, & Research*, *32*(2), 28–41. doi:10.1080/15566382.2004.12033805

Ray, D. C. (2011). *Advanced play therapy: Essential conditions, knowledge, and skills for child practice*. London: Routledge. doi:10.4324/9780203837269

Ray, D. C., Lee, K. R., Meany-Walen, K. K., Carlson, S. E., Carnes-Holt, K. L., & Ware, J. N. (2013). Use of toys in child-centered play therapy. *International Journal of Play Therapy*, *22*(1), 43–57. doi:10.1037/a0031430

Ray, D. C., Purswell, K. P., Haas, S. H., & Aldrete, C. (2017). Child-centered play therapy-research integrity checklist: Development, reliability, and use. *International Journal of Play Therapy*, *26*(4), 207–217. doi:10.1037/pla0000046

Reddy, L. A., Files-Hall, T. M., & Schaefer, C. E. (2005). Announcing empirically based play interventions for children. In L. A. Reddy, T. M. Files-Hall, & C. E. Schaefer (Eds.), *Empirically-based Play Interventions for Children* (pp. 3–10). Washington, DC: American Psychological Association. doi:10.1037/11086-001

Rozman, A. L. (2015). Art therapy with children in grief and loss groups. In C. Malchiodi (Ed.), *The Handbook of Art Therapy* (2nd ed.; pp. 422–432). New York, NY: Guilford Press.

Siddaway, A. P., Wood, A. M., Schulz, J., & Trickey, D. (2015). Evaluation of the CHUMS child bereavement group: A pilot study examining statistical and clinical change. *Death Studies*, *1*(39), 99–110. doi:10.1080/07481187.2014.913085 PMID:25153045

Sories, F., Maier, C., Beer, A., & Thomas, V. (2015). Addressing the needs of military children through family-based play therapy. *Contemporary Family Therapy*, *37*(3), 209–200. doi:10.100710591-015-9342-x

Steele, W., & Malchiodi, C. A. (2012). *Trauma-informed practiced with children and adolescents*. New York, NY: Routledge. doi:10.4324/9780203829493

Stutey, D. M., Helm, H. M., LoSasso, H., & Kreider, H. D. (2015). Play therapy and photo-elicitation: A narrative examination of children's grief. *International Journal of Play Therapy*, *25*(3), 154–165. doi:10.1037/a0039956

Swank, J. M. (2018). Peer feedback within a play therapy course: A qualitative exploration. *International Journal of Play Therapy*, *27*(1), 25–34. doi:10.1037/pla0000060

Sweeney, D. S., Baggerly, J. N., & Ray, D. C. (2014). *Group play therapy: A dynamic approach*. New York, NY: Routledge/Taylor & Francis Group. doi:10.4324/9780203103944

Thanasiu, P. L., Rust, K. L., & Walter, S. M. (2018). Service learning and live supervision as early components in play therapy training. *International Journal of Play Therapy*, *27*(2), 103–113. doi:10.1037/pla0000069

Tonkins, S. A., & Lambert, M. J. (1996). A treatment outcome study of bereavement groups for children. *Child & Adolescent Social Work Journal*, *1*(13), 3–21. doi:10.1007/BF01876592

Turner, S. R. (2017). *Play therapy for traumatic loss: Recovery from suicide and homicide*. Presented at the annual Texas Association for Play Therapy Conference, Austin, TX.

Van der Kolk, B. A. (2015). *The body keeps the score: Brain, body, and mind in the healing of trauma*. New York, NY: Penguin Books.

Webb, N. B. (2002). *Helping bereaved children: A handbook for practitioners*. New York, NY: Guilford Press.

Webb, N. B. (2003). Play and expressive therapies to help bereaved children: Individual, family, and group treatments. *Smith College Studies in Social Work*, *73*(3), 405–422. doi:10.1080/00377310309517694

Weber, A. M., & Haen, C. (2005). *Clinical applications of drama therapy in child and adolescent treatment*. London, England: Brunner-Routledge.

Wong, P. T. P. (2008). Transformation of grief through meaning: Meaning-centered counseling for bereavement. In A. Tomer, G. T. Eliason, & P. T. P. Wong (Eds.), *Existential and spiritual issues in death attitudes*. New York, NY: Lawrence Erlbaum.

Worden, J. W. (1996). *Children and grief: When a parent dies*. New York, NY: Guilford Press.

Worden, J. W. (2009). *Grief counseling and grief therapy: A handbook for the mental health practitioner* (4th ed.). New York, NY: Springer.

Yasenik, L., & Gardner, K. (2012). *Play therapy dimensions model: A decision-making guide for integrative play therapists*. New York, NY: Jessica Kingsley Publishers.

KEY TERMS AND DEFINITIONS

Bereavement: Bereavement is a period of mourning which occurs after any type of death loss, influenced by cultural and religious norms.

Group Play Therapy: Two or more children engaging in therapeutic play therapy.

Play Themes: Patterns of play which aid the therapist in conceptualizing play communication.

Play Therapy Supervision: The process in which a skilled and experienced play therapy practitioner develops, mentors, and monitors a supervisee's play therapy practice.

Self-Care: The intentional practice of supporting emotional, physical, and spiritual health to promote counselor wellness.

Support Groups: A support group is a group of individuals who come together to process their common experiences which may or may not be led by a licensed professional.

Termination: The ending phase of therapy.

Appendix

PLAY THERAPY FORMS

University play therapy clinics may provide a variety of services, therefore, may need several different types of session note templates. The following pages offer examples of session note forms that are used at Louisiana State University Health Science Center-New Orleans's Child and Family Counseling Clinic.

- Family Play Therapy Form
- Caregiver Consultation Form
- Professional Consultation Form
- Group Session Note
- Case Conceptualization Form

Family Play Therapy Session: Notes should include the client name as well as those family members present in the session. The note also includes a place for the therapist's name. The session summary space is allotted a narrative format to allow therapist the freedom to document the highlights or overview of the session. Each session note allows for the documentation of evidence of treatment goal progress and session goal progress. Participation of each individual family member is documented by circling the appropriate quality or level—the initials of the individual person may be used to indicate the similarities or differences. As with many mental health notes, the mood or affect of each member participating is also noted, again with the family member's initials showing the affect or mood of each. Circling the intervention provided allows clinicians the ability to track over time which interventions are working for the family. Lastly, the therapist's plan is noted by circling the appropriate strategy.

Caregiver Consultation Form: Should include the client and therapist name, as well as, the caregiver(s) present. The session summary space is allotted a narrative format to allow therapist the freedom to document the highlights or overview of the caregiver consultation session. Each caregiver consultation session note allows for the documentation of evidence of treatment goal progress and session goal progress. Participation of the caregiver(s) is documented by circling the appropriate quality or level. Additionally, the mood or affect of each member participating is also noted, again with the family member's initials showing the affect or mood of each. Circling the intervention provided allows clinicians the ability to track over time which interventions are working for the caregiver consultations. Lastly, the therapist's plan is noted by circling the appropriate strategy.

Professional Consultation Form: Should include the client and therapist name, as well as, the collateral contact name. The purpose of the consultation is also noted (and should be reflected on the release of information form-HIPPA). The consultation summary space is allotted a narrative format to allow therapist the freedom to document the highlights or overview of the consultation session. Finally, circling the intervention provided allows clinicians the ability to track over time which interventions are working for the client as reported by the collateral consultant.

Group Session Note: The individual group note should only include information about the specific client and should never include confidential information about other group members. In addition, play therapists may provide parents with an informational group handout for each week. The handout may provide education about group topics, elaborate on group goals, and share helpful tips that reinforce the goals of the weekly session for parents and teachers.

The individual client note should include the client name and the therapist's name. The session summary space should include the highlights or overview of the group session. Each session note allows for the documentation of both treatment goal and session goal progress. The client's level and quality of participation is documented by circling the appropriate term(s), and the play therapist may indicate changes in presentation during the session by indicating if they occurred upon entry or exit to group. Notation is made for how the group member interacted with their peers and the facilitator. Mood and affect are also documented by circling any term that applies. Lastly, the therapist's plan is noted by circling the appropriate strategy. If the group session is the client's last, the therapist should indicate whether or not it is a planned successful or unplanned termination.

Case Conceptualization Form: Case conceptualization forms may be helpful to beginning play therapists (Vaughn, Stigger, Dugan, 2017). This form allows the new play therapist to take large amounts of information gathered in an initial intake session and summarize in the areas of: source of information, chief complaint, histories (psychiatric, medical, family psychiatric, social, education, and developmental), psychological testing, assessment, and plan. Detailed information on types of information belonging into each category may be found in the referenced article.

Play Therapy Session Note: Include the child and therapist name, a session summary, and any disclosures made by the child (indicate if child or therapist initiated). Additionally, somatic complaints, tactical stimulation, or the number of bathroom breaks may be noted. Play therapists may also find it beneficial to document if limits were used, if so, what type (protection of child, therapist, or materials). The use of specific types of toys and play themes may also be listed. Additionally, Ray (2011) provides an overview of session progress worksheets in her text Advanced Play Therapy.

Figure 1.

Family Play Therapy Progress Note

Date:______________

Time:______________

Length: ______________

Client Name:____________________**Therapist(s):**____________________

Summary:____

Progress made toward session goals: YES NO AEB:____________________

Progress made toward treatment goals: YES NO AEB:____________________

Quality/ Level of Participation (circle all that apply):

Active/Engaged	Argumentative	Attention Seeking	Confused	Constructive Comments
Distracted	Guarded Inattentive	Minimal verbal participation	Monopolizing	No verbal participation
Removed from group	Resistant	Seemed to listen to others	Defensive	Receptive to feedback

Other:____

Mood/Affect (circle all that apply):

Angry	Anxious	Bright	Congruent	Defensive
Depressed	Excited	Flat	Guarded	Happy
Irritable	Sad	Tearful	Other	

Interventions Provided:

Support	Education	Problem Solving	Confrontation	Modeling
Role Play	Other:			

Plan (circle all that apply and explain):

Continue family therapy	Refer to individual therapy	Schedule Caregiver consultation	Schedule Collateral Consultation	Refer to:

____________________ __________

Signature Date

Appendix

Figure 2.

Professional Consultation Note

Date:_________________

Time:_________________

Length: _________________

Client Name:__________________________**Therapist(s):**____

Collateral Contact:______________________**Type: Phone Email Face to Face**

Purpose of Consult:____

Requested by:____

Release of Information sent/received: Yes No **Date of Expiration:**_______________________________________

Consultation Summary:

____

____

____

____

____

Progress made toward consult goals: YES NO AEB:____

Interventions Provided:

Support Education Problem Solving Confrontation Modeling

Role Play Other:

Plan (circle all that apply and explain):

Refer to family therapy	Refer to individual therapy	Schedule Caregiver consultation	Schedule Collateral Consultation	Continue Individual therapy	Refer to group therapy	Refer to:

_______________________________________ ____________

Signature Date

Figure 3.

Caregiver Consultation Note

Date:______________
Time:______________
Length: ______________

Client Name:______________________**Therapist(s):**______________________
Caregiver Present:____
Summary:____

____

____

____

Progress made toward consult goals: YES NO AEB:______________________

Progress made toward child/family treatment goals: YES NO AEB:______________________

Quality/ Level of Participation (circle all that apply):

Active/Engaged	Argumentative	Attention Seeking	Confused	Constructive Comments
Distracted	Guarded Inattentive	Minimal verbal participation	Monopolizing	No verbal participation
Removed from group	Resistant	Seemed to listen to others	Defensive	Receptive to feedback

Other:____

Mood/Affect (circle all that apply):

Angry	Anxious	Bright	Congruent	Defensive
Depressed	Excited	Flat	Guarded	Happy
Irritable	Sad	Tearful	Other	

Interventions Provided:

Support	Education	Problem Solving	Confrontation	Modeling
Role Play	Other:			

Plan (circle all that apply and explain):

Continue family therapy	Refer to individual therapy	Schedule Caregiver consultation	Schedule Collateral Consultation	Refer to:

______________________ ____________
Signature Date

Appendix

Figure 4.

Group Play Therapy Progress Note

Date:__________________

Time:__________________

Length:__________________

Client Name:__________________________**Therapist(s):**____________________________________

Summary:____

____

____

____

Progress made toward session goals: YES NO AEB:____

Progress made toward treatment goals: YES NO AEB:_______________________________________

Interventions Provided:

Support	Education	Problem Exploration	Confrontation	Role Play	CBT
Modeling	CC Play Therapy	Therapeutic Game	Art Activity	Sandtray	Other/Explain:

Quality/ Level of Participation (circle all that apply and indicate presentation upon entry and exit as applies):

Active/Engaged	Argumentative	Attention Seeking	Resistant to Feedback	Constructive Comments
Distracted	Guarded	Minimal or no verbal participation	Monopolizing	Cooperative
Removed from group/ Left group	Resistant to participate	Seemed to listen to others	Defensive	Receptive to feedback

Interaction with Peers (circle all that apply):

Attention seeking	Cooperative	Defensive/Hostile	Guarded	Manipulative

Interaction with Facilitator (circle all that apply):

Attention seeking	Cooperative	Defensive/Hostile	Guarded	Manipulative

Mood/Affect (circle all that apply):

Angry	Anxious	Bright	Congruent	Defensive
Depressed	Excited	Flat	Guarded	Happy
Irritable	Sad	Tearful	Confused	Other:

Plan (circle all that apply):

Continue group therapy	Refer to individual or family therapy	Schedule caregiver consultation	Schedule collateral consultation with:	Terminate	Refer to:

______________________________ __________

Signature Date

Figure 5.

Date: Case Activity Notes

Sources of Information	
Chief Complaint	
History of present illness	
Past psychiatric history	
Past medical history	
Family psychiatric history and medical history	
Social history	
Education history	
Developmental history	
Psychological testing	
Assessment	
Plan	

Name of Client:

Clinician's signature:

Supervisor's signature:

REFERENCES

Ray, D. C. (2011). *Advanced play therapy: Essential conditions, knowledge, and skills for child practice*. New York: Routledge. doi:10.4324/9780203837269

Vaughn, K., Stigger, B., & Dugan, E. (2017). A resource to efficient case conceptualization. *Play Therapy*, *12*(2), 24–28.

Compilation of References

Abramsky, S. (2012). The other America 2012. *Nation, 294*(20), 11-18. Retrieved from https://login.ezproxy.net.ucf.edu/login?auth=shibb&url=https://search-ebscohost- com.ezproxy.net.ucf.edu/login.aspx?direct=true&AuthType=ip,cookie,shib,sso,uid&db=ulh&AN=74602403&site=eds-live&scope=site

Ackerman, A. M. (2017). An integrated model for counselor social justice advocacy in child welfare. *The Family Journal (Alexandria, Va.), 25*(4), 389–397. doi:10.1177/1066480717736061

Aguilera, M. E. (2009). *An exploratory study of the developmental process of novice play therapists* (Doctoral dissertation). Retrieved from ProQuest dissertations & theses. (UMI Number 3376769)

Aguilera, M. E. (2010). An exploratory study of the developmental experience of novice play therapists. *Dissertation Abstracts International; Section A, 70,* 3352.

Allan, J. (1994). *Inscapes of the child's world: Jungian counseling in schools and clinics*. Dallas, TX: Spring Publications, Inc.

Allen, J., & Levin, S. (1993). Born on my bum: Jungian play therapy. In T. Kottman & C. Schaefer (Eds.), *Play therapy: A casebook for practitioners* (pp. 209–243). Northvale, NJ: Aronson.

Allen, V. B., Folger, W. A., & Pehrsson, D. E. (2007). Reflective process in play therapy: A practical model for supervising counseling students. *Education, 127*, 472–479.

American Association for Marriage and Family Therapy. (2012). *AAMFT code of ethics.* Alexandria, VA: Author.

American Association for Marriage and Family Therapy. (2015). Retrieved August 5, 2018 from https://www.aamft.org/Legal_Ethics/Code_of_Ethics.aspx

American Counseling Association. (2014). *2014 ACA Code of Ethics - As approved by the ACA Governing Council.* Retrieved August 5, 2018 from ttps://www.counseling.org/resources/ aca-code-of-ethics.pdf

American Counseling Association. (2014). *ACA code of ethics*. Alexandria, VA: Author.

American Counseling Association. (2014). *Code of ethics*. Alexandria, VA: Author.

American Marketing Association. (2013). *About marketing*. Retrieved from https:// www.ama.org/AboutAMA/Pages/Definition-of-Marketing.aspx

American Psychological Association. (2017). *Ethical Principles of Psychologists and Code of Conduct*. Retried on August 5, 2018 from http://www.apa.org/ethics/ code/ethics-code-2017.pdf

American Psychological Association. (2018). *Ethical principles of psychologists and code of conduct*. Washington, DC: Author.

American School Counseling Association. (2014). *State-by-state student-to-counselor ratio report 10 year trends*. Retrieved from https://www.schoolcounselor.org/asca/media/asca/Publications/ratioreport.pdf

American School Counseling Association. (2017). *The school counseling and comprehensive school counseling programs position statement*. Retrieved from https://www.schoolcounselor.org/asca/media/asca/PositionStatements/PS_ComprehensivePrograms.pdf

American School Counselor Association. (2012). *ASCA national model: A framework for school counseling programs. Executive summary*. Alexandria, VA: Author.

Anderson, S. A., Schlossberg, M., & Rigazio-DiGilio, S. (2000). Family therapy trainees' evaluations of their best and worst supervision experiences. *Journal of Marital and Family Therapy*, *26*(1), 79–91. doi:10.1111/j.1752-0606.2000.tb00278.x PMID:10685354

Asakura, K., & Maurer, K. (2018). Attending to social justice in clinical social work: Supervision as a pedagogical space. *Clinical Social Work Journal*, *46*(4), 289–297. doi:10.100710615-018-0667-4

Ashby, J. S., Kottman, T., & DeGraff, D. (2008). *Active interventions for kids and teens: Adding adventures and fun to counseling*. Alexandria, VA: American Counseling Association.

Association for Counselor Education and Supervision (ACES) Taskforce on Best Practices in Clinical Supervision. (2011, April). *Best practices in clinical supervision*. Retrieved June 30, 2013, from http://www.acesonline.net/wp-content/uploads/2011/10/ACES-Best-Practices-in-clinical-supervision-document-FINAL.pdf

Association for Play Therapy. (1997). A definition of play therapy. *The Association for Play Therapy Newsletter*, *16*(1), 7.

Association for Play Therapy. (2010). *Sample syllabus: Introductory graduate play therapy course*. Retrieved from https://cdn.ymaws.com/www.a4pt.org/resource/ resmgr/Sample_Play_Therapy_Course_S.pdf

Association for Play Therapy. (2013). *RPT/S credentialing guide: Registered play therapist (RPT) & Supervisor (RPT-S)*. Retrieved from http://c.ymcdn.com/sites/www.a4pt.org/resource/resmgr/RPT_and_RPT-S_Credentials/RPTS_Guide.pdf

Association for Play Therapy. (2016). *Play Therapy Best Practices*. Clovis, CA: Author.

Association for Play Therapy. (2016). *Play therapy best practices: Clinical, professional & ethical issues*. Clovis, CA: Author.

Association for Play Therapy. (2016). *Play therapy best practices: Clinical, Professional and Ethical Issues*. Retrieved from https://cdn.ymaws.com/www.a4pt.org/resource/resmgr/ publications/ Best_Practices__-_Sept_2016.pdf

Association for Play Therapy. (2016). *Play Therapy Best Practices: Clinical, Professional, and Ethical Issues*. Retrieved August 2, 2018 from https://cdn.ymaws.com/www.a4pt.org/ resource/ resmgr/publications/Best_Practices__-_Sept_2016.pdf

Association for Play Therapy. (2017a). *APT annual growth report by CEO*. Retrieved from https:// cdn.ymaws.com/www.a4pt.org/resource/resmgr/about_apt/Website_version.pdf

Association for Play Therapy. (2017b). *Credentialing guide: Registered play therapist (RPT) & supervisor (RPT-S)*. Retrieved from: https://cdn.ymaws.com/www.a4pt.org/resource/ resmgr/ Credentials/RPTS_Guide_Dec_2017.pdf

Association for Play Therapy. (2018a). *Approved center of play therapy education*. Retrieved from https://www.a4pt.org/page/ApprovedCenter

Association for Play Therapy. (2018b). *Approved provider guide*. Retrieved from https://www. a4pt.org/resource/resmgr/education_&_training/approved_provider_guide_-_au.pdf

Association for Play Therapy. (2018c). *Why play therapy?* Retrieved from https://www.a4pt.org/ page/WhyPlayTherapy

Association for Play Therapy. (2019). Retrieved from https://www.a4pt.org/ page/Credentials Homepage

Association for Play Therapy. (n.d.a). *About play therapy*. Retrieved from https://www.a4pt.org/ page/AboutAPT

Association for Play Therapy. (n.d.a). Retrieved from http://www.a4pt.org/page/educationtraining

Association for Play Therapy. (n.d.b). *Clarifying the use of play therapy*. Retrieved from https:// www.a4pt.org/page/ClarifyingUseofPT

Association for Play Therapy. (n.d.b). Retrieved from http://www.a4pt.org/page/ CredentialsHomepage

Association for Play Therapy. (n.d.c). *Find a play therapist*. Retrieved from https:// www.a4pt. org/page/TherapistDirectory

Association for Play Therapy. (n.d.d.). *Education and training*. Retrieved from https:// www. a4pt.org/general/custom.asp?page=EducationTraining

Association of Play Therapy. (2019). *Approved provider guide*. Retrieved from https://cdn.ymaws. com/www.a4pt.org/resource/resmgr/education_&_training/approved_provider_guide_-_au.pdf

Aubry, T. D., Hunsley, J., Josephson, G., & Vito, D. (2000). Quid pro quo: Fee for services delivered in a psychology training clinic. *Journal of Clinical Psychology, 56*(1), 23–31. doi:10.1002/(SICI)1097-4679(200001)56:1<23::AID-JCLP3>3.0.CO;2-8 PMID:10661366

Axline, V. (1947). *Play Therapy*. New York: Ballantine.

Axline, V. (1964). *Dibs in search of self*. New York, NY: Ballantine.

Axline, V. M. (1969). *Play therapy*. New York, NY: Ballantine Books.

Badenoch, B. (2008). *Being a brain-wise therapist*. New York, NY: Norton.

Baggerly, J. (2006). Service learning with children affected by pervert: Facilitating multicultural competence in counseling education students. *Journal of Multicultural Counseling and Development, 34*(4), 244-255. Retrieved from https://login.ezproxy.net.ucf.edu/login?auth=shibb&url=https://search-ebscohost-com.ezproxy.net.ucf.edu/login.aspx?direct=true&AuthType=ip,cookie,shib,sso,uid&db=tfh&AN=23054881&site=eds-live&scope=site

Baggerly, J., & Abugideiri, S. E. (2010). Grief counseling for Muslim preschool and elementary school children. *Journal of Multicultural Counseling and Development, 38*(2), 112–124. Retrieved from https://login.ezproxy.net.ucf.edu/login?auth=shibb&url=https://search- ebscohost-com.ezproxy.net.ucf.edu/login.aspx?direct= true&AuthType= ip, cookie,shib,sso,uid&db=eric&AN=EJ881625&site=eds-live&scope=site

Baggerly, J. (2006). Service learning with children affected by poverty: Facilitating multicultural competence in counseling education students. *Journal of Multicultural Counseling and Development, 34*(4), 244–255. doi:10.1002/j.2161-1912.2006.tb00043.x

Barnes, M. A. (1996). *The healing path with children: An exploration for parents and professionals*. Kingston, Ontario, Canada: Viktoria, Fermoyle, & Berrigan.

Barnett, J. E., Cornish, J. A. E., Goodyear, R. K., & Lichtenberg, J. W. (2007). Commentaries on the ethical and effective practice of clinical supervision. *Psychology: Research and Practice, 38*, 268–275.

Barrett, K. M., Lester, S. V., & Durham, J. C. (2011). Child maltreatment and the advocacy role of professional school counselors. *Journal for Social Action in Counseling and Psychology, 3*(2), 86–103.

Bartle-Haring, S., Silverthorn, B. C., Meyer, K., & Toviessi, P. (2009). Does live supervision make a difference? A multilevel analysis. *Journal of Marital and Family Therapy, 35*(4), 406–414. doi:10.1111/j.1752-0606.2009.00124.x PMID:19785698

Beddoe, L., Ackroyd, J., Chinnery, S., & Appleton, C. (2011). Live supervision of students in field placement: More than just watching. *Social Work Education, 30*(5), 512–528. doi:10.1080/02615479.2010.516358

Bergman, A., Axberg, U., & Hanson, E. (2017). When a parent dies: A systematic review of the effects of support programs for parentally bereaved children and their caregivers. *BMC Palliative Care*, *16*(39). doi:10.118612904-017-0223-y PMID:28797262

Bernard, J. M., & Goodyear, R. K. (2014). *Fundamentals of Clinical Supervision* (5th ed.). Boston: Pearson.

Bernard, J. M., & Goodyear, R. K. (2018). *Fundamentals in Clinical Supervision* (6th ed.). New York, NY: Pearson Publishing.

Bernard, J. M., & Goodyear, R. K. (2018). *Fundamentals of clinical supervision* (6th ed.). Upper Saddle River, NJ: Pearson Education.

Bertolino, B. (2018). *Effective counseling and psychotherapy: An evidence-based approach*. New York, NY: Springer. doi:10.1891/9780826141132

Bitko, R. H., Holbrook, J. R., Robinson, L. R., Kaminski, J. W., Ghandour, R., Smith, C., & Peacock, G. (2016). Health care, family, and community factors associated with mental, behavioral, and developmental disorders in early childhood: United States, 2011-2012. *MMWR. Morbidity and Mortality Weekly Report*, *65*(9), 221–226. doi:10.15585/mmwr.mm6509a1 PMID:26963052

Blanco, P. J., Muro, J. H., & Stickley, V. K. (2014). Understanding the concept of genuineness in play therapy: Implications for the supervision and teaching of beginning play therapists. *International Journal of Play Therapy*, *23*(1), 44–54. doi:10.1037/a0035478

Bodrova, E., & Leong, D. J. (2015). Vygotskian and post-Vygotskian views on children's play. *American Journal of Play*, *7*, 371–388.

Borders, L. D., & Brown, L. L. (2005). *The new handbook of counseling supervision*. New York, NY: Routledge.

Borders, L. D., & Leddick, G. (1987). *Handbook of counseling supervision*. Alexandria, VA: American Counseling Association.

Boylston, W., & Tuma, J. (1972). Training of mental health professionals through the use of the 'bug in the ear'. *The American Journal of Psychiatry*, *129*(1), 92–95. doi:10.1176/ajp.129.1.92 PMID:5034190

Bradway, K. (1979). Sandplay in psychotherapy. *Art Psychotherapy*, *6*(2), 85–93. doi:10.1016/0090-9092(79)90003-6

Bratton, S., Ray, D., & Landreth, G. (2010). Play therapy. In A. Gross & M. Hersen (Eds.), Handbook of clinical psychology: Vol. 2. Children and adolescents. New York, NY: John Wiley & Sons.

Bratton, S. C., Landreth, G. L., Kellam, T., & Blackard, S. R. (2006). *Child parent relationship therapy (CPRT) treatment manual: A 10-session filial therapy model for training parents*. New York, NY: Routledge Taylor and Francis Group. doi:10.4324/9780203956793

Bratton, S., Ceballos, P., & Sheely, A. (2008). Expressive arts in a humanistic approach to play therapy supervision: Facilitating therapist self-awareness. In A. A. Drewes & J. A. Mullen (Eds.), *Supervision can be playful: Techniques for child and play therapist supervisors* (pp. 211–232). Lanham, MD: Rowman & Littlefield.

Bratton, S., Landreth, G., & Homeyer, L. (1993). An intensive three day play therapy supervision/ training model. *International Journal of Play Therapy*, *2*(2), 61–78. doi:10.1037/h0089366

Bratton, S., Ray, D., Rhine, T., & Jones, L. (2005). The efficacy of play therapy with children: A meta-analytic review of treatment outcomes. *Professional Psychology, Research and Practice*, *36*(4), 376–390. doi:10.1037/0735-7028.36.4.376

Bray, B. (2014, November 17). Storytelling and hope in Ferguson. *Counseling Today*. Retrieved from https://ct.counseling.org/2014/11/storytelling-and-hope-in- ferguson/

Brear, P., Dorrian, J., & Luscri, G. (2008). Preparing our future counseling professionals: Gatekeeping and implications for research. *Counselling & Psychotherapy Research*, *8*(2), 93–101. doi:10.1080/14733140802007855

Brody, V. (1992). The dialogue of touch: Developmental play therapy. *International Journal of Play Therapy*, *1*(1), 21–30. doi:10.1037/h0090232

Brody, V. (1997). *The dialogue of touch: Developmental play therapy*. Northvale, NJ: J. Aronson.

Bromfield, R. (1995). The use of puppets in play therapy. *Child & Adolescent Social Work Journal*, *12*(6), 435–444. doi:10.1007/BF01875812

Brown, E. C., & Gibbons, M. M. (2018). Addressing needs of children of incarcerated parents with child-centered play therapy. *Journal of Child and Adolescent Counseling*, *4*(2), 134–145. doi:10.1080/23727810.2017.1381931

Brubaker, M. D., Puig, A., Reese, R. F., & Young, J. (2010). Integrating social justice into counseling theories pedagogy: A case example. *Counselor Education and Supervision*, *50*(2), 88–102. Retrieved from https://login.ezproxy.net.ucf.edu/ login?auth=shibb&url= https://search-ebscohost-com.ezproxy.net.ucf.edu/login.aspx?direct= true&AuthType=ip,cookie, shib,sso,uid &db=eric&AN=EJ911809&site=eds- live&scope=site

Bubenzer, D. L., Mahrle, C., & West, J. D. (1987). *Live counselor supervision: Trainee acculturation and supervisor interventions*. Paper presented at the American Association for Counseling and Development Annual Convention, New Orleans, LA.

Buhler, C. (1951). The world test, a projective technique. *Journal of Child Psychiatry*, *2*, 4–23.

Buhler, C., & Manson, M. (1956). The picture world test: A new projective technique. *The Journal of Psychology*, *42*(2), 303–316. doi:10.1080/00223980.1956.9713043

Bureau of Labor Statistics. (2018). *Occupational outlook handbook*. Retrieved August 1, 2018, from https://www.bls.gov/ooh/

Burke, N. J., Hellman, J. L., Scott, B. G., Weems, C. F., & Carrion, V. G. (2011). The impact of adverse childhood experiences on an urban pediatric population. *Child Abuse & Neglect*, *35*(6), 408–413. doi:10.1016/j.chiabu.2011.02.006 PMID:21652073

Burnes, T. R., & Singh, A. A. (2010). Integrating social justice training into the practicum experience for psychology trainees: Starting earlier. *Training and Education in Professional Psychology*, *4*(3), 153–162. doi:10.1037/a0019385

Carlozzi, A. F., Romans, J. S. C., Boswell, D. L., Ferguson, D. B., & Whisenhunt, B. J. (1997). Training and supervision practices in counseling and marriage and family therapy programs. *The Clinical Supervisor*, *15*(1), 51–60. doi:10.1300/J001v15n01_04

Carmichael, K. (2006). *Play therapy: An introduction*. Upper Saddle River, NJ: Pearson Education, Inc.

Carnes-Holt, K., & Bratton, S. C. (2014). The efficacy of child parent relationship therapy for adopted children with attachment disruptions. *Journal of Counseling and Development*, *92*(3), 328–337. doi:10.1002/j.1556-6676.2014.00160.x

Carter, R., & Mason, P. (1998). The selection and use of puppets in counseling. *Professional School Counseling*, *1*(5), 50–53.

Cattanach, A. (2003). *Introduction to play therapy*. Hove, NY: Brunner-Routledge.

Cattanach, A. (2007). *Narrative approaches in play with children*. London: Jessica Kingsley.

Ceballos, P. L., Parikh, S., & Post, P. B. (2012). Examining social justice attitudes among play therapists: Implications for multicultural supervision and training. *International Journal of Play Therapy*, *21*(4), 232–243. doi:10.1037/a0028540

Centers for Disease Control and Prevention. (2019). *Asthma: Management and treatment*. Retrieved from https://www.cdc.gov/niosh/index.htm

Centers for Disease Control and Prevention. (2019). *Workplace Safety and Health Topics*. Retrieved from https://www.cdc.gov/niosh/index.htm

Champe, J., & Kleist, D. M. (2003). Live supervision: A review of the research. *The Family Journal (Alexandria, Va.)*, *11*(3), 1–8. doi:10.1177/1066480703252755

Chang, C. Y., Barrio Minton, C. A., Dixon, A. L., Myers, J. E., & Sweeney, T. J. (2012). *Professional counseling excellence through leadership and advocacy*. New York, NY: Routledge. doi:10.4324/9780203829165

Chang, C. Y., Crethar, H. C., Ratts, M. J., & Editors, G. (2010). Social justice: A national imperative for counselor education and supervision. *Counselor Education and Supervision*, *50*(2), 82–87. doi:10.1002/j.1556-6978.2010.tb00110.x

Chang, C., Ritter, K., & Hays, D. (2005). Multicultural trends and toys in play therapy. *International Journal of Play Therapy*, *14*(2), 69–85. doi:10.1037/h0088903

Clark, G. (2016). Using technology to enhance supervision at the University of Southern California. In S. Goss, K. Anthony, L. S. Stretch, & D. M. Nagel (Eds.), *Technology in mental health: Applications in practice, supervision and training* (pp. 366–377). Springfield, IL: Charles C. Thomas.

Clark, P., & Kimberly, C. (2014). Impact of fees among low-income clients in a training clinic. *Contemporary Family Therapy*, *36*(3), 363–368. doi:10.100710591-014-9303-9

Clute, M. A., & Kobayashi, R. (2013). Are children's grief camps effective? *Journal of Social Work in End-of-Life & Palliative Care*, *9*(1), 43–57. doi:10.1080/15524256.2013.758927 PMID:23438644

Cohen, J. A., Mannariron, A. P., & Knudsen, K. (2004). Treating childhood traumatic grief: A pilot study. *Journal of the American Academy of Child and Adolescent Psychiatry*, *43*(10), 1225–1233. doi:10.1097/01.chi.0000135620.15522.38 PMID:15381889

Colby, S. L., & Ortman, J. M. (2015). *Projections of the size and composition of the U.S. population: 2014 to 2060, current population reports* (Report No. P25-1143). Washington, DC: U.S. Census Bureau.

Cole. (2016). Can focusing on customer experience unify marketing and sales functions. *Marketing News*. Retrieved from https://www.ama.org/publications/MarketingNews/ Pages/experiential-view-unify-the-entire-prospect-to-customer-lifecycle.aspx

Coleman, V., Parmer, T., & Barker, S. (1993). Play therapy for multicultural populations: Guidelines for mental health professionals. *International Journal of Play Therapy*, *2*(1), 63–74. doi:10.1037/h0089381

Constantine, M. G., Hage, S. M., Kindaichi, M. M., & Bryant, R. M. (2007). Social justice and multicultural issues: Implications for the practice and training of counselors and counseling psychologists. *Journal of Counseling and Development*, *85*(1), 24–29. doi:10.1002/j.1556-6678.2007.tb00440.x

Corey, M. S., Corey, G., & Corey, C. (2017). *Groups: Process and Practice* (10th ed.). NY: Brooks/Cole Publishers.

Costas, M., & Landreth, G. (1999). Filial therapy with nonoffending parents of children who have been sexually abused. *International Journal of Play Therapy*, *8*(1), 43–66. doi:10.1037/h0089427

Council for Accreditation for Counseling and Related Programs. (2016). *2016 CACREP Standards*. Retrieved from http://www.cacrep.org/wp-content/uploads/2018/05/2016-Standards-with-Glossary-5.3.2018.pdf

Council for Accreditation of Counseling and Related Educational Programs (CACREP). (n.d.). *2009 Standards*. Available: www.cacrep.org/wp-content/uploads/2017/07/2009-Standards.pdf

Council for Accreditation of Counseling and Related Educational Programs (CACREP). (n.d.). *2016 Standards*. Available: https://www.cacrep.org/for-programs/2016-cacrep-standards/

Council for Accreditation of Counseling and Related Educational Programs. (2016). *2016 CACREP standards*. Retrieved from CACREP website: http://www.cacrep.org/wp-content/uploads/2017/08/2016-Standards-with-citations.pdf

Council for Accreditation of Counseling and Related Educational Programs. (2017). *CACREP/CORE merger: July 2017 announcement*. Retrieved from https://www.cacrep.org/news-and-events/cacrepcore-updates/

Crenshaw, D. A. (1995). *Bereavement: Counseling the grieving throughout the life cycle*. New York, NY: Continuum Press.

Currier, J. M., Irish, J. E. F., Neimeyer, R. A., & Foster, J. D. (2015). Attachment, continuing bonds, and complicated grief following a violent loss: Testing a moderated model. *Death Studies*, *39*(1), 201–210. doi:10.1080/07481187.2014.975869 PMID:25551174

Currier, J. M., Neimeyer, R. A., & Berman, J. S. (2008). The effectiveness of psychotherapeutic interventions for the bereaved: A comprehensive quantitative review. *Psychological Bulletin*, *134*(5), 648–661. doi:10.1037/0033-2909.134.5.648 PMID:18729566

Davis, E., & Pereira, J. (2014). Child-centered play therapy: A creative approach to culturally competent counseling. *Journal of Creativity in Mental Health*, *9*(2), 262–274. doi:10.1080/15401383.2014.892863

Davis, N. (1996). *Once upon a time: Therapeutic stories that teach and heal*. Royal Oak, MI: Self-Esteem Shop.

De Domenico, G. (2000). *An experiential Sandtray-Worldplay home study course for individuals and groups (Module 1)*. Oakland, CA: Vision Quest Images.

De Domenico, G. (2000). *Sandtray-Worldplay: A comprehensive guide to the use of sandtray in psychotherapy and transformational settings*. Oakland, CA: Vision Quest Images.

Dean, J. K. (2009). *Quantifying social justice advocacy competency: Development of the social justice advocacy scale* (Doctoral dissertation). Retrieved from http://digitalarchive.gsu.edu/cps_diss/40

Deaver, S. P., & Shiflett, C. (2011). Art-based supervision techniques. *The Clinical Supervisor*, *30*(2), 257–276. doi:10.1080/07325223.2011.619456

DeKruyf, L., Auger, R., & Trice-Black, S. (2013). The role of school counselors in meeting students' mental health needs: Examining issues of professional identity. *Professional School Counseling*, *16*(5), 271–282. doi:10.1177/2156759X0001600502

Department of Justice. (2010). *2010 ADA standards for accessible design*. Retrieved from https://www.ada.gov/regs2010/2010ADAStandards/2010ADAStandards.pdf

DiClemente, C. C., Prochaska, J. O., & Gilbertini, M. (1985). Self-efficacy and the stages of self-change of smoking. *Cognitive Therapy and Research*, *9*(2), 181–200. doi:10.1007/BF01204849

Dixon, A. L., Tucker, C., & Clark, M. A. (2010). Integrating Social Justice Advocacy with National Standards of Practice: Implications for School Counselor Education. *Counselor Education and Supervision, 50*(2), 103–115. Retrieved from https://login.ezproxy.net.ucf.edu/login?auth=shibb&url=https://search-ebscohost- com.ezproxy.net.ucf.edu/login.aspx?direct=true&AuthType=ip,cookie,shib,sso,uid&db=e ric&AN=EJ911810&site=eds-live&scope=site

Dollarhide, C. T., Smith, A. T., & Lemberger, M. E. (2007). Critical incidents in the development of supportive principals: Facilitating school counselor-principal relationships. *Professional School Counseling, 10*(4).

Doll, B., & Doll, C. (1997). *Bibliotherapy with young people: Librarians and mental heath Professionals working together*. Englewood, CA: Libraries Unlimited, Inc.

Donald, E. J., Culbreth, J. R., & Carter, A. W. (2015). Play therapy supervision: A review of the literature. *International Journal of Play Therapy, 24*(2), 59–77. doi:10.1037/a0039104

Dopp, A. R., & Cain, A. C. (2012). The role of peer relationships in parental bereavement during childhood and adolescence. *Death Studies, 36*(2), 41–60. doi:10.1080/07481187.2011.573175 PMID:24567994

Dowdney, L. (2000). Annotation: Childhood bereavement following parental death. *Journal of Child Psychology and Psychiatry, and Allied Disciplines, 4*(7), 819–830. doi:10.1111/1469-7610.00670 PMID:11079425

Drewes, A. A. (2005). Appendix: Multicultural play therapy resources. In E. Gil & A. A. Drewes (Eds.), *Cultural issues in play therapy* (pp. 72–95). New York, NY: Guilford Press.

Drewes, A. A. (2008). Culturally competent supervision of child and play therapists. In A. A. Drewes & J. A. Mullen (Eds.), *Supervision can be playful: Techniques for child and play therapist supervisors* (pp. 77–92). Lanham, MD: Jason Aronson.

Drewes, A. A., & Mullen, J. A. (2008). *Supervision can be playful: Techniques for child and play therapist supervisors*. Lanham, MD: Jason Aronson, Inc.

Duncan, B. L., Miller, S. D., Sparks, J., Claud, D., Reynolds, L., Brown, J., & Johnson, L. (2003). The Session Rating Scale: Preliminary psychometric properties of a "working" alliance measure. *Journal of Brief Therapy, 3*, 3–12.

Edgar-Bailey, M., & Kress, V. E. (2010). Resolving child and adolescent traumatic grief: Creative techniques and interventions. *Journal of Creativity in Mental Health, 5*(2), 158–176. doi:10.1080/15401383.2010.485090

Elliott, V. S. (2016). Ethical challenges and considerations in the treatment of children. *Modern Psychoanalysis, 41*(2), 93–112. Retrieved from http://dewey.umhb.edu:2048/login?url=http://search.ebscohost.com/login.aspx?direct=true&db=pbh&AN=131626916&site=eds-live

Ellis, M. V. (2010). Bridging the science and practice of clinical supervision: Some discoveries, some misconceptions. *The Clinical Supervisor, 29*(1), 95–116. doi:10.1080/07325221003741910

Fall, M., Drew, D., Chute, A., & Moore, A. (2007). The voices of registered play therapists as supervisors. *International Journal of Play Therapy*, *16*(2), 133–146. doi:10.1037/1555-6824.16.2.133

Feen-Calligan, H., McIntyre, B., & Sands-Goldstein, M. (2009). Art therapy applications of dolls in grief recovery, identity, and community service. *Art Therapy: Journal of the American Art Therapy Association*, *26*(4), 167–173. doi:10.1080/07421656.2009.10129613

Felitti, V., Anda, R., Nordenberg, D., Williamson, D., Spitz, A., Edwards, V., & Marks, J. (1998). Relationship of childhood abuse and household dysfunction to many of the leading causes of death in adults: The adverse childhood experiences (ACE) study. *American Journal of Preventive Medicine*, *14*(4), 245–258. doi:10.1016/S0749-3797(98)00017-8 PMID:9635069

Field, N. P., & Filanosky, C. (2010). Continued bonds, risk factors for complicated grief, and adjustment to bereavement. *Death Studies*, *34*(1), 1–29. doi:10.1080/07481180903372269 PMID:24479173

Figures at a Glance. (2018, June 19). Retrieved from http://www.unhcr.org/figures-at-a glance.htm

Findling, J. H., Bratton, S. C., & Henson, R. K. (2006). Development of the Trauma Play Scale: An observation-based assessment of the impact of trauma on the play therapy behaviors of young children. *International Journal of Play Therapy*, *15*(1), 7–36. doi:10.1037/h0088906

Fontes, C., Coral, T., & Toso, L. (2015). The therapeutic toy in a pediatric critical care environment: Integrative Review. *Journal of Nursing*, *9*(8), 8899–8907.

Gallant, J., & Thyer, B. (1989). The "Bug-in-the-ear" in clinical Supervision. *The Clinical Supervisor*, *7*(2-3), 43–58. doi:10.1300/J001v07n02_04

Garcia, F. (2012). Healing good-byes and healthy hellos: Learning and growing from painful endings and transitions. *Transactional Analysis Journal*, *42*(1), 53–61. doi:10.1177/036215371204200107

Gardner, R. (1973). *The Talking, Feeling, and Doing Game*. Cresskill, NJ: Creative Therapeutics.

Gardner, R. A. (2001). The talking, feeling, and doing game. In C. E. Schaefer & S. E. Reid (Eds.), *Gameplay: Therapeutic use of childhood games* (2nd ed.; pp. 78–105). New York: Wiley.

Gaskill, R. L., & Perry, B. D. (2017). The neurobiological power of play: Using the neurosequential model of therapeutics to guide play in the healing process. In C. A. Malchiodi & D. A. Crenshaw (Eds.), *Creative arts and play therapy for attachment problems* (pp. 178–196). New York, NY: Guilford Press.

Gass, M. A., Gillis, H. L., & Russel, K. C. (2018). *Adventure therapy: Theory, research, and practice*. New York, NY: Routledge.

Gibbs, K. A., & Green, E. J. (2008). Sanding in supervision. In A. A. Drewes & J. A. Mullen (Eds.), *Supervision can be playful: Techniques for child and play therapist supervisor* (pp. 27–38). Plymouth, UK: Jason Aronson.

Gilchrist, L., & Stringer, M. (1992). Marketing counseling: Guidelines for training and practice. *Counselor Education and Supervision, 31,* 154-162.

Gil, E. (2005). From sensitivity to competence in working across cultures. In E. Gil & A. A. Drewes (Eds.), *Cultural issues in play therapy* (pp. 3–25). New York, NY: Guilford Press.

Gil, E. (2006). *Helping abused and traumatized children.* New York: Guilford Press.

Gil, E. (2015). *Play in family therapy* (2nd ed.). New York: The Guilford Press.

Gil, E., & Crenshaw, D. (2015). *Termination challenges in child psychotherapy.* New York, NY: Guilford Press.

Gil, E., & Shaw, J. A. (2009). Prescriptive Play Therapy. In K. O'Conner & L. Braverman (Eds.), *Play therapy theory and practice: comparing theories and techniques* (2nd ed.; pp. 451–487). Hoboken, NJ: John Wiley & Sons, Incorporated.

Giordano, M. A. (2000). *Effectiveness of a child-centered self-reflective play therapy supervision model* (Doctoral dissertation). Retrieved from ProQuest dissertations & theses. (UMI Number 3064391)

Gladding, S. T. (2015). *Family therapy: History, theory, and practice* (6th ed.). Upper Saddle River, NJ: Pearson.

Glance, D., Fanning, G., Schoepke, A., Soto, W., & Williams, M. A. (2012). *Gatekeeping in counselor education.* Retrieved from http://www.counseling.org/resources/library/vistas/ vistas12/ Article_11.pdf

Glazer, H. R., & Stein, D. (2015). Mindfulness and the play-therapist supervisor: A study in transformative learning. *International Journal of Play Therapy, 24*(1), 41–53. doi:10.1037/ a0038663

Glosoff, H. L., & Durham, J. C. (2010). Using supervision to prepare social justice counseling advocates. *Counselor Education and Supervision, 50*(2), 116–129. doi:10.1002/j.1556-6978.2010. tb00113.x

Goodyear, R. K. (2014). Supervision as pedagogy: Attending to its essential instructional and learning processes. *The Clinical Supervisor, 33*(1), 82–99. doi:10.1080/07325223.2014.918914

Graham, C. (2018). Developing the dream: Play in private practice. *Play Therapy, 13*(3), 24–27.

Grainge, A. S., Bulmer, C., Fleming, M., & Allan, R. (2013). Using live supervision to deliver family intervention training. *Mental Health Practice, 16*(9), 12–18. doi:10.7748/mhp2013.06.16.9.12.e828

Graves-Alcorn, S. L., & Green, E. J. (2014). The Expressive Arts Therapy Continuum: History and Theory. In E. J. Green & A. A. Drewes (Eds.), *Integrating expressive arts and play therapy with children and adolescents* (pp. 1–16). Hoboken, NJ: John Wiley & Sons, Incorporated.

Green, E. J., & Connolly, M. E. (2009). Jungian family sandplay with bereaved children: Implications for play therapists. *International Journal of Play Therapy, 18*(2), 84–98. doi:10.1037/a0014435

Green, E. J., & Myrick, A. C. (2014). Treating complex trauma in adolescents: A phase-based, integrative approach for play therapists. *International Journal of Play Therapy*, *23*(3), 131–145. doi:10.1037/a0036679

Guerney, B. G. Jr, Guerney, L., & Andronico, M. (1966, March). Filial therapy. *Yale Scientific Magazine*, *40*(6), 14, 20.

Guerney, L. (1978). Training and evaluation of students as consultants in an adult-child relationship enhancement program. *Professional Psychology*, *9*, 193–198.

Haen, C. (2015). Vanquishing monsters: Group drama therapy for treating trauma. In C. Malchiodi (Ed.), *Creative interventions traumatized children* (pp. 235–257). New York, NY: Guilford Press.

Haidt, J., Koller, S. H., & Dias, M. G. (1993). Affect, culture, and morality, or is it wrong to eat your dog? *Journal of Personality and Social Psychology*, *65*(4), 613–628. doi:10.1037/0022-3514.65.4.613 PMID:8229648

Haine, R. A., Wolchik, S. A., Sandler, I., Millsap, R. E., & Ayers, T. S. (2006). Positive parenting as a protective resource for parentally bereaved children. *Death Studies*, *30*(1), 1–28. doi:10.1080/07481180500348639 PMID:16296557

Hanson, M. J. (2004). Ethnic, cultural, and language diversity in service settings. In E. E. Lynch & M. J. Hanson (Eds.), *Developing cross-cultural competence: A guide for working with with children and their families*. Baltimore, MD: Brookes Publishing Company.

Harris, Z. L., & Landreth, G. L. (1997). Filial therapy with incarcerated mothers: A five week model. *International Journal of Play Therapy*, *6*(2), 53–73. doi:10.1037/h0089408

Hartwig, E. K., & Bennett, M. M. (2017). Four approaches to using sandtray in play therapy supervision. *International Journal of Play Therapy*, *26*(4), 230–238. doi:10.1037/pla0000050

Hays, D. G., Dean, J. K., & Chang, C. Y. (2007). Addressing privilege and oppression in counselor training and practice: A qualitative analysis. *Journal of Counseling and Development*, *85*(3), 317–324. doi:10.1002/j.1556-6678.2007.tb00480.x

Helm, H. M., O'Halloran, M. S., & Kahlo, D. (2010). Funding training clinics. In A. K. Mobley & J. E. Myers (Eds.), *Developing and maintaining counselor education laboratories* (2nd ed.). Alexandria, VA: Association of Counselor Education and Supervision.

Heppner, P. P., Kivlighan, D. M., Burnett, J. W., Berry, T. R., Goedinghaus, M., Doxsee, D. J., …Wallace, D. L. (1994). Dimensions that characterize supervisor interventions delivered in the context of live supervision of practicum counselors. *Journal of Counseling Psychology, 41*(2), 227-235.

Herman, J. L. (2015). *Trauma and recovery: The aftermath of violence from domestic violence to political terror*. New York, NY: Basic Books. (Original work published 1997)

Hill, N. E., & Torres, K. (2010). Negotiating the American dream: The paradox of aspirations and achievement among Latino students and engagement between their families and schools. *The Journal of Social Issues*, *66*(1), 95–112. doi:10.1111/j.1540-4560.2009.01635.x

Hill, N. R., Harrawood, L. K., Vereen, L. G., & Doughty, E. A. (2012). Advocacy training: Curriculum for professional and client advocacy. In C. C. Chang, C. A. Barrio Minton, A. L. Dixon, J. E. Meyers, & T. J. Sweeney (Eds.), *Professional counseling excellence through leadership and advocacy* (pp. 267–289). New York, NY: Routledge.

Hinman, C. (2003). Multicultural considerations in the delivery of play therapy services. International Journal of Play Therapy, 12, 107-122. doi:10.1037/h0088881

Hittner, J., & Fawcett, M. (2011, October 27). Developing a counselor education training clinic: The first year. In *Ideas and research you can use: VISTAS 2012*. Retrieved from: https://www.counseling.org/resources/library/vistas/vistas12/Article_22.pdf

Hittner, J., & Fawcett, M. (2012). *Developing a Counselor Education Training Clinic: The First Year.* Retrieved from https://www.counseling.org/knowledge-center/vistas/by-subject2/vistas-education-and-supervision/docs/default-source/vistas/vistas_2012_article_22

Hoge, M. A., Huey, L. Y., & O'Connell, M. J. (2004). Best practices in behavioral health workforce education and training. *Administration and Policy in Mental Health*, *32*(2), 91–106. doi:10.1023/B:APIH.0000042742.45076.66 PMID:15586846

Holland, J. (2001). *Understanding children's experiences of parental bereavement*. London, England: Jessica Kingsley Publishers.

Homeyer, L., & Sweeney, D. (2017). *Sandtray: A practical manual* (3rd ed.). New York, NY: Routledge.

Hopmeyer, E., & Werk, A. (1994). A comparative study of family bereavement groups. *Death Studies*, *18*(3), 243–256. doi:10.1080/07481189408252657 PMID:10135136

Huang, Ln. N. (1998). Southeast Asian refugee children and adolescents. In J. T. Gibbs & L. N. Huang (Eds.), Children of color: Psychological interventions with culturally diverse youth (pp. 264-304). San Francisco, CA: Josey-Bass Publishers.

Huang, L., Macbeth, G., Dodge, J., & Jacobstein, D. (2004). Transforming the workforce in children's mental health. *Administration and Policy in Mental Health*, *32*(2), 167–187. doi:10.1023/B:APIH.0000042745.64582.72 PMID:15586849

Hudak, D. (2000). The therapeutic use of ball play in psychotherapy with children. *International Journal of Play Therapy*, *9*(1), 1–10. doi:10.1037/h0089437

Hudspeth, E. F. (2015). An Introduction to Clinical Supervision in Play Therapy: Research, Practice, and Application. *International Journal of Play Therapy*, *24*(2), 55–58. doi:10.1037/pla0000011

Hunt, C., & Sharpe, L. (2008). Within-session supervision communication in the training of clinical psychologists. *Australian Psychologist*, *43*(2), 121–126. doi:10.1080/00050060801933402

Hunt, Q. A., & Hertlein, K. M. (2015). Conceptualizing suicide bereavement through an attachment lens. *The American Journal of Family Therapy*, *41*(1), 16–27. doi:10.1080/01926187.2014.975651

Iqbal, A. (2015). The ethical considerations of counselling psychologists working with trauma: Is there a risk of vicarious traumatisation? *Counselling Psychology Review*, *30*(1), 44–51. Retrieved from https://www.researchgate.net/publication/284154295_The_ethical_considerations_of_counselling_psychologists_working_with_trauma_Is_there_a_risk_of_vicarious_traumatisation

Irvin, E. C. (1993). Using puppets in assessment. In C. E. Schaefer & D. M. Cangelosi (Eds.), *Play therapy techniques* (pp. 69–81). Northvale, NJ: Jason Aaronson.

Jakob, M., Weck, F., & Bohus, M. (2013). Live supervision: From the one-way mirror to video-based online supervision. *Verhaltenstherapie*, *23*, 170–180. doi:10.1159/000354234

Jandorf, L., Gutierrez, Y., Lopez, J., Christie, J., & Itzkowitz, S. H. (2005). Use of a patient navigator to increase colorectal cancer screening in an urban neighborhood health clinic. *Journal of Urban Health*, *82*(2), 216–224. doi:10.1093/jurban/jti046 PMID:15888638

Jones, L., & Rubin, L. (2005). PT 101: Teaching introduction to play therapy at the graduate level. *International Journal of Play Therapy*, *6*, 1–20. doi:10.1037/h0088899

Judi's House/JAG Institute for Grieving Children and Families. (2018). *Understanding childhood grief in the U.S.* Retrieved from https://www.judishouse.org/cbem/

Kagan, S., & Lusebrink, V. (1978). The expressive therapies continuum. *Art Psychotherapy*, *5*(4), 171–180. doi:10.1016/0090-9092(78)90031-5

Kalff, D. M. (2004). *Sandplay: A psychotherapeutic approach to the psyche*. Cloverdale, CA: Temenos Press.

Kao, S. C., & Landreth, G. L. (1997). Evaluating the impact of child-centered play therapy training. *International Journal of Play Therapy*, *6*(2), 1–20. doi:10.1037/h0089405

Kestly, T. A. (2016). Presence and play: Why mindfulness matters. *International Journal of Play Therapy*, *25*(1), 14–23. doi:10.1037/pla0000019

Kieling, C., Baker-Henningham, H., Belfer, M., Conti, G., Ertem, I., Omigbodun, O., & Rahman, A. (2011). Child and adolescent mental health worldwide: Evidence for action. *Lancet*, *378*(9801), 1515–1525. doi:10.1016/S0140-6736(11)60827-1 PMID:22008427

Killian, T., Cardona, B., & Hudspeth, E. F. (2017). Culturally responsive play therapy with Somali refugees. *International Journal of Play Therapy, 26*(1) 23-32. https://doi-org.ezproxy.net.ucf.edu/10.1037/pla0000040

Kimberlin, C. L., & Winterstein, A. G. (2008). Validity and reliability of measurement instruments used in research. *American Journal of Health-System Pharmacy*, *65*(23), 2276–2284. doi:10.2146/ajhp070364 PMID:19020196

King, J., Prout, B., Stuhl, A., & Nelson, R. (2016). Scrapbooking as an intervention to enhance coping in individuals experiencing grief and loss. *Therapeutic Recreation Journal*, *50*(2), 181–185. doi:10.18666/TRJ-2016-V50-I2-7308

Klein, M. (1955). The psychoanalytic play technique. *The American Journal of Orthopsychiatry*, *25*(2), 223–237. doi:10.1111/j.1939-0025.1955.tb00131.x PMID:14376493

Klitzke, M. J., & Lombardo, T. W. (1991). A "bug-in-the-eye" is better than a "bug-in-the-ear": A teleprompter technique for on-line therapy skills training. *Behavior Modification*, *15*(1), 113–117. doi:10.1177/01454455910151007 PMID:2003846

Knell, S. (1998). Cognitive-behavioral play therapy. *Journal of Clinical Child Psychology*, *27*(1), 28–33. doi:10.120715374424jccp2701_3 PMID:9561934

Knell, S. M. (1995). *Cognitive-behavioral play therapy*. Northvale, NJ: Jason Aronson Inc.

Knell, S. M. (1999). Cognitive behavioral play therapy. In S. W. Russ & T. Ollendick (Eds.), *Handbook of psychotherapies with children and families* (pp. 385–404). New York, NY: Plenum. doi:10.1007/978-1-4615-4755-6_20

Knell, S. M. (2009). Cognitive behavioral play therapy. In K. J. O'Connor & L. D. Braverman (Eds.), *Play therapy theory and practice: Comparing theories and techniques* (pp. 203–236). Hoboken, NJ: Wiley.

Knell, S. M. (2009). Cognitive-Behavioral Play Therapy. In K. O'Conner & L. Braverman (Eds.), *Play therapy theory and practice: comparing theories and techniques* (2nd ed.; pp. 203–236). Hoboken, NJ: John Wiley & Sons, Incorporated.

Knopf, D., Park, M. J., & Paul Mulye, T. (2008). *The mental health of adolescents: A national profile, 2008*. San Francisco, CA: University of California, National Adolescent Health Information Center.

Koltz, R. L., & Feit, S. S. (2012). A phenomenological study : The experience of live supervision during a pre-practicum counseling techniques course. *Qualitative Report*, *17*(80), 1–24.

Koltz, R. L., & Feit, S. S. (2012). A phenomenological study: The experience of live supervision during a pre-practicum counseling techniques course. *Qualitative Report*, *17*(80), 1–24.

Koppelman, J. (2004). *The provider system for children's mental health: Workforce capacity and effective treatment* (NHPF Issue Brief No. 801). Washington, DC: National Health Policy Forum.

Kottman, T. (2011). *Play Therapy: Basics and beyond* (2nd ed.). Alexandria, VA: American Counseling Association.

Kottman, T. (2011). *Play therapy: Basics and beyond.* Alexandria, VA: American Counseling Association.

Kottman, T., & Meany-Walen, K. (2015). *Partners in Play: An Adlerian approach to play therapy* (3rd ed.). Alexandria, VA: American Counseling Association. doi:10.1002/9781119272205

Kottman, T., & Meany-Walen, K. (2016). *Partners in play: An Adlerian approach to play therapy* (3rd ed.). Alexandria, VA: American Counseling Association.

Kottman, T., & Meany-Walen, K. K. (2018). *Doing play therapy: From building the relationship to facilitating change*. New York: The Guilford Press.

Kranz, P. L., Ramirez, S. Z., Flores-Torres, L., Steele, R., & Lund, N. L. (2005). Physical settings, materials, and related Spanish terminology recommended for play therapy with first-generation Mexican-American children. *Education, 126*(1), 93-99. Retrieved from https://login.ezproxy.net.ucf.edu/login?auth=shibb&url=https://search-ebscohost- com.ezproxy.net.ucf.edu/login.aspx?direct=true&AuthType=ip,cookie,shib,sso,uid&db=e ric&AN=EJ725160&site=eds-live&scope=site

Kranz, P. L., & Lund, N. L. (1994). Recommendations for supervising play therapists. *International Journal of Play Therapy, 3*(2), 45–52. doi:10.1037/h0089168

Kristensen, P., Weisaeth, L., & Heir, T. (2012). Bereavement and mental health after sudden and violent losses: A review. *Psychiatry, 75*(1), 76–97. doi:10.1521/psyc.2012.75.1.76 PMID:22397543

Kubler-Ross, E. (1969). *On death and dying*. New York, NY: MacMillan Press.

Landgarten, H. (1987). *Family art psychotherapy: A clinical guide and casebook*. New York, NY: Brunner/ Mazel Publishers.

Landis, L. L., & Young, M. E. (1994). The reflecting team in counselor education. *Counselor Education and Supervision, 33*(3), 210–218. doi:10.1002/j.1556-6978.1994.tb00287.x

Landreth, G. (2003). *Toys & materials for play therapy*. Denton, TX: Play Therapy Institute.

Landreth, G. (2012). *Play therapy: The art of the relationship* (3rd ed.). New York, NY: Routledge Taylor and Francis Group. doi:10.4324/9780203835159

Landreth, G., & Bratton, S. (2006). *Child parent relationship therapy (CPRT): A 10-session filial therapy model*. New York, NY: Routledge Taylor and Francis Group.

Lebby, K. (2018a, October). *Year in review*. CEO keynote presented at the Annual Association for Play Therapy International Conference, Phoenix, AZ.

Lebby, K. (2018b, December). From the CEO [Editorial]. *Play Therapy, 13*(4), 2.

LeBlanc, M., & Ritchie, M. (2001). A meta-analysis of play therapy outcomes. *Counselling Psychology Quarterly, 14*(2), 149–163. doi:10.1080/09515070110059142

Lee, A. C. (2009). Psychoanalytic Play Therapy. In K. O'Conner & L. Braverman (Eds.), *Play therapy theory and practice: comparing theories and techniques* (2nd ed.; pp. 25–81). Hoboken, NJ: John Wiley & Sons, Incorporated.

Lee, C. C. (2012). Social justice as the fifth force in counseling. In C. C. Chang, C. A. Barrio Minton, A. L. Dixon, J. E. Meyers, & T. J. Sweeney (Eds.), *Professional counseling excellence through leadership and advocacy* (pp. 109–120). New York, NY: Routledge.

Lee, R. E., & Everett, C. A. (2004). *The integrative family therapy supervisor: A primer*. New York, NY: Brunner-Routledge.

Lee, R. E., Nichols, D. P., Nichols, W. C., & Odom, T. (2004). Trends in family therapy supervision: The past 25 years and into the future. *Journal of Marital and Family Therapy*, *30*(1), 61–69. doi:10.1111/j.1752-0606.2004.tb01222.x PMID:14763209

Leick, N., & Davidsen-Nielsen, M. (1991). *Healing pain: Attachment, loss, and grief therapy*. New York, NY: Routledge.

Levinger, A. (1994). Co-play therapy. *International Journal of Play Therapy*, *3*(2), 53–62. doi:10.1037/h0089127

Levinson, E. M., Black, L., Rafoth, M. A., & Slonim, J. E. (2010). Community collaboration and university-based clinics in school counseling. In E. M. Levinson (Ed.), *Handbook of education, training, and supervision of school psychologists in school and community* (Vol. 2, pp. 291–305). New York, NY: Routledge.

Lin, D., & Bratton, S. (2015). A meta-analytic review of child-centered play therapy approaches. *Journal of Counseling and Development*, *93*(1), 45–58. doi:10.1002/j.1556-6676.2015.00180.x

Lowenfeld, M. (1939). The world pictures of children: A method of recording and studying them. *The British Journal of Medical Psychology*, *18*(1), 65–101. doi:10.1111/j.2044-8341.1939.tb00710.x

Lowenfeld, M. (1950). The nature and use of the Lowenfeld World Technique in work with children and adults. *The Journal of Psychology*, *30*(2), 325–331. doi:10.1080/00223980.1950.9916070

Lusebrink, V. (1992). A systems-oriented approach to the expressive therapies: The expressive therapies continuum. *The Arts in Psychotherapy*, *18*(5), 395–404. doi:10.1016/0197-4556(91)90051-B

Lusebrink, V. B. (1990). *Imagery and visual expression in therapy*. New York, NY: Plenum Press.B. doi:10.1007/978-1-4757-0444-0

Machiodi, C. A. (2015). Neurobiology, creative interventions, and childhood trauma. In C. Malchiodi (Ed.), *Creative interventions traumatized children* (pp. 3–23). New York, NY: Guilford Press.

Machuca, R., Johnson, T., & Moro, R. (2016). Tablet-based live supervision: Eye-Bug Supervision. VISTAS 2016 Summer Ed.

Machuca, R., Johnson, T., & Moro, R. R. (2015). Tablet-assisted live supervision: Eye-bug supervision. In *Ideas and research you can use: VISTAS 2016, Article 55*. Retrieved from https://www.counseling.org/docs/default-source/vistas/article_5547f227f16116603abcacff0000bee5e7.pdf?sfvrsn=4

MacKay, L. M. (2017). Differentiation of self: Enhancing therapist resilience when working with relational trauma. *Australian and New Zealand Journal of Family Therapy*, *38*(4), 637–656. doi:10.1002/anzf.1276

Malchiodi, C. A. (2011). *Handbook of Art Therapy* (2nd ed.). New York, NY: Guilford Press.

Malchiodi, C. A. (2014). *Creative interventions with traumatized children*. New York, NY: Guilford Press.

McGoldrick, M., Gerson, R., & Petry, S. (2008). *Genograms: Assessment and intervention* (3rd ed.). New York, NY: W. W. Norton.

McNeill, B. W., Stoltenberg, C. D., & Romans, J. C. S. (1992). The integrated developmental model of supervision: Scale development and validation procedures. *Professional Psychology, Research and Practice*, *23*(6), 504–508. doi:10.1037/0735-7028.23.6.504

Meany-Walen, K. K., Lindo, N. A., Turley, E., Chung, C., Akay, S., Cheng, Y. J., & Chen, S. Y. (2013). Evaluating the impact of intensive supervision of child-centered play therapy training. *British Journal of Play Therapy*, *9*, 16–25.

Meany-Walen, K., Cobie-Nuss, A., Eittreim, E., Teeling, S., Wilson, S., & Xander, C. (2018). Play therapists' perceptions of wellness and self-care practices. *International Journal of Play Therapy*, *27*(3), 176–186. doi:10.1037/pla0000067

Mellin, E. A., Hunt, B., & Lorenz, D. C. (2009). Rehabilitation counselor preparation for working with youth with psychiatric disabilities. *Rehabilitation Education*, *23*(1), 33–42. doi:10.1891/088970109805059191

Mellin, E. A., & Pertuit, T. L. (2009). Research priorities for mental health counseling with youth: Implications for counselor preparation, professional development, and research. *Counselor Education and Supervision*, *49*(2), 137–155. doi:10.1002/j.1556-6978.2009.tb00093.x

Mersky, J. P., Topitzes, J., & Reynolds, A. J. (2013). Impacts of adverse childhood experiences on health, mental health, and substance use in early adulthood: A cohort study of an urban, minority sample in the U.S. *Child Abuse & Neglect*, *37*(11), 917–925. doi:10.1016/j.chiabu.2013.07.011 PMID:23978575

Miller, S. D. (2018). *Performance Metrics-Licenses for the ORS & SRS*. Available: https://scott-d-miller-ph-d.myshopify.com/collections/performance-metrics/products/performance-metrics-licenses-for-the-ors-and-srs

Miller, K. L., Miller, S. M., & Evans, W. J. (2002). Computer-assisted live supervision in college counseling centers. *Journal of College Counseling*, *5*(2), 187–192. doi:10.1002/j.2161-1882.2002.tb00221.x

Miller, S. D., Duncan, B. L., Brown, J., Sparks, J., & Claud, D. (2003). The Outcome Rating Scale: A preliminary study of the reliability, validity, and feasibility of a brief visual analog measure. *Journal of Brief Therapy*, *2*, 91–100.

Mobley, A. K., & Myers, J. E. (2010). *Developing and Maintaining Counselor Education Laboratories* (2nd ed.). Retrieved from https://www.acesonline.net/resources/developing-and-maintaining-counselor-education-laboratories

Moncada, F. (1962). *Asi juegan los ninos: Recopilacion de juegos infantiles*. Mexicao, D. F., Mexico: Editorial Avante.

Moody, S., Kostohryz, K., & Vereen, L. (2014). Authentically engaged learning through live supervision: A phenomenological study. *Counselor Education and Supervision, 53*(1), 19–33. doi:10.1002/j.1556-6978.2014.00046.x

Moustakas, C. E. (1959). *Psychotherapy with children*. Harper and Row.

Moustakas, C. E. (1997). *Relationship play therapy*. Northvale, NJ: Jason Aronson Incorporated.

Mullen, J. A. (2016). Play therapy supervision. In K. J. O'Connor, C. H. Schaefer, & L. D. Braverman (Eds.), *Handbook of play therapy* (2nd ed.; pp. 549–560). Hoboken, NJ: John Wiley & Sons.

Mullen, J. A., Luke, M., & Drewes, A. A. (2007). Supervision can be playful, too: Play therapy techniques that enhance supervision. *International Journal of Play Therapy, 16*(1), 69–85. doi:10.1037/1555-6824.16.1.69

Munns, E. (2000). *Theraplay: Innovations in attachment-enhancing play therapy*. Northvale, NJ: Jason Aronson Incorporated.

Muro, J. H., Holliman, R. P., Blanco, P. J., & Stickley, V. K. (2015). Exploring play therapy training: An investigation on the impact of practice on attitudes, knowledge, and skills with master's level students. *International Journal of Play Therapy, 24*(4), 234–247. doi:10.1037/a0039811

Muro, J., Stickely, V., Muro, L., Blanco, P., & Tsai, M. (2015). Considerations for elementary schools and university collaborations: A guide to implementing counseling research. *The Journal of Research Administration, 46*(1), 102–117.

Murrell, E., Steel, Z., Gaston, J., & Proudfoot, H. (2002). Training the clinical psychologist: Profile of a university-based clinic. *Australian Psychologist, 37*(2), 123–128. doi:10.1080/00050060210001706766

National Association for Social Work. (2015). *Standards and indicators for cultural competence in social work practice*. NASW Press. Retrieved from https://www.socialworkers.org/ LinkClick.aspx?fileticket= 7dVckZAYUmk%3d&portalid=0

National Association of Social Workers. (2008). *Code of ethics of the national association of social workers*. Washington, DC: Author.

National Association of Social Workers. (2017). Retrieved August 3, 2018 from www.socialworks.org/About/ethics/Code-of-Ethics

National Board for Certified Counselors. (2016). Retrieved August 3, 2018 from http://www.nbcc.org/Assets/Ethics/NBCCCodeofEthics.pdf/

Neimeyer, R. A., Burke, L. A., Mackay, M. M., & van Dyke Stringer, J. G. (2010). Grief therapy and the reconstruction of meaning: From principles to practice. *Journal of Contemporary Psychotherapy*, *40*(2), 73–83. doi:10.100710879-009-9135-3

Nemiroff, M. A., & Annunziata, J. (1990). *A child's first book about play therapy*. Washington, DC: American Psychological Association.

Neukrug, E. S. (1991). Computer-assisted live supervision in counselor skills training. *Counselor Education and Supervision*, *31*(2), 132–138. doi:10.1002/j.1556-6978.1991.tb00151.x

O'Connor, K. (2005). Addressing diversity issues in play therapy. *Professional Psychology: Research and Practice, 36*(5), 566-573. https://doi-rg.ezproxy.net.ucf.edu/10.1037/0735-7028.36.5.566

O'Connor, K. (1994). Ecosystemic play therapy. In K. O'Connor & C. Schafer (Eds.), *Handbook of play therapy: Advances and innovations* (Vol. 2, pp. 61–84). New York: Wiley.

O'Connor, K. (2000). *The play therapy primer* (2nd ed.). New York, NY: Wiley.

O'Connor, K. (2005). Addressing diversity issues in play therapy. *Professional Psychology, Research and Practice*, *36*(5), 566–573. doi:10.1037/0735-7028.36.5.566

O'Connor, K. (2016). Ecosystemic play therapy. In K. J. O'Connor, C. E. Schaefer, & L. D. Braverman (Eds.), *Handbook of play therapy* (2nd ed.; pp. 195–225). Hoboken, NJ: Wiley.

O'Connor, K. J. (2009). Ecosystemic Play Therapy. In K. O'Conner & L. Braverman (Eds.), *Play therapy theory and practice: comparing theories and techniques* (2nd ed.; pp. 367–450). Hoboken, NJ: John Wiley & Sons, Incorporated.

O'Connor, K., & Braverman, L. (2009). *Play therapy theory and practice: Comparing theories and techniques* (2nd ed.). Hoboken, NJ: John Wiley and Sons, Incorporated.

O'Guinn, Semenik, & Close Scheinbaum. (2015). Advertising and integrated brand promotion. Boston, MA: Cengage.

Oaklander, V. (1988). *Windows to our children: A Gestalt approach to working with children and adolescents*. Gouldsboro, ME: The Gestalt Journal Press.

Oaklander, V. (2006). *Hidden treasures: A map to the child's inner self*. New York, NY: Routledge.

Odom, S. L., Pungello, E. P., & Gardner-Neblett, N. (Eds.). (2012). Translating contemporary developmental and health science: Designing an early childhood program for young children and their families living in poverty. In Infants, toddlers, and families living in poverty: Research implications for early child care (pp. 353–371). New York, NY: Guilford Press.

Office of Environmental Health Hazard Assessment (OEHHA). (2019). *Proposition 65 Warnings Website*. Retrieved from https://www.p65warnings.ca.gov/

Office of Human Research Protections. (2018). *45 CF 46*. Available: https://www.hhs.gov/ohrp/regulations-and-policy/regulations/45-cfr-46/index.html

Pallant, J. (2016). *SPSS Survival Manual*. London, UK: Open University Press.

Pardeck, J. T., & Pardeck, J. A. (1993). *Bibliotherapy: A clinical approach to helping children*. London: Gordon and Breach Science Publishers.

Parikh, S. B., Cebellow, P., & Post, P. (2013). Application: Theory to culturally competent practice: Factors related to play therapists' social justice advocacy attitudes. *Journal of Multicultural Counseling and Development*, *41*(4), 240–252. doi:10.1002/j.2161-1912.2013.00039.x

Patterson, L., Stutey, D. M., & Dorsey, B. (2018). Play therapy with African American children exposed to adverse childhood experiences. *International Journal of Play Therapy, 27*(4), 215-226. https://doi-org.ezproxy.net.ucf.edu/10.1037/pla0000080

Peabody, M. A. (2015). Building with purpose: Using LEGO SERIOUS PLAY in play therapy supervision. *International Journal of Play Therapy*, *24*(1), 30–40. doi:10.1037/a0038607

Perou, R., Bitsko, R. H., Blumberg, S. J., Pastor, P., Ghandour, R. M., Gfroerer, J. C., … Huang, L. N. (2013, May). Mental health surveillance among children-United States, 2005-2011. *MMWR Supplements, 17*(62), 1-35. Retrieved from: https://www.cdc.gov/mmwr/preview/mmwrhtml/su6202a1.htm?s_cid=su6202a1_w

Perryman, K. L., Moss, R. C., & Anderson, L. (2016). Sandtray supervision: An integrated model for play therapy supervision. *International Journal of Play Therapy*, *25*(4), 186–196. doi:10.1037/pla0040288

Perryman, K., & Doran, J. (2010). Guidelines for incorporating play therapy in the schools. In A. A. Drewes & C. E. Schaefer (Eds.), *School-based play therapy* (2nd ed.; pp. 61–86). Hoboken, NJ: John Wiley & Sons. doi:10.1002/9781118269701.ch3

Piaget, J., & Inhelder, B. (1969). *The psychology of the child* (2nd ed.). New York, NY: Basic Books.

Porges, S. W. (2011). *The Polyvagal Theory: Neurophysiological foundations of emotions, attachment, communication, and self-regulation*. New York, N.Y: W. W. Norton.

Post, P., & Tillman, L. S. (2015). Cultural issues in play therapy. In D. A. Crenshaw & A. L. Stewart (Eds.), *Play therapy: A comprehensive guide to theory and practice* (pp. 406–510). New York, NY: The Guilford Press.

President's New Freedom Commission on Mental Health. (2003). *Achieving the promise: Transforming mental health care in America* (DHHS Publication No. SMA-03-3832). Retrieved from https://govinfo.library.unt.edu/mentalhealthcommission/reports/FinalReport/downloads/FinalReport.pdf

Prigerson, H. G., Maciejewski, P., Reynolds, C. III, Bierhals, A., Newsom, J., Fasiczka, A., ... Miller, M. (1995). Inventory of complicated grief. *Psychiatry Research*, *59*(1-2), 65–79. doi:10.1016/0165-1781(95)02757-2 PMID:8771222

Prochaska, J. O., & DiClemente, C. C. (1982). Transtheoretical therapy: Toward a more integrative model of change. *Psychotherapy (Chicago, Ill.)*, *19*(3), 276–288. doi:10.1037/h0088437

Prochaska, J. O., & DiClemente, C. C. (1983). Stages and process of self-change of smoking: Toward and integrative model for change. *Journal of Consulting and Clinical Psychology*, *51*(3), 390–395. doi:10.1037/0022-006X.51.3.390 PMID:6863699

Prochaska, J. O., & DiClemente, C. C. (1992). Stages of change in the modification of problem behaviors. *Progress in Behavior Modification*, *28*, 184–218. PMID:1620663

Prochaska, J. O., Velicer, W. F., Rossi, J. S., Goldstein, M. G., Marcus, B. H., Rakowski, W., ... Rossi, S. R. (1994). Stages of change and decisional balance for 12 problem behaviors. *Health Psychology*, *13*(1), 39–46. doi:10.1037/0278-6133.13.1.39 PMID:8168470

Public Relations Society of America. (n.d.). *About public relations*. Retrieved from https:// www.prsa.org/all-about-pr/

Purswell, K. E., & Stulmaker, H. L. (2015). Expressive arts in supervision: Choosing developmentally appropriate interventions. *International Journal of Play Therapy*, *24*(2), 103–117. doi:10.1037/a0039134

Ramirez, O. (1998). Mexican American children and adolescents. In J. T. Gibbs & L. N. Huang (Eds.), *Children of color: Psychological interventions with culturally diverse youth* (pp. 215–239). San Francisco, CA: Josey-Bass Publishers.

Rashkin, R. (2005). *Feeling better: A kid's book about therapy*. Washington, DC: Imagination Press.

Ratts, M. J., Singh, A. A., Nassar-McMillan, S., Butler, S. K., & McCullough, J. R. (2015). *Multicultural and social justice counseling competencies*. Retrieved from https://www.counseling.org/docs/default-source/competencies/multicultural-and-social-justice-counseling-competencies.pdf?sfvrsn=8573422c_20

Ratts, M. J., Singh, A. A., Nassar-McMillan, S., Butler, S. K., & McCullough, J. R. (2016). Multicultural and social justice counseling competencies: Guidelines for the counseling profession. *Journal of Multicultural Counseling and Development*, *44*(1), 28–48. doi:10.1002/jmcd.12035

Ray, D. C., & McCullough, R. (2016). *Evidence-based practice statement: Play therapy* [Research report]. Retrieved from http://www.a4pt.org/?page=EvidenceBased

Ray, D. (2004). Supervision of basic and advanced skills in play therapy. *Journal of Professional Counseling, Practice, Theory, & Research*, *32*(2), 28–41. doi:10.1080/15566382.2004.12033805

Ray, D. (2011). *Advanced play therapy: essential conditions, knowledge, and skills for child practice*. New York: Routledge Taylor and Francis Group. doi:10.4324/9780203837269

Ray, D. (2012). *Advanced play therapy: Essential conditions, knowledge, and skills for child practice*. New York, NY: Routledge.

Ray, D. C. (2010). Challenges and barriers to implementing play therapy in schools. In A. A. Drewes & C. E. Schaefer (Eds.), *School-based play therapy* (2nd ed.; pp. 87–106). Hoboken, NJ: John Wiley & Sons. doi:10.1002/9781118269701.ch4

Ray, D. C. (2018, March). The evidence-based determination: A moving target. *Play Therapy, 13*(1), 21.

Ray, D. C. (Ed.). (2016). *A therapist's guide to child development: The extraordinary normal years*. New York, NY: Routledge.

Ray, D. C., Minton, C. A. B., Schottelkorb, A. A., & Brown, A. G. (2010). Single-case design in child counseling research: Implications for counselor education. *Counselor Education and Supervision, 49*(3), 193–208. doi:10.1002/j.1556-6978.2010.tb00098.x

Ray, D. C., Purswell, K., Haas, S., & Aldrete, C. (2017). Child-centered play therapy-research integrity checklist: Development, reliability, and use. *International Journal of Play Therapy, 26*(4), 207–217. doi:10.1037/pla0000046

Ray, D. C., & Schottelkorb, A. A. (2010). Single-case design: A primer for play therapists. *International Journal of Play Therapy, 19*(1), 39–53. doi:10.1037/a0017725

Ray, D., Armstrong, S., Balkin, R., & Jayne, K. (2015). Child centered play therapy in the schools: Review and meta-analysis. *Psychology in the Schools, 52*(2), 107–123. doi:10.1002/pits.21798

Ray, D., Lee, K., Meany-Walen, K., Carlson, S., Carnes-holt, K., & Ware, J. (2013). Use of toys in child-centered play therapy. *International Journal of Play Therapy, 22*(1), 43–57. doi:10.1037/a0031430

Reddy, L. A., Files-Hall, T. M., & Schaefer, C. E. (2005). Announcing empirically based play interventions for children. In L. A. Reddy, T. M. Files-Hall, & C. E. Schaefer (Eds.), *Empirically-based Play Interventions for Children* (pp. 3–10). Washington, DC: American Psychological Association. doi:10.1037/11086-001

Reichelt, S., & Skjerve, J. (2002). Correspondence between supervisors and trainees in their perception of supervision events. *Journal of Clinical Psychology, 57*(7), 759–772. doi:10.1002/jclp.2003 PMID:12205716

Ronnestad, M. H., & Skovholt, T. M. (2013). *The developing practitioner: Growth and stagnation of therapists and counselors*. New York, NY: Routledge.

Rozman, A. L. (2015). Art therapy with children in grief and loss groups. In C. Malchiodi (Ed.), *The Handbook of Art Therapy* (2nd ed.; pp. 422–432). New York, NY: Guilford Press.

Rubin, J. (1999). *Art therapy: An introduction*. Philadelphia, PA: Brunner/Mazel.

Rubin, J. (2010). *Introduction to art therapy: Sources and resources*. New York: Routledge.

Ruff, W. G., & Shoho, A. R. (2005). Understanding instructional leadership through the mental models of three elementary school principals. *Educational Administration Quarterly, 41*(3), 554–577. doi:10.1177/0013161X04269621

Russ, B. R. (2016). *Counselor preparation and adolescent youth: A study of clinical mental health counselors* (Doctoral dissertation). Western Michigan University. Retrieved from http://scholarworks.wmich.edu/dissertations/2463

Sacks, V., & Murphey, D. (2018, February). *The prevalence of adverse childhood experiences, nationally, by state, and by race/ethnicity* (Research Brief #2018-03). Retrieved from https://www.childtrends.org/wp-content/uploads/2018/02/ACESBrief_ChildTrends_February2018.pdf

Sanok, J. (2018, January 17). *How to attract your ideal client* [Webinar]. Retrieved from: https://24b71c9a-dc9b-4e8e-b130-25cb723ebb1c.webinarninja.com/webinars/16578

Saraceno, B., van Ommeren, M., Batniji, R., Cohen, A., Gureje, O., Mahoney, J., & Underhill, C. (2007). Barriers to improvement of mental health services in low-income and middle-income countries. *Lancet*, *370*(9593), 1164–1174. doi:10.1016/S0140-6736(07)61263-X PMID:17804061

Saxena, S., Thornicroft, G., Knapp, M., & Whiteford, H. (2007). Resources for mental health: Scarcity, inequity, and inefficiency. *Lancet*, *370*(9590), 878–889. doi:10.1016/S0140-6736(07)61239-2 PMID:17804062

Sayed, M. A. (2003). Psychotherapy of Arab patients in the West: Uniqueness, empathy, and “otherness.” *American Journal of Psychotherapy, 57*(4), 445–459. Retrieved from https://login.ezproxy.net.ucf.edu/login?auth=shibb&url=https://search-ebscohost- com.ezproxy.net.ucf.edu/login.aspx?direct=true&AuthType=ip,cookie,shib,sso,uid&db=l sdbip&AN=PREV200400136507&site=eds-live&scope=site

Schaefer, C. & Peabody, M. A. (2016, June). Glossary of play therapy terms. *Play Therapy*, 20-24.

Schaefer, C. (2001). Prescriptive play therapy. *International Journal of Play Therapy*, *10*(2), 57–73. doi:10.1037/h0089480

Schaefer, C. E., & Drewes, A. A. (Eds.). (2014). *The therapeutic powers of play: 20 core agents of change* (2nd ed.). Hoboken, NJ: Wiley.

Scherl, C., & Haley, J. (2000). Computer monitor supervision: A clinical note. *The American Journal of Family Therapy*, *28*(3), 275–282. doi:10.1080/01926180050081702

Schottelkorb, A. A., Doumas, D. M., & Garcia, R. (2012). Treatment for childhood refugee trauma: A randomized, controlled trial. *International Journal of Play Therapy*, *21*(2), 57–73. doi:10.1037/a0027430

Shapiro, L. (1993). *The book of psychotherapeutic games: A review of the most popular games use din psychotherapy.* The Center for Applied Psychology Incorporated.

Siddaway, A. P., Wood, A. M., Schulz, J., & Trickey, D. (2015). Evaluation of the CHUMS child bereavement group: A pilot study examining statistical and clinical change. *Death Studies*, *1*(39), 99–110. doi:10.1080/07481187.2014.913085 PMID:25153045

Smith-Adcock, S., Davis, E., Pereira, J., Allen, C., Socarras, K., Bodurtha, K., & Smith-Bonahue, T. (2012). Preparing to play: A qualitative study of graduate students' reflections on learning play therapy in an elementary school. *International Journal of Play Therapy*, *21*(2), 100–115. doi:10.1037/a0026931

Smith-Adcock, S., Shin, S. M., & Pereira, J. (2015). Critical incidents in learning child-centered play therapy: Implications for teaching and supervision. *International Journal of Play Therapy*, *2*(2), 78–91. doi:10.1037/a0039122

Smith, N., & Landreth, G. (2003). Intensive filial therapy with child witnesses of domestic violence: A comparison with individual and sibling group play therapy. *International Journal of Play Therapy*, *12*(1), 67–88. doi:10.1037/h0088872

Solomon, J., & George, C. (1999). *Attachment disorganization*. New York: Guilford.

Sories, F., Maier, C., Beer, A., & Thomas, V. (2015). Addressing the needs of military children through family-based play therapy. *Contemporary Family Therapy*, *37*(3), 209–200. doi:10.100710591-015-9342-x

Spruill, D. A., & Benshoff, J. M. (2000). Helping beginning counselors develop a personal theory of counseling. *Counselor Education and Supervision*, *40*(1), 70–80. doi:10.1002/j.1556-6978.2000.tb01800.x

Stadler, H. (1988). Marketing counseling: Caveat emptor. *Counselor Education and Supervision*, *27*(4), 320–322. doi:10.1002/j.1556-6978.1988.tb00774.x

Stanley, J. (1999). *Reading to heal: How to use bibliotherapy to improve your life*. Boston, MA: Element Books, Inc.

Stauffer, S. (2008). Trauma and disorganized attachment in refugee children: Integrating theories and exploring treatment options. *Refugee Survey Quarterly, 27,* 150-163. https://doi- org.ezproxy.net.ucf.edu/10.1093/rsq/hdn057

Steele, J. M., Bischof, G. H., & Craig, S. E. (2014). Political ideology and perceptions of social justice advocacy among members of the American Counseling Association. *International Journal for the Advancement of Counseling*, *36*(4), 450–467. doi:10.100710447-014-9217-0

Steele, W., & Malchiodi, C. A. (2011). *Trauma-informed practices with children and adolescents*. New York, NY: Routledge.

Steele, W., & Malchiodi, C. A. (2012). *Trauma-informed practiced with children and adolescents*. New York, NY: Routledge. doi:10.4324/9780203829493

Stewart, A., & MacIntyre, G. (2013, April). Advocacy: Models and effectiveness. *Insights, 20.* Retrieved from https://www.iriss.org.uk/sites/default/files/iriss-insight-20.pdf

Stoltenberg, C. D. (1981). Approaching supervision from a developmental perspective: The counselor complexity model. *Journal of Counseling Psychology*, *28*(1), 59–65. doi:10.1037/0022-0167.28.1.59

Stoltenberg, C. D. (1997). The integrated developmental model of supervision. *Psychotherapy in Private Practice*, *16*(2), 59–69. doi:10.1300/J294v16n02_07

Stulmaker, H. L., Lertora, I., & Garza, Y. (2015). Facilitating empathic perspective taking in beginning child-centered play therapists: The role of supervision. *International Journal of Play Therapy*, *24*(4), 177–189. doi:10.1037/a0039330

Stutey, D. M., Helm, H. M., LoSasso, H., & Kreider, H. D. (2015). Play therapy and photo-elicitation: A narrative examination of children's grief. *International Journal of Play Therapy*, *25*(3), 154–165. doi:10.1037/a0039956

Substance Abuse and Mental Health Services Administration. (2014). *SAMHSA's concept of trauma and guidance for a trauma-informed approach* (HHS Publication No. SMA 14-4884). Retrieved from https://store.samhsa.gov/system/files/sma14-4884.pdf

Sue, D. W., Arredondo, P., & McDavis, R. J. (1992). Multicultural counseling competencies and standards: A call to the profession. *Journal of Counseling and Development*, *70*(4), 477–486. doi:10.1002/j.1556-6676.1992.tb01642.x

Sue, D., & Sue, D. (2003). *Counseling the culturally diverse: Theory and practice* (4th ed.). New York, NY: Wiley.

Swank, J. M. (2018). Peer feedback within a play therapy course: A qualitative exploration. *International Journal of Play Therapy*, *27*(1), 25–34. doi:10.1037/pla0000060

Sweeney, D., Baggerly, J., & Ray, D. (2014). Group play therapy: A dynamic approach. New York: Routledge: Taylor & Francis Group. doi:10.4324/9780203103944

Tanner, Z., & Mathis, R. D. (1995). A child-centered typology for training novice play therapists. *International Journal of Play Therapy*, *4*(2), 1–13. doi:10.1037/h0089316

Teufel, L. A. (2007). *Clinical supervision of child and adolescent counselors in residential foster care: A collective case study*. Graduate Thesis and Dissertations. Retrieved from Scholar Commons. http://scholarcommons.usf.edu/etd/2383

Thanasiu, P. L., Rust, K. L., & Walter, S. M. (2018). Service learning and live supervision as early components in play therapy training. *International Journal of Play Therapy*, *27*(2), 103–113. doi:10.1037/pla0000069

Thomas, D. A. (2015). Intentionality in supervision: Supervising play therapy interns and practitioners. In *Ideas and research you can use*: *VISTAS Online, Article 38*. Retrieved from: https://www.counseling.org/docs/default-source/vistas/article_387a5c21f16116603abcacff0000bee5e7.pdf?sfvrsn=6

Thomas, J. T. (2010). *The ethics of supervision and consultation: Practical guidance for mental health professionals*. Washington, DC: American Psychological Association. doi:10.1037/12078-000

Tolan, P. H., & Dodge, K. A. (2005). Children's mental health as a primary care and concern: A system for comprehensive support and service. *The American Psychologist*, *60*(6), 601–614. doi:10.1037/0003-066X.60.6.601 PMID:16173893

Tonkins, S. A., & Lambert, M. J. (1996). A treatment outcome study of bereavement groups for children. *Child & Adolescent Social Work Journal*, *1*(13), 3–21. doi:10.1007/BF01876592

Torres-Harding, S. R., Siers, B., & Olson, B. D. (2012). Development and psychometric evaluation of the social justice scale (SJS). *American Journal of Community Psychology*, *50*(1-2), 77–88. doi:10.100710464-011-9478-2 PMID:22080396

Toscani, F. (1998). Sandrama: Psychodramatic sandtray with a trauma survivor. *The Arts in Psychotherapy*, *25*(1), 21–29. doi:10.1016/S0197-4556(97)00058-0

Trice-Black, S., Riechel, M. E. K., & Shillingford, M. (2013). School Counselors' Constructions of Student Confidentiality. *Journal of School Counseling*, *11*(12), n12.

Trusty, J., & Brown, D. (2005). Advocacy competencies for professional school counselors. *Professional School Counseling*, *8*(3), 259–265.

Tsai, M.-H., & Ray, D. (2011). Play therapy outcome prediction: An exploratory study at a university-based clinic. *International Journal of Play Therapy*, *20*(2), 94–108. doi:10.1037/a0023441

Turner, S. R. (2017). *Play therapy for traumatic loss: Recovery from suicide and homicide.* Presented at the annual Texas Association for Play Therapy Conference, Austin, TX.

U.S. Department of Health and Human Services. (2002). *Trends in the well-being of America's children and youth. Section 1. Population, family, and neighborhood.* Retrieved from https://aspe.hhs.gov/report/trends-well-being-americas-children-and-youth-2002

U.S. Public Health Service. (2000). *Report of the surgeon general's conference on children's mental health: A national action agenda.* Washington, DC: Department of Health and Human Services.

United Nations. (1989). Convention on the Rights of the Child. *Treaty Series*, *1577*, 3.

United States Access Board. (1990). *Chapter 4: Entrances, Doors, and Gates.* Retrieved from https://www.access-board.gov/guidelines-and-standards/buildings-and-sites/about-the- ada-standards/guide-to-the-ada-standards/chapter-4-entrances,-doors,-and-gates

United States Census Bureau. (2010). *Poverty: 2008 and 2009-American survey briefs.* Retrieved from www.census.gov/prod/2010pubs/acsbr09-1.pdf

United States Department of Health and Human Services. (2019). *HIPAA for professionals.* Retrieved from https://www.hhs.gov/hipaa/for-professionals/index.html

United States Department of Labor. (2019). *Occupational Safety and Health Administration: Universal Precautions.* Retrieved from: https://www.osha.gov/SLTC/etools/ hospital/ hazards/univprec/univ.html

Van der Kolk, B. A. (2015). *The body keeps the score: Brain, body, and mind in the healing of trauma*. New York, NY: Penguin Books.

Van Velsor, P., & Orozco, G. L. (2007). Involving low-income parents in the schools: Community centric strategies for school counselors. *Professional School Counseling, 11*(1).

VanderGast, T. S., Culbreth, J. R., & Flowers, C. (2010). An exploration of experiences and preferences in clinical supervision with play therapists. *International Journal of Play Therapy, 19*(3), 174–185. doi:10.1037/a0018882

VanderGast, T. S., & Hinkle, M. S. (2015). So happy together? Predictors of satisfaction with supervision for play therapist supervisees. *International Journal of Play Therapy, 24*(2), 92–102. doi:10.1037/a0039105

VanderGast, T. S., Post, P. B., & Kascsak-Miller, T. (2010). Graduate training in child-parent relationship therapy with a multicultural immersion experience: Giving away the skills. *International Journal of Play Therapy, 19*(4), 198–208. doi:10.1037/a0021010

VanFleet, R. (2014). Selection of toys. In *Filial therapy: Strengthening parent- child relationships through play* (3rd ed.; pp. 23–25). Sarasota, FL: Professional Resource Press.

VanFleet, R., Sywulak, A. E., & Sniscak, C. C. (2010). *Child-centered play therapy*. New York, NY: Guilford Press.

Vargas, L. A., & Koss-Chioino, J. D. (1992). *Working with culture: Psychotherapeutic interventions with ethnic minority children and adolescents*. San Francisco, CA: Jossey- Bass, Inc.

Vaughn, K., Stigger, B., & Dugan, E. (2017). A resource to efficient case conceptualization. *Play Therapy, 12*(2), 24–28.

Vernon, A. (2009). *Counseling children and adolescents* (4th ed.). Denver, CO: Love Publishing.

Verschueren, K., & Koomen, H. M. Y. (2012). Teacher-child relationships from an attachment perspective. *Attachment and Human Development, 14*(3), 205–211. doi:10.1080/14616734.2012.672260 PMID:22537520

Vygotsky, L. S. (2016). Play and its role in the mental development of the child (N. Veresov & M. Barr, Trans.). *International Research in Early Childhood Education, 7*(2), 3-25.

Vygotsky, L. S. (1978). Interaction between learning and development. In M. Cole, V. John-Steiner, S. Scribner, & E. Souberman (Eds.), *Mind in society: The development of higher psychological processes* (pp. 79–91). Cambridge, MA: Harvard University Press.

Wadeson, H. (1980). *Art psychotherapy*. New York: John Wiley and Sons.

Webb, N. B. (2002). *Helping bereaved children: A handbook for practitioners*. New York, NY: Guilford Press.

Webb, N. B. (2003). Play and expressive therapies to help bereaved children: Individual, family, and group treatments. *Smith College Studies in Social Work, 73*(3), 405–422. doi:10.1080/00377310309517694

Weber, A. M., & Haen, C. (2005). *Clinical applications of drama therapy in child and adolescent treatment*. London, England: Brunner-Routledge.

Whealin, J. M., & Ruzek, J. (2008). Program evaluation for organizational cultural competence in mental health practices. *Professional Psychology, Research and Practice, 39*(3), 320–328. doi:10.1037/0735-7028.39.3.320

Wong, P. T. P. (2008). Transformation of grief through meaning: Meaning-centered counseling for bereavement. In A. Tomer, G. T. Eliason, & P. T. P. Wong (Eds.), *Existential and spiritual issues in death attitudes*. New York, NY: Lawrence Erlbaum.

Worden, J. W. (1996). *Children and grief: When a parent dies*. New York, NY: Guilford Press.

Worden, J. W. (2009). *Grief counseling and grief therapy: A handbook for the mental health practitioner* (4th ed.). New York, NY: Springer.

World Healthcare Organization. (2007). *Standard precautions in health care*. Retrieved from http://www.who.int/csr/resources/publications/EPR_AM2_E7.pdf

Wright, A. C., & Jaffe, K. J. (2014). *Six steps to successful child advocacy: Changing the world for children*. Thousand Oaks, CA: Sage. doi:10.4135/9781483387888

Wyatt, R. C., & Seid, E. L. (2008). Instruction's manual for Adlerian play therapy with Terry Kottman, PhD. Mill Valley, CA: Psychotherapy.net.

Yasenik, L., & Gardner, K. (2012). *Play therapy dimensions model: A decision-making guide for integrative play therapists*. New York, NY: Jessica Kingsley Publishers.

Yerushalmi, K. (2001). Participant supervision in co-therapy. *The Israel Journal of Psychiatry and Related Sciences, 38*(2), 102–114. PMID:11475912

Yogman, M., Garner, A., Hutchinson, J., Michnick Golinkoff, R., & Committee on Psychosocial Aspects of Child and Family Health, Council on Communications and Media. (2018). The power of play: A pediatric role in enhancing development in young children. *Pediatrics, 142*(3), e20182058. Retrieved from http://pediatrics.aappublications.org/content/pediatrics/142/3/e20182058.full.pdf

Yu, A. (2012). *iSupe: An innovation in live supervision*. Presented at the *Eighth International Interdisciplinary Conference on Clinical Supervision*, Garden City, NY.

Yuanhong, J., Ramirez, S., & Kranz, P. (•••). Physical settings and materials recommended for play therapy with Japanese children. *Journal of Instructional Psychology, 34*(4), 53–61.

Zilberstein, K., & Abel, S. K. (2014). *Calming stormy feelings: A child's introduction to psychotherapy*. Bloomington, IN: AuthorHouse.

Index

I

L

M

N

O

P

R

www.ingramcontent.com/pod-product-compliance
Lightning Source LLC
LaVergne TN
LVHW081339300926
849161LV00008B/2015
* 9 7 8 1 5 2 2 5 8 2 2 6 7 *